Over 400

Beauty Solutions

...from tip to toe

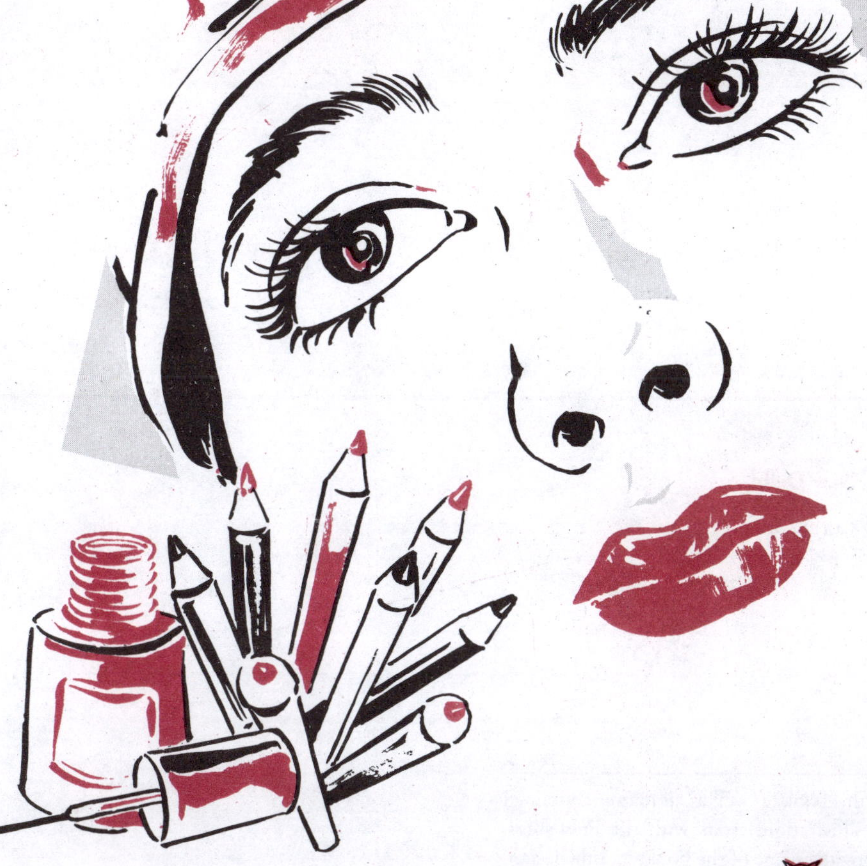

by

Tanushree Podder

PUSTAK MAHAL

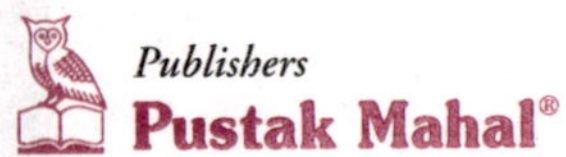

Publishers
Pustak Mahal®

Administrative office and sale centre
J-3/16 , Daryaganj, New Delhi-110002
☎ 23276539, 23272783, 23272784 • *Fax:* 011-23260518
E-mail: info@pustakmahal.com • *Website:* www.pustakmahal.com

Branches
Bengaluru: ☎ 080-22234025 • *Telefax:* 080-22240209
E-mail: pustak@airtelmail.in • pustak@sancharnet.in
Mumbai: ☎ 022-22010941, 022-22053387
E-mail: rapidex@bom5.vsnl.net.in
Patna: ☎ 0612-3294193 • *Telefax:* 0612-2302719
E-mail: rapidexptn@rediffmail.com

ISBN 978-81-223-0627-9

Edition: 2013

Printed at : Super Fine Book Binding Works, Tronica City (U.P.)

Dedication

I dedicate this book to my parents.
To my mother, who was a beautiful person with a beautiful soul. She has given me all the patience and love that I needed to bring out this book.

To my father to whom I owe all the grit, tenacity and hard work that is required to create a book.

Acknowledgement

I would like to thank all the beautiful people of my family for the support and encouragement they have given me in bringing out this book. Beauty is not just a beautiful face or figure, it is the entire persona, a beautiful soul within a beautiful body. And my family comprises of beautiful people in the truest sense.

A special round of thanks goes to my dear husband who was a model of endurance and patiently bore the irregular pace of life while I was busy with the book. Without his understanding and help, this book would not have seen the light of day. I can't forget to thank little Ankita, my ten-year-old daughter, who was the moving force behind this book. She pushed me and goaded me into finishing the book in a record time. The sheer enthusiasm and energy of this girl drove me into a spin of activity.

Preface

"A thing of beauty is a joy for ever," said Keats. Beauty has been the prerogative of the fairer sex since ages. In recent times, beauty and body care have become more important because they boost one's self-confidence, improve presentability and enhance chances in career development. As it is said—'A good face is a letter of recommendation.'

Many books have been written on the subject of beauty to help beauty-conscious generation of men and women to look good and feel good about oneself.

The book makes an endeavour to help the readers to use the art of make-up to camouflage one's flaws and highlight the good features. It provides information on the new products that have flooded the market with emphasis on their intended use.

It is a book for those who want to be beautiful people. Some are lucky enough to be born beautiful while others can equip themselves with the vast treasure of knowledge provided in this book.

Contents

Introduction *9-10*

CHAPTER I: *Hair* *11-36*

- Basic Hair Facts 12
- Diet and Hair 18
- Brushes and Combs 20
- Hair Fashion 24
- Colouring Tips 28
- Face Shapes and Hair Styles 31
- Your Figure and Hairstyle 33
- Camouflaging the Flaws 34

CHAPTER II: *Styling the Hair* *37-66*

- When to Go In for a Cut? 44
- Caring for the Hair Pieces 44
- Grey Hair 45
- Dandruff and Other Problems 46
- Shampoo Facts 57
- Hair Conditioners 62

CHAPTER III: *Skin* *67-86*

Basic Facts 68
Skin Care 71
Problem Skin 74
Glowing Complexion 82
Scars and Spots 84

CHAPTER IV: ***Ageing*** **87-106**

- Blemishes and Dark Circles 91
- Superfluous Hair 94
- Stretch Marks 96
- Body Weight and Exercises 97
- Body Odour & Perfumes 101
- Emotions and the Skin 103
- Sensitive Skin 104
- Teeth 105

CHAPTER V: ***Make-Up*** **107-128**

- Manicure and Pedicure 121

CHAPTER VI: ***Herbal Beauty Solutions*** **129-152**

- Herbal Hair Care 130
- Herbal Hair Oils 140
- Herbal Skin Solutions 141
- For Sparkling Teeth 151
- For Pedicure and Manicure 152

Introduction

Ever since God created Woman, she has been interested in looking good. Down the ages, women have devised various ways and means to improve their appearance. They have experimented with various potions and lotions so that they could preserve their beauty and enhance it. Cleopatra has been known to have used asses' milk for bathing, all for the sake of a beautiful and smooth skin.

This is the era of youthful looks, energy and vivacity. Whether it is a man or a woman, everyone wants to project a pleasing personality. While in a job or social interchange, appearance plays an important role. The cult of beauty is no longer the prerogative of the idle, rich women but a social fact, not a luxury but an obligation and not a necessity but a priority for every woman, whatever be her standing in the society.

Beauty gives confidence to a person. In this world of tough competition in every sphere, beauty is one more weapon, which comes handy when you are fighting for the top notches, whether in a career or personal life. This is the age of beautiful and smart people. The new millennium will see hordes of confident and beautiful people marching forth with renewed energy, vivacity and verve. We want you to be a part of that lot.

Some women are lucky to be born beautiful while others can make use of the vast treasure of knowledge that has come forth in this century, to make themselves beautiful. I believe that every woman is beautiful in some way or the other. Each of us has a specific quality and beauty, it is just a matter of highlighting that plus point and bring it forth for the world to notice. And all it takes is some effort and interest, to create a beautiful presence.

In this book, you have within your reach, a thousand tips and hints, which will help you revive your beauty and create a new persona. The queries that have always bothered

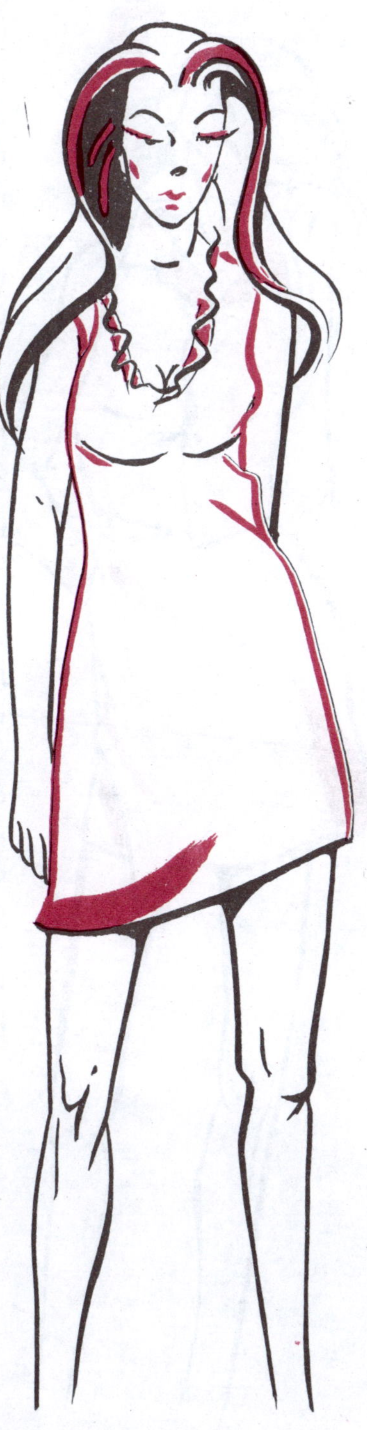

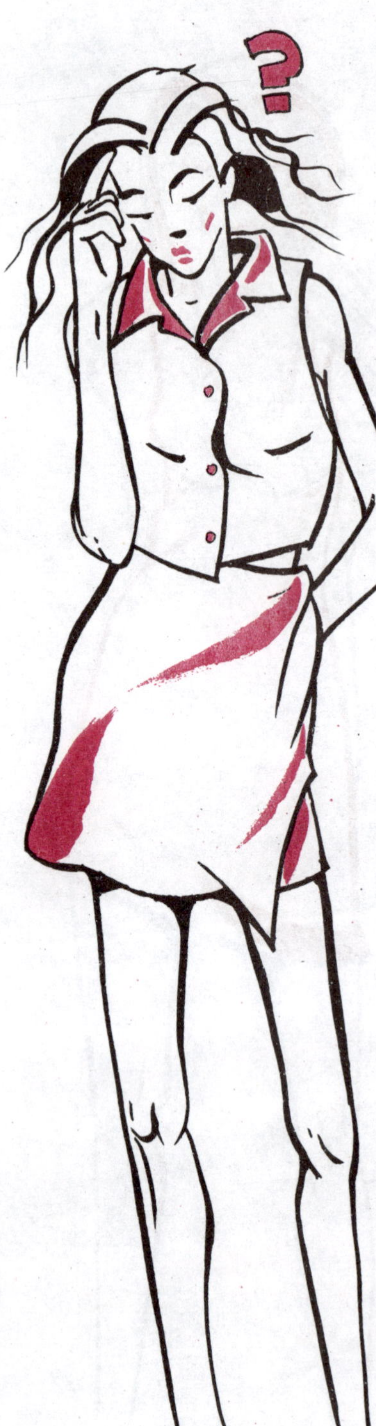

you and the answers you have sought after are now within your reach. These solutions will help you unravel your hidden beauty and personality. The ideas given here are tried and tested for efficacy. They have been around for ages but in fragmented form. These fragments have now been collated to put in use by the busy young women who do not have the time to pore through hundreds of books on beauty, hair care and skin care to take care of themselves. Almost all topics related to a beautiful appearance have been brought under an umbrella.

A book like this takes a long time to take shape. There are hundreds of questions that occur to the mind. Some have easy solutions and some defy solutions. Painstakingly and patiently, I have tried to sift out the mundane and give place to the relevant. The types of questions given here are asked by women of almost all age groups, all over the world. Beauty has a strange unifying quality, women the world over face similar problems of the hair and skin. I have come across various doubts and confusions that persist in the minds of women whenever new products are launched with a great fanfare. The information given by the companies can be misleading or exaggerated and there is always a lingering fear about the efficacy of the cosmetics. The changing pace of the world requires quick solution to almost all problems. It has been my endeavour to hand over the answers in a platter to those eager minds that are clouded by hundreds of questions. Here is wishing you a beautiful beginning!

—Tanushree Podder

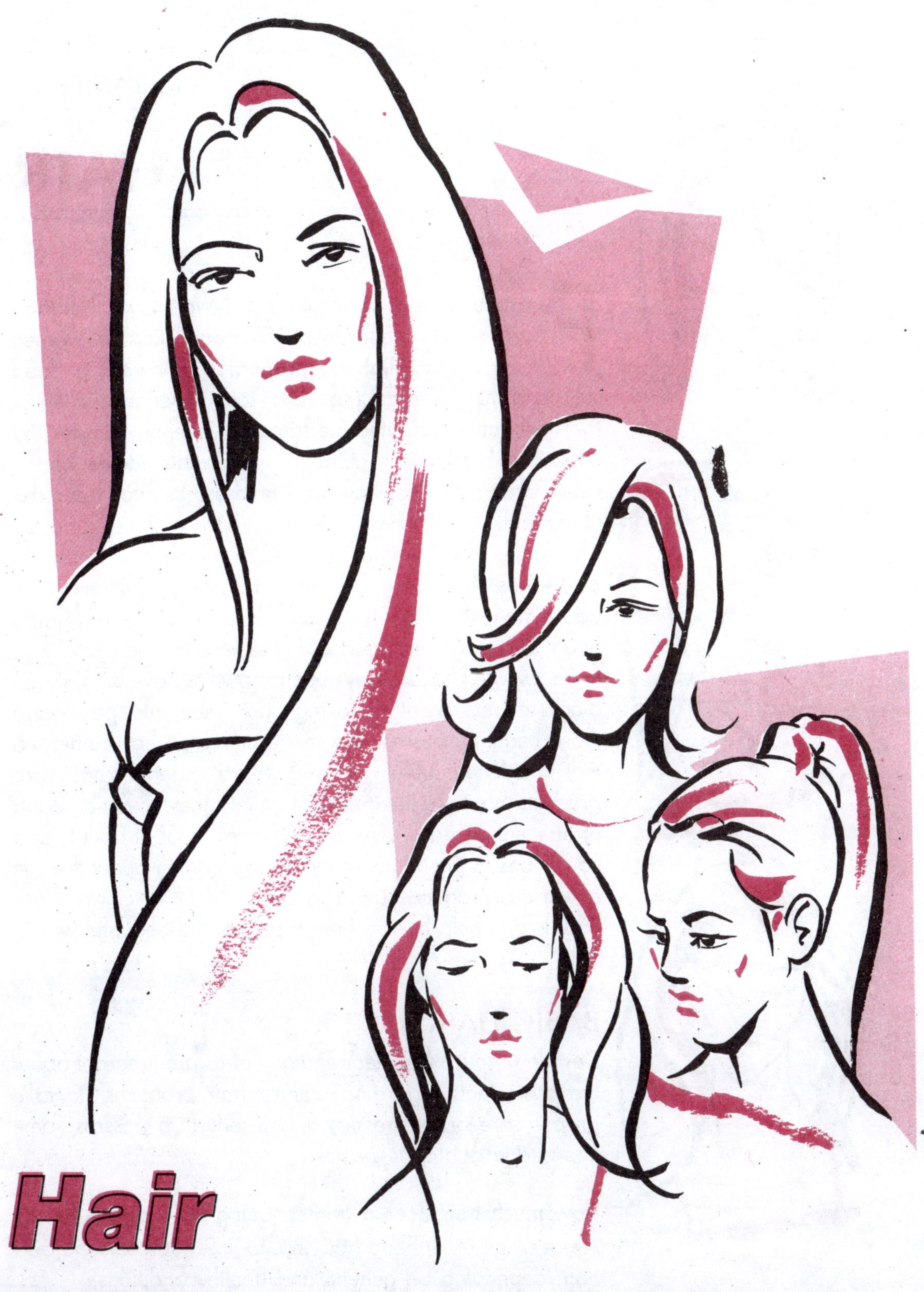

Hair

CHAPTER I

HAIR

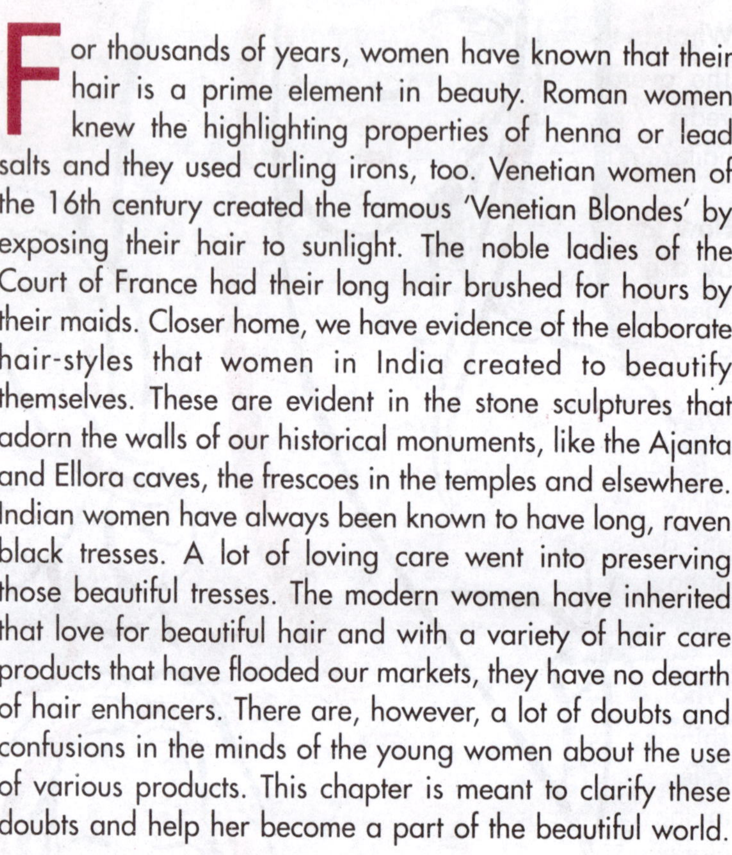

For thousands of years, women have known that their hair is a prime element in beauty. Roman women knew the highlighting properties of henna or lead salts and they used curling irons, too. Venetian women of the 16th century created the famous 'Venetian Blondes' by exposing their hair to sunlight. The noble ladies of the Court of France had their long hair brushed for hours by their maids. Closer home, we have evidence of the elaborate hair-styles that women in India created to beautify themselves. These are evident in the stone sculptures that adorn the walls of our historical monuments, like the Ajanta and Ellora caves, the frescoes in the temples and elsewhere. Indian women have always been known to have long, raven black tresses. A lot of loving care went into preserving those beautiful tresses. The modern women have inherited that love for beautiful hair and with a variety of hair care products that have flooded our markets, they have no dearth of hair enhancers. There are, however, a lot of doubts and confusions in the minds of the young women about the use of various products. This chapter is meant to clarify these doubts and help her become a part of the beautiful world.

BASIC HAIR FACTS

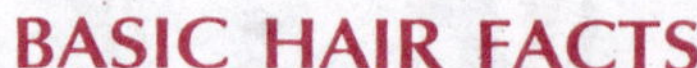

Despite so much knowledge, many of us are ignorant about the basic facts regarding hair or hair problems. To take proper care of the tresses, it is essential to possess some knowledge about the basics.

How much hair does a human being have on his head?
An average adult head has around 1,20,000 to 1,50,000 hair, depending on genetic and health conditions.

What is the average rate of growth of human hair?

Hair grows approximately by 1.25 cm every month.

What is the growth period of our hair?

Our hair grows for about 1000 days and rests for 100 days.

What is the average life span of a strand of hair?

The average life span of a strand of hair is about five years. After that the hair follicles begin to shrink and the hair remains static until it falls off or is brushed out.

How long does it take for the fallen hair to be replaced by a new one?

The replacement of fallen hair, in normal conditions, takes a few months.

What is the average hair fall in a day?

It is normal for about 100 hair to fall everyday. This figure varies according to health, nutrition and stress factors. But one does not have to get unduly worried about the amount of hair fall, as they keep getting replaced in due course of time.

What then, is the cause for thinning of hair?

Thinning of hair is caused due to non-replacement of the fallen hair. This could happen when new hair does not form in the hair follicle. This again could be caused due to inadequate blood supply to the scalp, glandular or hormonal changes, bad health or stress.

What is hair made up of and what is its structure?

Hair is made up of a strong protein called 'keratin', which contains 21 different amino acids. The hair shaft consists of the cuticle, the cortex and the medulla. The cuticle is the outer layer of the hair shaft, and is made up of multiple layers of translucent cells, which overlap each other like shingles on a roof. When the layers are smooth and flat against each other, the hair reflects more light and looks

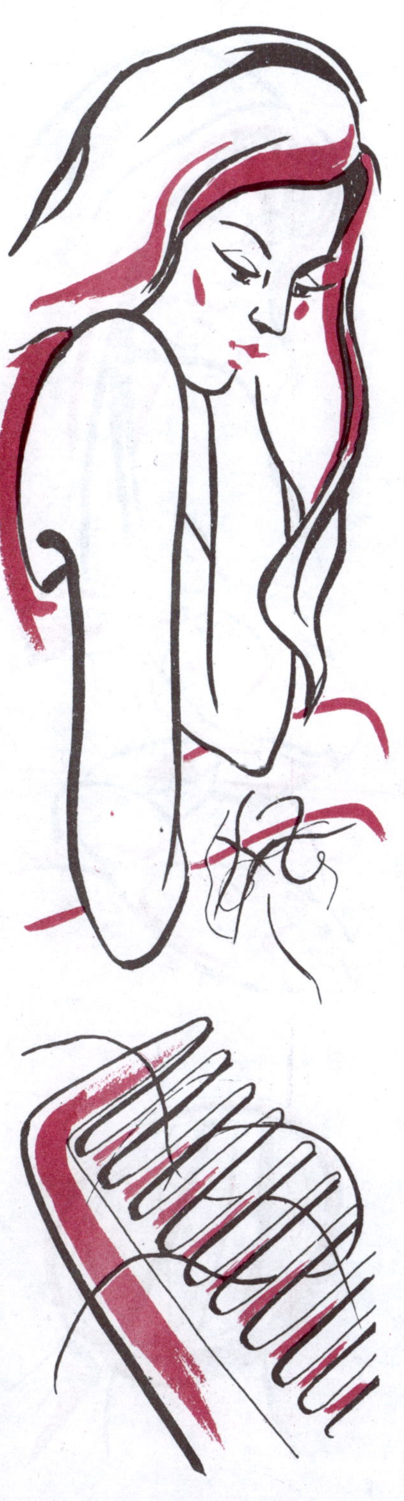

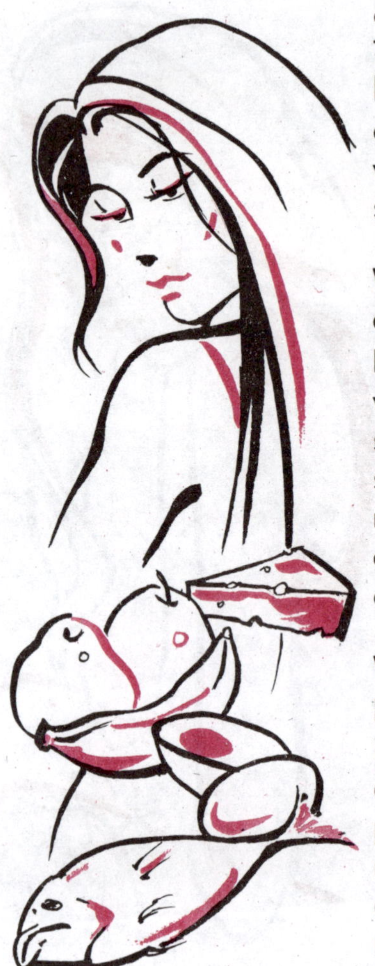

shiny. The middle layer of an individual hair is called the cortex, which comprises three quarters of the hair shaft. The pigment or melanin, gives hair its colour and it is located in the cortex. There are two types of melanin: eumelanin, which is the black pigment, and the pheomelanin which gives red or yellow pigment. The core of the hair shaft is called the medula.

What is the composition of keratin? And what nutritional care can be taken to avoid deficiencies?

Hair protein, keratin is composed of long molecular chains within the cortex. These chains form a twisted rope-like structure which has a network of cross-bonds. These provide stability, strength and elasticity to the hair. Since hair is made from a form of protein, it is necessary to ensure that one gets a high protein diet, adequate intake of Vitamin B complex and minerals.

What are the sources for these nutritional elements?

Brewer's yeast is a rich source of Vitamin B Complex. Liver is another such source. Minerals like iron, copper and iodine are also necessary for healthy hair. Iron and copper are present in meat, leafy vegetables and certain fruits. One must take fresh salads, meat, fresh fish, and liver, eggs and cheese in order to consume adequate amount of these necessary nutrients.

What are the phases in the life span of a hair, before it falls?

Normal human hair goes through three phases during its lifetime.

Anagen: this is the phase of growth

Catagen: this is the transitional phase

Telogen: this is the resting phase of the hair.

What does the thickness of hair depend on?

The thickness of hair depends on the number of hair follicles on one's scalp.

Can this number be changed in any way?

No, the number of hair follicles are determined before the birth of a child. Factors like genetics contribute to this decision. The number cannot be increased by any means including the application of any type of hair oil.

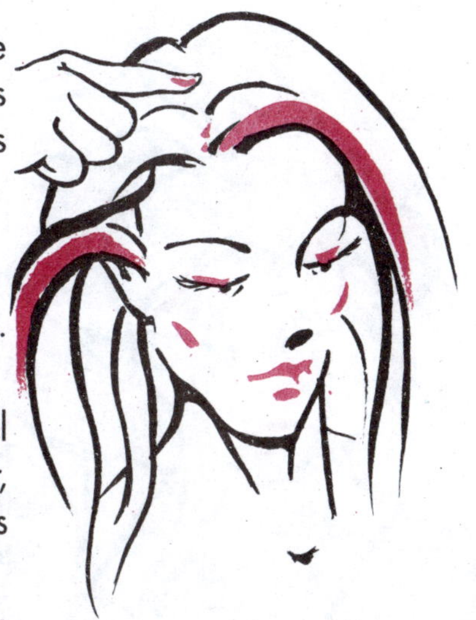

What causes hair loss?

There are five major factors which could lead to hair loss. They are due to:

1. High fever, frequent childbirth, haemorrages, surgical shock, and severe mental stress and strain. However, these factors are reversible and hair growth resumes after 3-4 months.
2. Diffuse Alopecia, which is endocrinal in origin. This can be due to hypo or hyper thyroidism, diabetes mellitus (not properly controlled), pregnancy or oral contraceptives.
3. Drugs like thallium, anti-thyrotoxicosis, anti cancer drugs, heavy metals like Bismuth, excess intake of vitamin A. While the first four causes are irreversible; the last one is reversible.
4. Nutritional deficiencies of proteins, iron, zinc etc. This factor is totally reversible.
5. Chronic diffuse Alopecia, which is androgenic in origin. This is genetically determined like the baldness seen in males. This can neither be prevented nor cured.

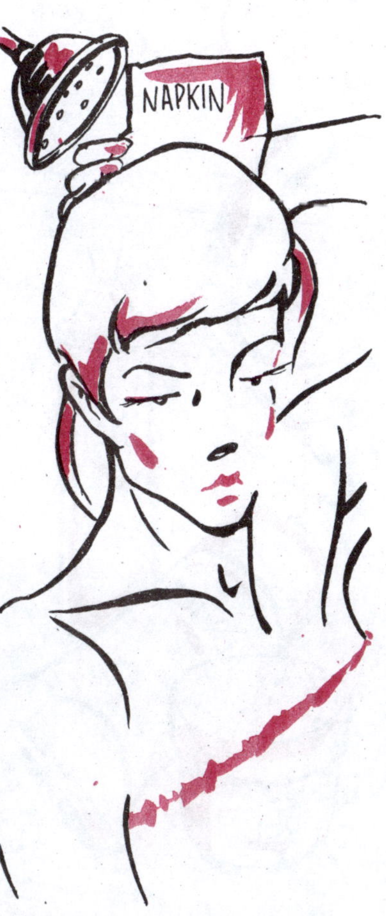

How can I determine whether my scalp is in good health?

To find out if you have a healthy scalp, press down on each side of your parting and examine the area that is visible. A healthy scalp is very supple and its colour is the same as your complexion. If you move the scalp by using your fingertips, it should move easily. This would indicate that the moisture content is right and the scalp is in good condition. Whereas, a tense scalp and one which does not seem pliable, is not a very healthy one.

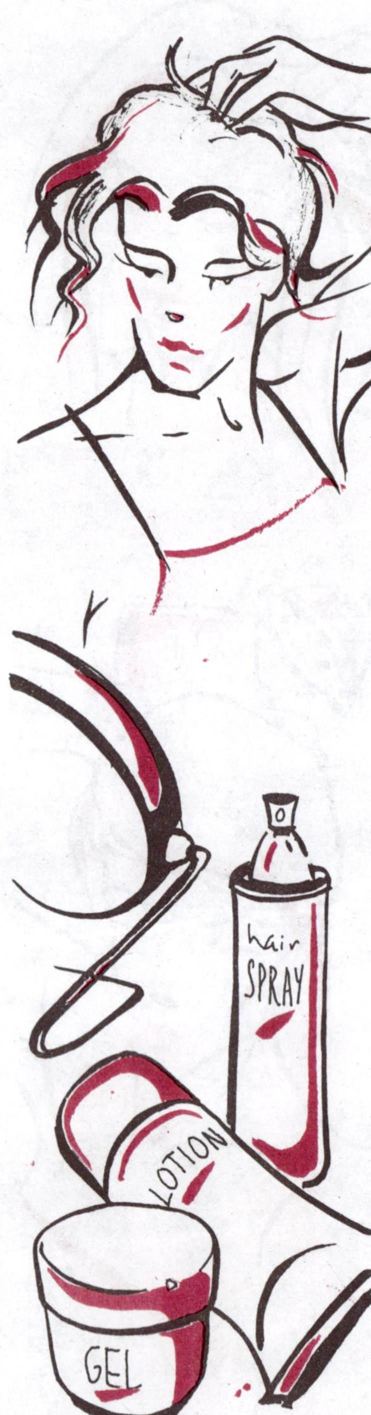

What are the categories of hair and how does one find out the type of hcir one has?

The two types of hair are: dry and oily. In general, an oily scalp tends to exist in combination with thin and fine hair. While the dry scalp generally goes with rough and thicker hair. To find out the type of hair you have, rub a soft paper napkin on the scalp after a shampoo. If the paper shows up an oily patch, your hair is definitely of the oily type whereas a dry one would reflect the dryness of the scalp.

How can I find out about the condition of my hair?

If your hair is supple, shiny, falls out at the rate of not more than 30 a day, needs shampooing only once every week, can hold a 'set', feels soft to touch and doesn't produce any static electricity, it is in good health.

If the hair is dull, difficult to style, doesn't hold a 'set', splits at the ends, produces a lot of static electricity or tangles easily then it is too dry.

If the hair is oily, greasy just 2 days after a shampoo, sticks together, won't keep any style, is dull and looks neglected, it is too oily.

If it has splits at the ends, falls out in bunches and has dandruff, looks patchy or appears 'moth eaten' whenever you give it a permanent or a colour rinse then it is unhealthy.

What are the most common scalp problems?

The three most common problems are: dandruff, dry scalp and oily scalp.

Dandruff, the most common problem, is caused because of a greasy scalp, which sheds its skin cells in quick succession.

The dry scalp is caused due to environmental factors and chemical treatments used for styling the hair. The main reason for the dryness being the depletion of moisture level.

Oily scalp is caused by the overproduction of sebum, by the oil glands in the scalp. This could also be due to the inadequate rinsing out of the hair.

What are the hair problems commonly faced by the girls in their twenties?

In the twenties, the skin, hair as well as the general health is at its peak. The hormonal changes that the teenager faces, also disappear by this time. The hair requires very little worry but there are several points that one must bear in mind. Most young girls in this age group, go on crash diets which effect their general health, skin as well as the hair since vital nutrients are often missing from their diets. They also try to experiment with different types of hairstyles and use various treatments, which may not be good for the hair, in the longer run. One must remember the importance of clean hair and a balanced diet. Don't forget to oil the hair before a shampoo. If you have permed or colour-treated your hair, use a shampoo formulated for these conditions. It is easy to ignore the warnings but the damage will be realised during the later years of life.

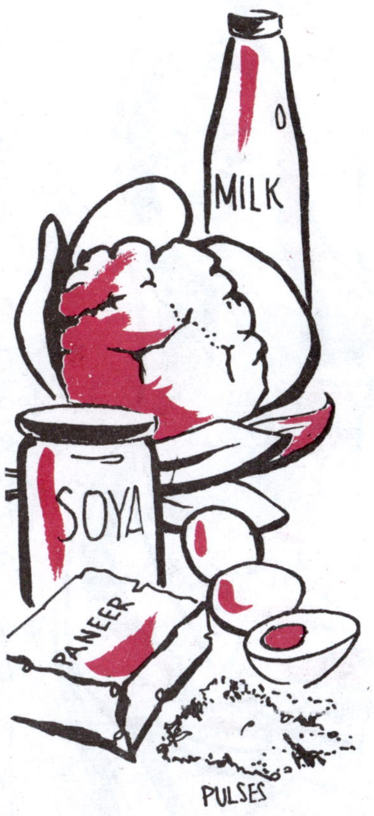

I am a thirty-year-old, working woman with a hectic schedule. I also smoke about one pack a day. I am worried about the health of my hair. Could you enumerate the problems that I could face and the care I should take of my hair?

By the time a woman is in her thirties, the decline of the hair as well as the skin has begun. The skin is not as elastic and the hair as bouncy and healthy as it was during the twenties. Exercise and diet play a very important role in the maintenance of hair as well as skin. You will have to cut down on your smoking since it deprives the cells of oxygen and makes the hair smell of tobacco. You will realise that your hair is drier than it was. This is indicative of the fact that the hair is not getting enough moisture. Stress is another factor that will effect the hair as well as the scalp. Learn to relax and maintain composure. Yoga could be a good therapy.

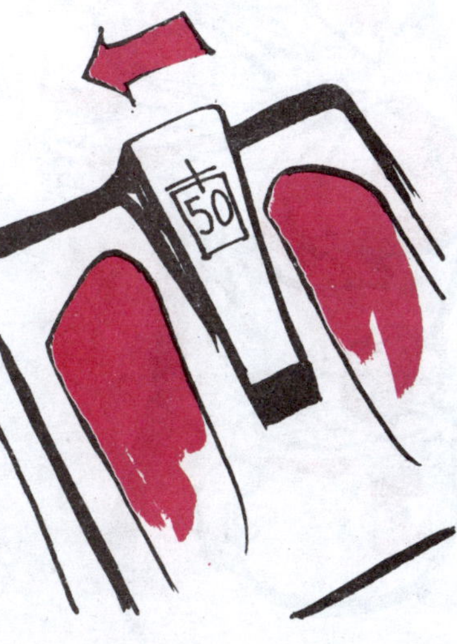

I am in my early forties and I find that my hair is looking too lifeless and dull. How can I counteract the effects of ageing on my hair?

Problems like dry hair and scalp are common at your age. You have to take these in your stride. What you can do is

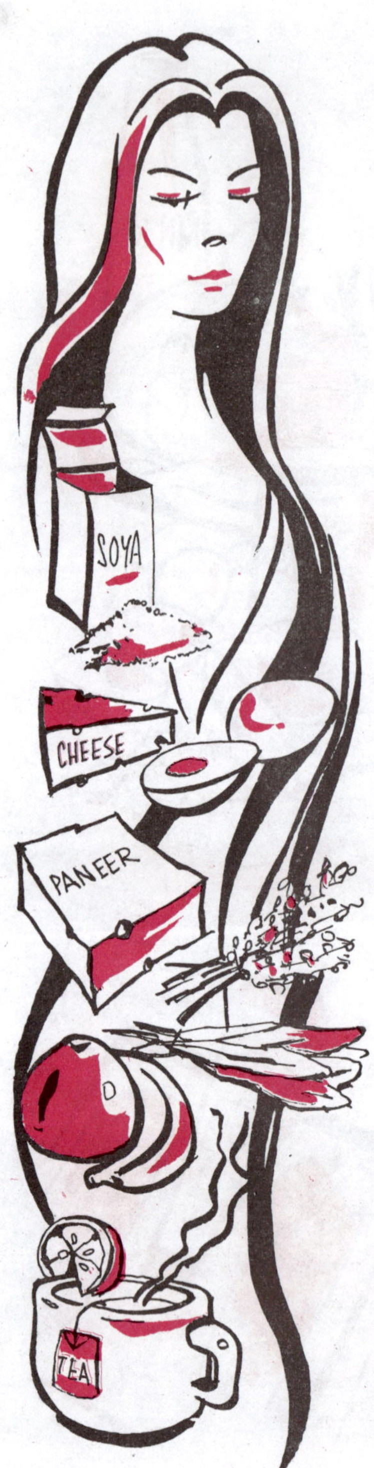

to keep a watch on your diet so that you are getting all the vital nutrients. Exercise is a must so work out a regular form of exercise even if it is just a walk in the morning or the evening. Use sprays that add shine and bounce to lifeless hair, without reducing it to a flat and oily mess. Stick to styles that are soft and easy to manage. Avoid tight curls and pulled back styles. They emphasise the lines and wrinkles that one wants to hide.

DIET AND HAIR

Diet plays a very important role in deciding the condition of one's hair. Good nutrition, which contains all the essential elements, is a must if one wants the hair to be in an optimum condition. Apart from the grooming and care, one has to be extremely careful about including various nutrients in the diet. Before one goes on a dieting spree for weight reduction, one must work out a proper nutritious diet in consultation with an expert dietician or else the damage done to the hair and health will cause a lot of heartache.

I have been dieting for the last six months and now I have noticed that the hair looks very dull and limp. I am losing a lot of hair, too. What could have gone wrong?

There are a lot of problems which arise when a person goes on a low cal diet. Without even being aware of the problem, one can develop deficiencies related to vitamin, mineral and proteins. Iron deficiency is the one, which causes the maximum damage to the hair and also results in low haemoglobin levels. This reduces the oxygen carrying capacity of the blood. Too little oxygen weakens the hair follicles leading to scalp dryness and hair loss. No matter which diet form you are undertaking, just remember to introduce the right amount of valuable nutrients otherwise you are bound to lose hair as well as effect the skin.

What are the steps to be taken in order to prevent a deficiency in nutrition, while one is on a diet?

The low protein content in fad diets and fasting for prolonged periods of time could lead to nutritional deficiencies. Fad diets, which work on the premise that one needs to eat only fruits and no cereals or the ones that say that only rice and vegetables are required, can cause a heavy damage. If these diets are followed for more than three to four weeks, the body is compelled to break down upon its own lean tissue. As a result the dispensable protein in the hair and the skin are the first ones to be affected. I would suggest that one should include good sources of proteins like 'paneer', sprouts, pulses and soya bean in his diet. In fact, soya bean contains the entire chain of amino acids, which is similar to the egg protein. The other foods like sprouts and dals have to be combined with other elements in order to provide the required amount of protein. Minerals and vitamin supplements like zinc, vitamin B, calcium and iron are also essential for the body.

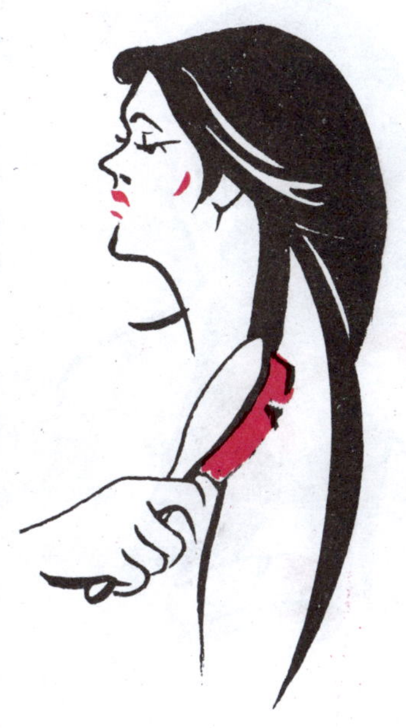

I am a thirty three-year-old woman with two children. I have undertaken a weight reduction programme because I was overweight. But the condition of my hair, which was already thin, has become worse. It is falling by dozens. How could I arrest the fall?

Any weight reduction programme, which is undertaken by a person, must be worked out carefully. If you are depriving your body of the required essential elements, your physical state will suffer and so will the hair and the skin. Crash diets proposed by several inexperienced persons can work adversely on the health. It is essential to work out the daily caloric and nutritional requirements in consultation with an experienced nutritionist before going on any diet or weight reduction programme. The health of the hair depends on the nutritional state of the dieter. However, a nutritious diet can significantly improve the condition of your hair.

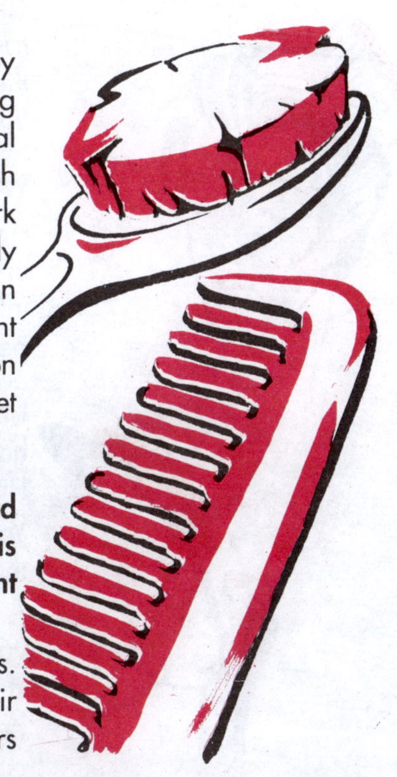

I hate taking milk and milk products. Lately I have noticed deterioration in the quality of my hair. How important is calcium for the hair and how can I take this element without taking milk?

Calcium is extremely important for the bones and tissues. Any deficiency of calcium will definitely damage your hair too. The requirement of calcium in adults above 25 years

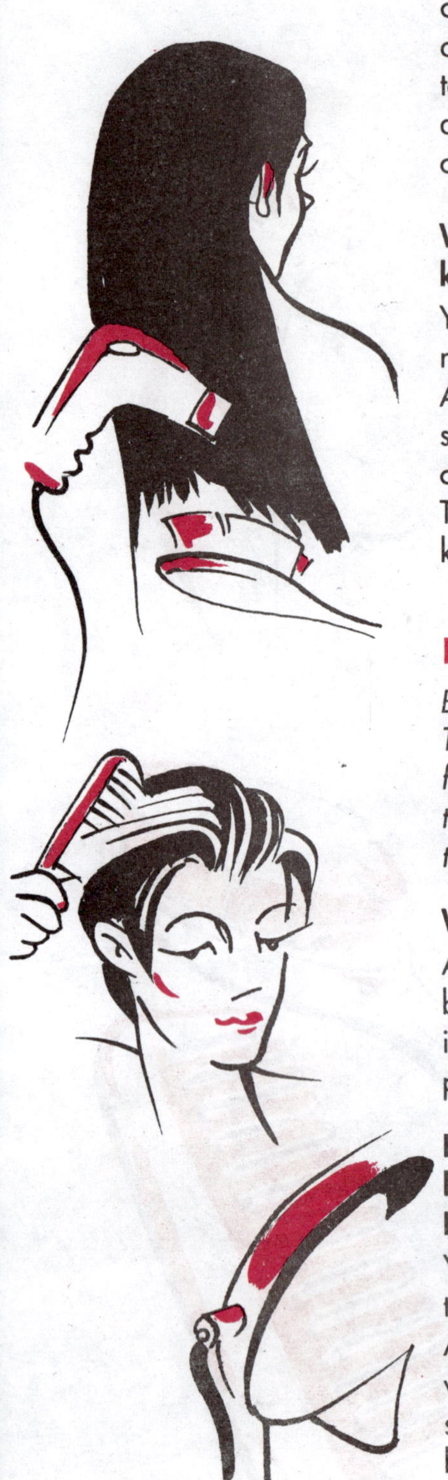

of age is about 800mg. This can be obtained from $2^1/_2$ cups of milk every day. If you don't like milk, you will have to obtain it from fresh, green leafy vegetables like spinach, amaranth and methi. You could also try taking curd or cheese or soya milk.

What diet could one take during the summer in order to keep the hair looking good?

You could take fresh fruit juices and plenty of water to replenish the water content in the body lost due to sweat. Also avoid heavy, starchy meals. Include salads, fruits, sprouts and yoghurt in your daily diet. Substitute your cup of tea with iced tea, lemon juice and a dash of honey. These will ensure that you get adequate nutrients while keeping the unnecessary elements out.

BRUSHES AND COMBS

Brushes and combs are necessary, elements in hair care. These should be kept scrupulously clean, not shared with friends and changed whenever they are worn out. Choosing the right kind of brush is a very important factor and several things must be kept in mind while selecting the right one.

What is a boar bristle brush?

A boar bristle brush is one in which the filament or the bristle comes from a wild boar. Usually the bristles are re-inforced with a heat resistant nylon to help the bristle penetrate the hair.

I have heard that it is important to use the right kind of hairbrush otherwise the hair roots could get damaged. How far is it true? What kind of hairbrush should I use?

You are right. Using the wrong kind of brush could damage the hair. You should have two hairbrushes in your hair kit. A medium sized oval one for general grooming and adding volume to your style. Also a round brush to smoothen and straighten the hair. A brush should have an easy grip and be almost weightless. A heavy and an awkward brush could make it difficult for you to style the hair.

Which is a better hairbrush—the one with natural bristles or the one with plastic bristles?

Natural bristles come from the wild boar and are softer and more flexible than nylon bristles and help to distribute the hair's natural oils throughout the hair. The bristles also help close the cuticles of the hair while brushing, giving the hair a nice, healthy shine. These types of brushes are gentler on the hair and scalp. Using a boar bristle brush usually eliminates split ends-related hair damage. A brush that slides through wet hair with little effort is the best. You may have noticed that the professional hair stylists use sturdy plastic brushes. Take care to choose a brush with pure bristles or a combination brush for general styling. Avoid brushes with sharp, rigid bristles as these can tear the hair and damage the scalp.

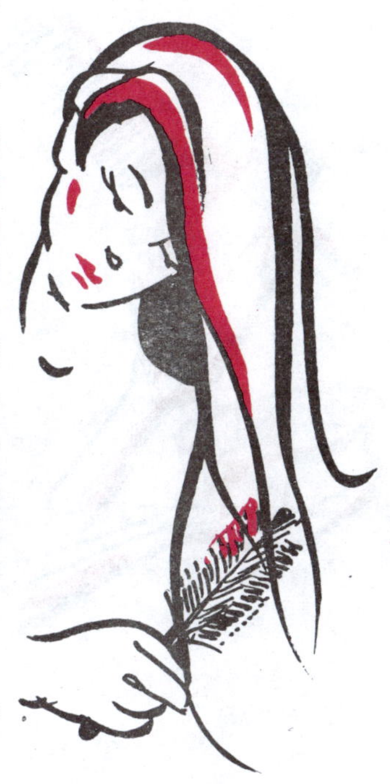

What kind of brush does one need while blow drying the hair?

For straightening hair, use a round brush with densely packed and firm boar bristles, the bigger the brush the straighter the hair. Avoid a style that needs precision drying if you are not very dexterous. A plastic brush with wide spaced bristles achieves movement and lift while a vent brush allows air to circulate directly at the root level. Fine hair needs soft bristles to protect it while firm bristles will smooth thick or curly hair. Damaged or fragile hair needs a gentle brush made of pliable plastic.

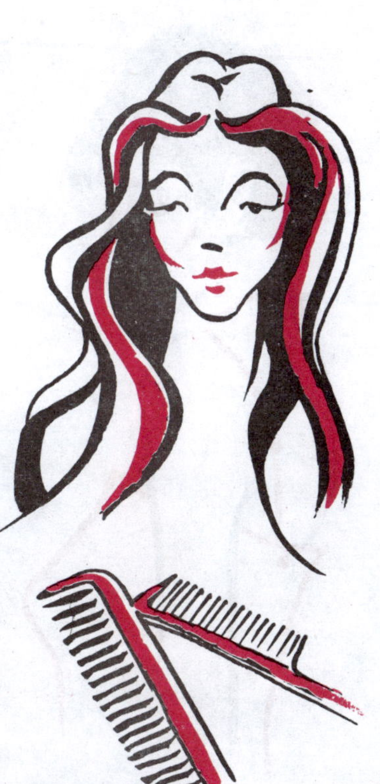

How often does one need to clean the hair brush?

Personal hairbrushes should be washed on a routine basis, depending on the build up of natural oils from the scalp and the use of styling products. A dirt-clogged hairbrush does not glide smoothly through the hair. To keep the brush clean, comb out loose hair and swirl it in warm water with a mild shampoo or one tablespoon of washing soda. You may add a few drops of antiseptic lotion. Rinse well with clean water and leave it to dry naturally.

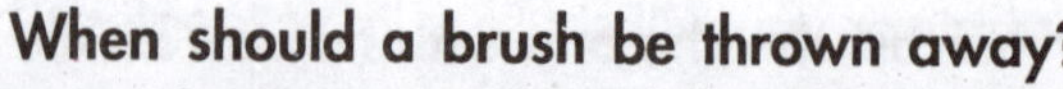

When should a brush be thrown away?

A brush should be thrown away when the bristles begin to lose their stiffness or when the brush loses its effectiveness.

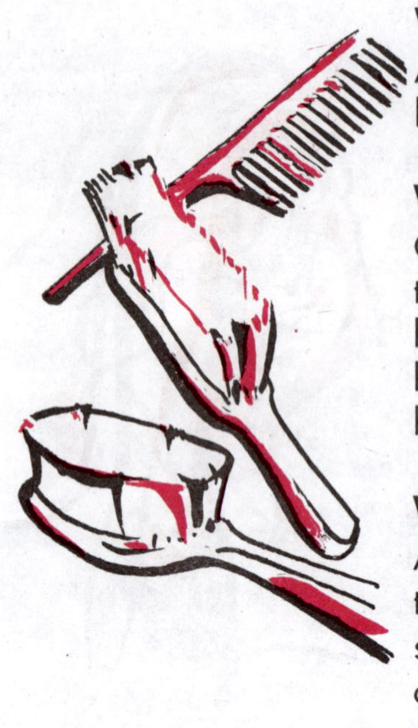

When should combs be used?

Combs are best used on damp, towel-dried hair for combing through the tangles. Combs are also used for sectioning the hair and can also be used on dry, short hair to fix a hairstyle. Wide toothed combs are best for detangling the hair.

What type of brush can be used to make the hair shine?

A boar bristle brush makes the hair shine because it helps to pick up and distribute the hair and the natural oils of the scalp along the hair shaft as well as pull dirt or dust particles off the hair.

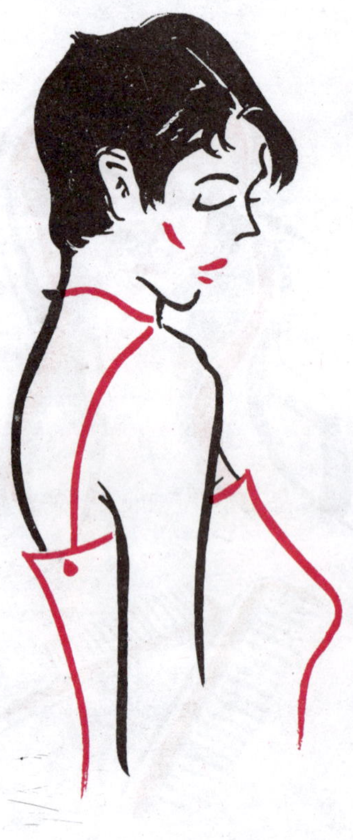

Someone told me that I should brush my hair at least for 15 minutes every night. Does this procedure make the hair grow?

Brushing stimulates the blood circulation in the scalp, bringing more blood towards the scalp, which stimulates hair growth. The more often you brush, the more oils you distribute from your scalp to the hair strands. This in turn conditions and protects the hair. As a result, hair is stronger and healthier. Maybe that is why our grandmothers used to swear by the 100 strokes before going to bed.

When should one use a boar bristle brush and when should nylon bristle brush be used?

A nylon bristle brush is best used on thick hair and to help the hair to detangle. Use a boar bristle brush for brushing out a style to create a fuller look. Boar bristle brushes are the best to use at night to brush hair out for a healthy shine.

When is a full, round, spiral brush used?

A full, round spiral brush is used on most textures and lengths of hair but it is best suited on short or layered hair. Because of the spiral, be careful not to completely rotate the brush in your hair or you will cause a lot of tangles. The diameter of the barrel determines the size of the resulting curl. Never pull the brush out of the hair after you have finished styling.

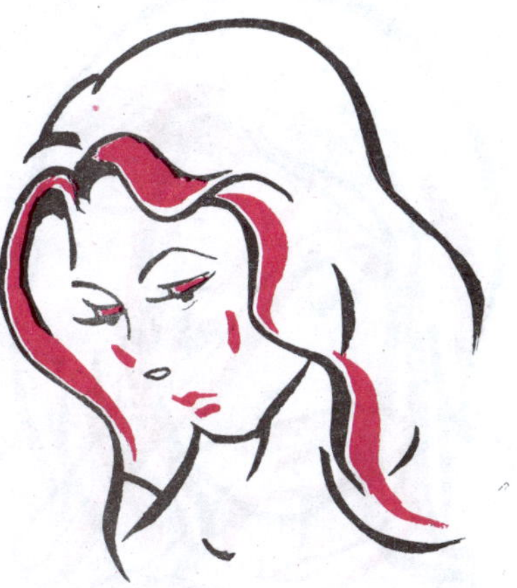

I have very thick and straight hair. What kind of brush can I use?

For thick and straight hair, a rubber cushion brush with nylon bristles and ball-tip end, is the best. The rubber cushion helps in making brushing easier, while the nylon bristles provide the strength to move the brush through thick hair. The ball-tips reduce the drag and resistance.

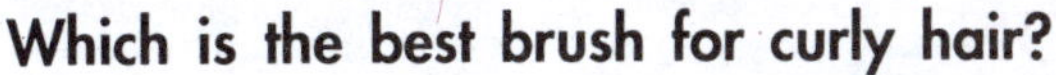

Which is the best brush for curly hair?

Generally, curly hair should not be brushed unless you intend to straighten it out. The best brush in that case is a natural boar bristle brush.

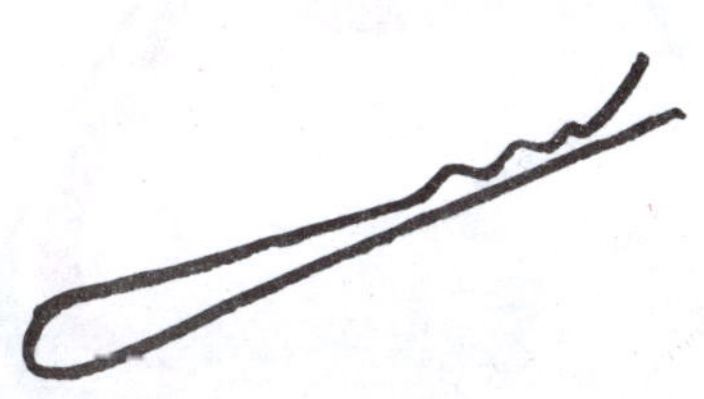

Which is the suitable brush for fine, thin hair?

You could use a wide-spaced, ball-tipped bristle brush. This will prevent breakage and add lift and volume while blow-drying.

What kind of comb should be used for 'teasing' the hair?

A special comb with small-serrated teeth between the longer teeth is generally used as a teasing comb. The smaller teeth on the teasing comb pack hair towards the roots to create fullness and volume in the hair. The best comb for teasing depends on the thickness of the hair. For fine, thin hair; use a comb with tightly spaced teeth to achieve volume and lift. For thicker, coarser hair, a comb with medium to wide spaced teeth with serrated edges is most effective.

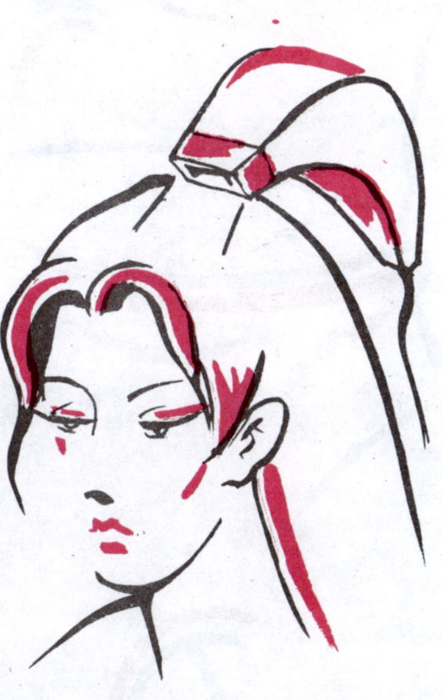

Does one have to change the brush according to the season?

Yes, it is best to switch to a natural bristle hairbrush for the winter. Nylon brushes can stir up static electricity. If you still find it in the hair, try spraying the brush lightly with a hairspray.

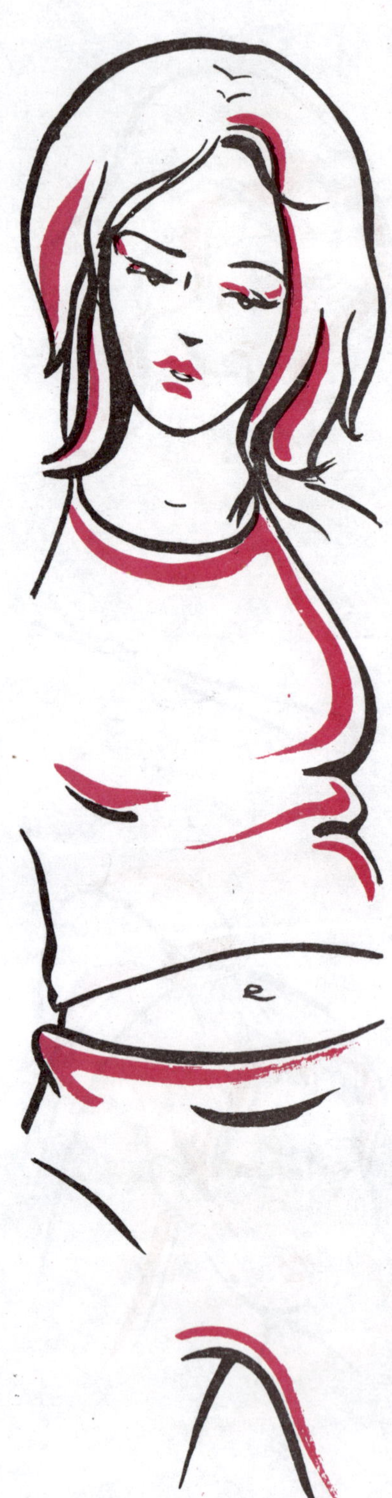

How can I straighten my thick and wavy hair at home?
You can straighten coarse, thick and wavy hair by blow drying. The hair must be completely blown dry before you try to coax out the curls. When the hair is totally dry, use a flat paddle brush that helps to smoothen hair strands down. Do one section at a time, using a blow dryer on medium setting and the paddle brush. Start at the back of the head, near the nape. Brush underneath the hair, close to the roots, then over the surface for a smooth finish. Try using a light spritz on your brush while going over the hair to help hold it.

HAIR FASHION

Fashions keep changing with time but the essential and basic factors remain unchanged. For centuries there have been women with scanty hair who have used different types of hair-pieces to add artificial volume to their scanty hair. Only the technology keeps changing. The type of hairstyle may change but the requirement of basic implements remains unchanged.

I have very scanty hair and I want to use a hairpiece. What is the best way to fasten a hairpiece to my natural hair?
Secure the hairpiece with bobby pins or hair extension clips that can be easily sewn into your own hairpiece. Many new types of hairpieces come with their own clips that lock the hairpiece on to your hair.

What is a ratt? How can one use a ratt for a French roll?
A ratt is a hair foundation made of a sponge type of material and used to create fullness and sophisticated hair roll, like the French roll. These can be used on all types of hair, from extra thick to extra fine hair. Ratts are made from featherweight foam for comfort and durability. You can even sleep on them. To use a ratt, position the foundation on to the hair, where you want the roll. Fasten each end of the foundation to the hair with a bobby pin. Push the pin

through the foundation or pin over the foundation by squeezing the end. Smooth hair over the foundation and tuck the ends of hair under the foundation with a comb or brush. Fasten with hairpins. Voila! You have a neat French roll.

Should I use hairpins or bobby pins for a French Twist and chignons? What is the difference?

Hair pins are open at the end and are used to hold large amounts of hair in place. Bobby pins are crimped at the end to hold small amounts of hair tightly. Both are used to create the base of support for either a French twist or to hold a chignon ratt in place.

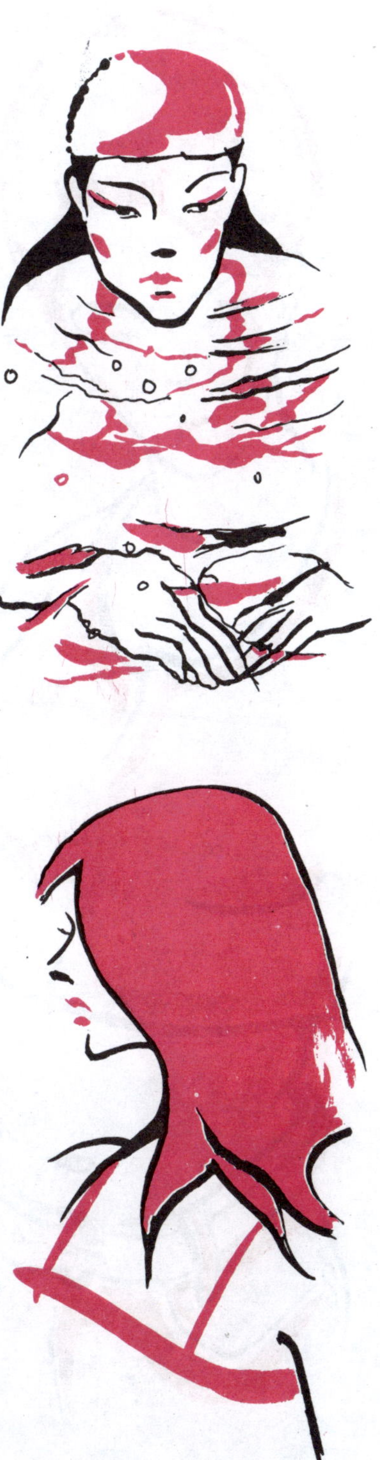

What is the proper method of blow drying the hair?

Hair should be towel-dried before blow-drying. Use high heat and speed to remove excess moisture from the hair. Select lower temperatures and speeds for finishing hairstyles. Lower heat and speeds should be used for drying and styling permed, colour treated or fragile hair. Whenever you brush hair and partly blow dry it against its natural growth pattern, you will add bulk and body to the style. After partially drying hair in this manner, then brush hair and blow dry it in the direction you want your finished style.

However, it is best not to use a blow dryer frequently. In the longer run, it can be damaging for the hair.

I have medium to long hair and would like to wear it in a chignon. How do I create this chic look?

You must purchase a doughnut shaped ratt, then pull your hair back in a ponytail. Now pull the ponytail through the doughnut hole. Shape the hair around the ratt and secure ends under the ratt with hairpins. To hold stray hair in place, spray lightly with a light hairspray. If the hair is thin, tease it lightly before shaping it around the ratt, smoothing hair as you tuck ends under it.

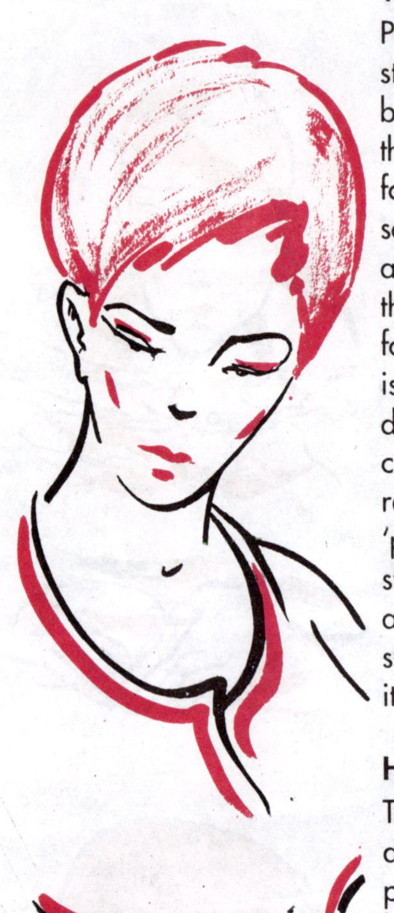

What is a perm? How does it work?

Permanent waves i.e. perm (in short) changes the hair from straight to wavy. They are created by breaking the cross bonds of hydrogen and cystine or sulphur bonds. When the hair takes its new shape, the bonds must be re-established for the curls to be permanent. The classic permanent wave solution of 'cold wave' lotion generally consists of thioglycolic acid plus ammonia. When the hair is wrapped on the rod, this solution is applied. A certain amount of time is required for the hair to take on the shape and size of the rod. This is called the 'processing time'. The stylist must be able to determine how much time is needed to achieve the type of curl desired, otherwise the hair can be over-processed, resulting in too curly or frizzy hair. Once the hair is 'processed', the stylist applies a neutraliser while the hair is still on the rods. The neutraliser provides a dual chemical action, neutralising and oxidising, which results in the hair staying curled. After all the neutraliser penetrates the hair, it is carefully unwrapped and rinsed thoroughly with water.

How many types of basic perms are available these days?

There are two basic types of perms: the acidic and the alkaline. Acid perms have the most gentle formula. They produce soft, natural, yet long lasting curls on non-resistant hair. Alkaline perms, also called 'cold waves', have more strength and produce firmer, more resilient curl when used on resistant or hard-to-curl hair types. Exothermic perms are alkaline perms that have heat activators, which provide more snap to the curl. New perm technology is producing almost damage-free perms that are ammonia-free and lower in thioglycolic acid. These new perms result in beautiful springy curls.

What is a reverse perm?

A reverse perm is actually the process of taking the curls out of the hair. It can be used to change a naturally tight curl to a looser curl or to straighten the hair.

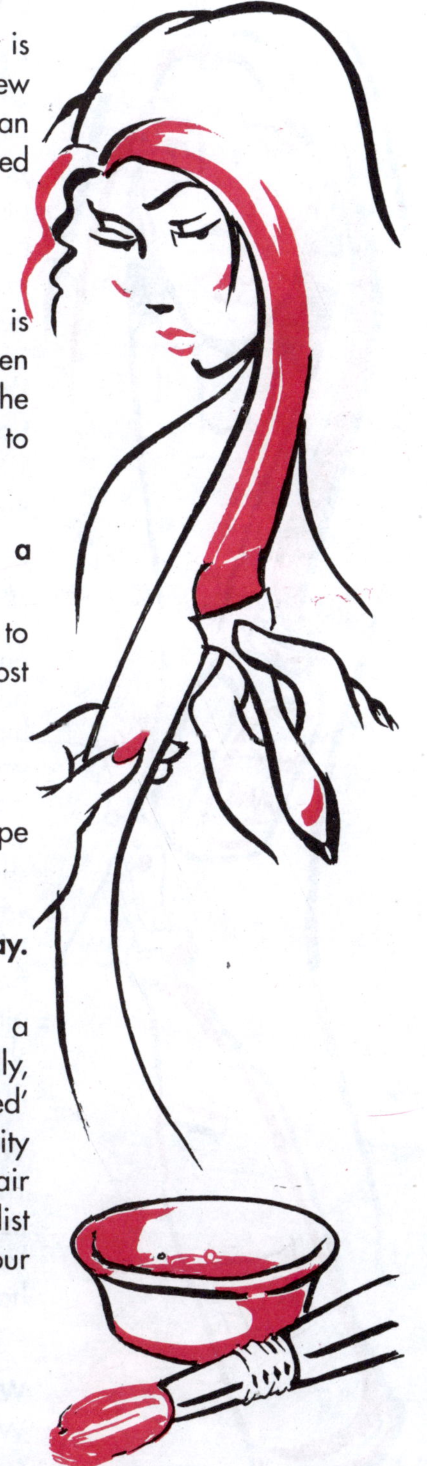

What is a spiral perm?

A spiral perm means that shoulder length or longer hair is rolled on the perm rod vertically, resulting in a corkscrew type of curl. Spiral perms can also be used to crease an explosion of curls. For a traditional perm, the hair is rolled horizontally.

What is meant by the term 'root perm'?

A root perm is used only at the root area of the hair. It is used to perm new growth on the hair that has been previously permed or to add extra lift at the root area. The previously permed ends are protected with products to prevent the waving lotion from penetrating the ends.

What is the difference between a home perm and a professional perm?

Home perms are usually milder formulas that take longer to process. Professional perms have the advantage of the most current technology and the experience of a stylist.

What is a cold wave?

'Cold wave' is the term used for an alkaline wave. This type of perm does not require any added heat to process.

I am a swimmer and have to get into the pool everyday. Can I go in for a perm and will it last?

Yes, you can get your hair permed and it will last for a reasonable duration of time. If you swim in a pool daily, your hair should be classified as 'chemically damaged' because it is being exposed to a high level of alkalinity every day. Take care to remove the chlorine from the hair after swimming, by using a good shampoo. The hairstylist will give you a perm after examining the condition of your hair.

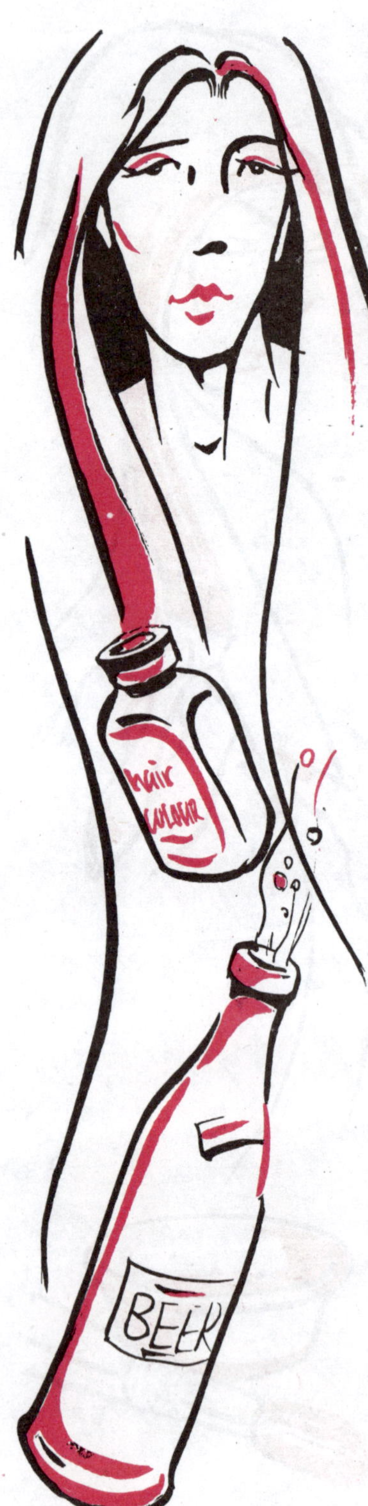

COLOURING TIPS

Even in the eras gone by, women have loved to bring a change in the way their hair looks. They have resorted to using various types of dyes to colour their hair. In the recent years, it has become a fashion to colour the hair and to highlight it with different tints. Although these products have recently made an inroad into the Indian markets, the clamour for these products point to the awakening of interest in the Indian fairer sex.

I want to join the latest bandwagon of hair colouring. Can you educate me a little about the process?

There are two types of hair colourants: the permanent and the semi-permanent. If you have more than 25% grey hair, you may go in for a permanent colour to cover it. If you want your hair lightened, permanent colour is generally a 'must'. Permanent hair colour grows out before it washes out. But, if you just want to experiment and try out something different, you could try a temporary rinse which adds highlights to darker shades. A temporary rinse lasts until your next shampoo. For a longer lasting colour, your stylist may use a semi-permanent hair colour, which lasts through six shampoos, at least. If the hair is fragile or not in good shape, a semi-permanent or an in-between colour generally will be gentler than permanent hair colour. The in-between type of colour is between the permanent and the semi-permanent and does not contain any ammonia. It lasts almost as long as the permanent colour i.e. through 25-30 shampoos. The most stressful process on the hair is a double process in which hair is bleached first and then coloured.

What is a 'base colour'?

The term 'base colour' refers to the tone of the colour to be used. Tones range from warmest red to the coolest tones like ash grey. Tone is an indicator of how warm or cool hair colour is, and it is often referred to as the hair's base colour.

What is meant by the term 'lifting'?

When your hair colour is 'lifted', it means that your natural colour is lightened so that the new colour can be deposited into the hair shaft.

What is the difference between 'single process' and 'double process'?
When permanent colour is deposited in one step, the process is a one-step or 'single process'. A 'double process' involves first lightening the hair with bleach, which changes the level of the hair colour. The second process is the application of the new colour to achieve the new, desired tone.

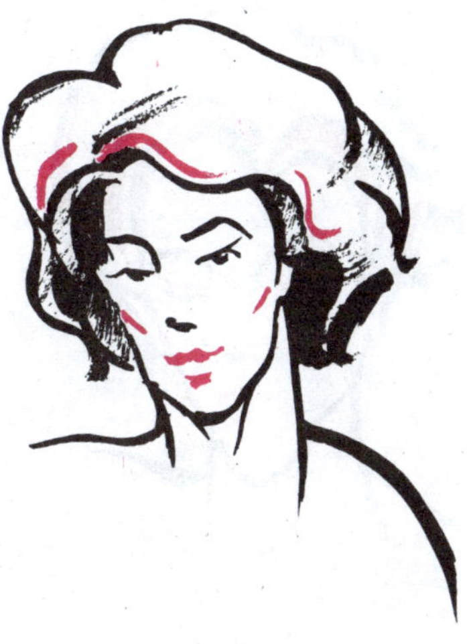

I have heard the term 'toner' being used by hairstylists while colouring the hair. What is meant by this term?
When a colourant is used after bleaching, it is often called a 'toner'. Generally, the toner is a permanent colour, but semi-permanent and the new 'in-between' types of colour products can also be used as toners.

What guidelines should be followed in choosing a hair colour?
Choose a colour close to your natural shade. Consider your skin tone and eye colour. Hair colour with warm tones like red, gold and auburn shades are more compatible with warm skin tones and brown eyes. Cool tone colours like lighter gold or ash is more suitable for the fair skinned people.

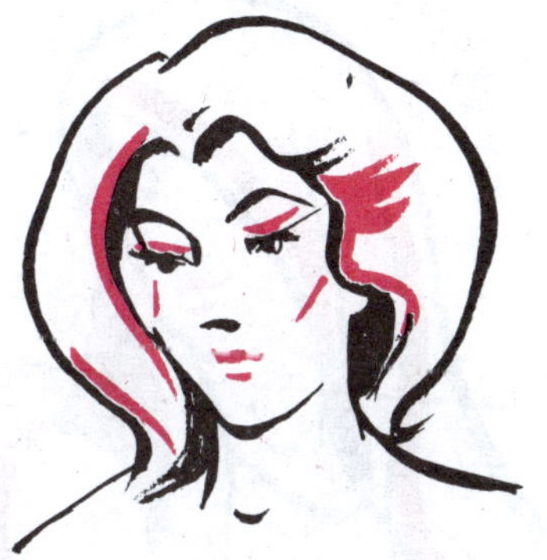

What is the difference between frosting, tipping and streaking?
Frosting involves pulling several fine strands of hair through a 'frosting cap' and using bleach to remove the colour. Tipping is a process in which only the tip ends of different strands of hair are bleached. Streaking or painting means to apply colour or bleach with a colourbrush much like painting. These processes are also known as highlighting which can also be done with squares of foil or other material.

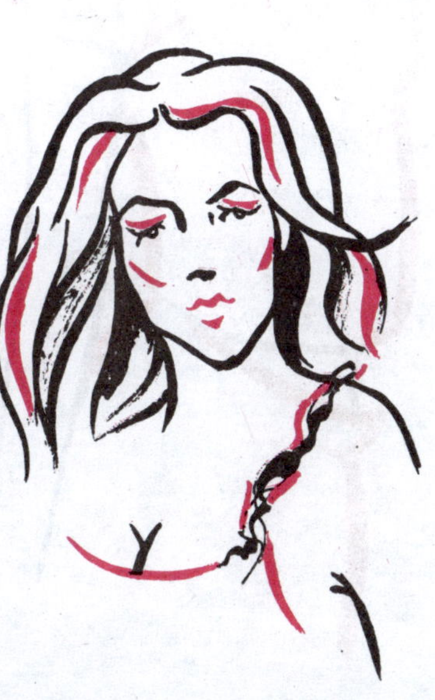

How often can one colour the hair?
Hair can be coloured as long as the hair fibre is strong and the scalp is not sensitive. If hair is spongy or breaks easily, use a semi-permanent hair colour formulated for damaged hair. Also, begin a rigorous conditioning programme immediately. Generally, touch-ups should be done every four to five weeks, depending on the growth of the hair.

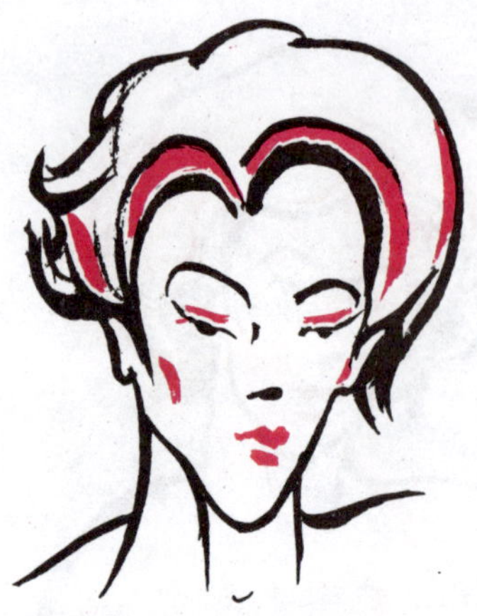

As soon as you find that the roots have started looking different from the rest of the hair, it is time to go in for a touch-up.

How long does a colour rinse last?

A rinse is considered temporary hair colour, which means that the colour does not penetrate the hair shaft. Colour rinses generally last only through one or two shampoos. Although there is no chemical reaction, if hair is damaged and porous, the colour can penetrate and stain the hair.

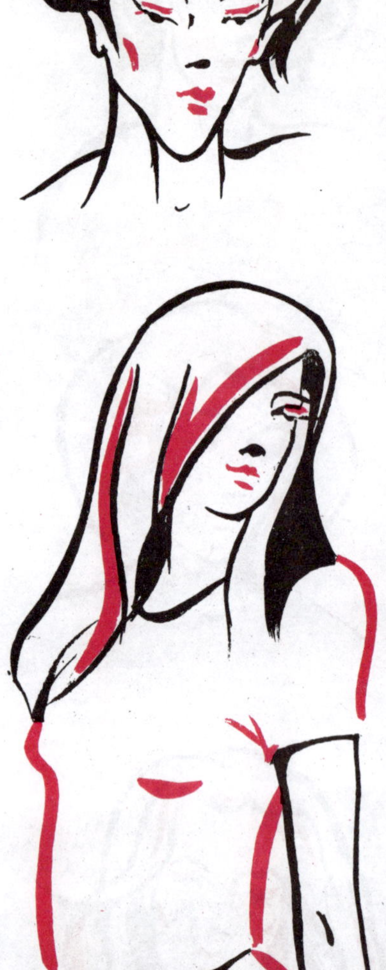

Does the difference in temperature affect hair colour?

Most professional hair colour products are tested at high as well as low temperatures. Prolonged exposures to either extreme, however, may cause the product to deteriorate.

If you feel that your hair colour does not last through the temperature difference, change the brand.

Does hard water affect the hair colour?

Hard water contains a lot of minerals, which can discolour the hair or cause it to fade more quickly.

Is there a hair colour product that also acts as a conditioner?

Most of the hair colour products these days contain conditioning ingredients, especially the semi-permanent and long lasting semi-permanents. The hair feels softer and shinier after colouring because of this.

Could I be allergic to hair colour? How does one find out about the allergy?

One could be allergic to certain ingredients contained in any hair product. To be allergic means a state of hypersensitivity in an individual whenever he is exposed to those substances which cause the allergy. The symptoms of this type of allergy may be: congestion of the mucous membrane, swelling of the face, an asthma attack in an asthmatic, a rash, peeling skin or some sort of reddening, an attack of hives or a liver upset. One may, especially if one has any of the tendencies quoted above, experience more or less violent reactions after using a hair preparation.

I have heard that perming and chemical dyeing can cause damage to the hair. I want to get my hair permed, what should I do?
All types of chemical treatments and perming cause damage to the hair and should be avoided as far as possible. If at all, you have decided to get your hair permed, ensure that your hair is in an optimum condition to bear the brunt.

Can beer be used on the hair?
Definitely. Beer is a good hair conditioner. To use it, shampoo your hair and pour some beer over it. Leave it on for about five minutes and then rinse thoroughly.

How can one add volume to shoulder length hair?
To add volume to shoulder length hair, blow dry upside down and then mist it with hair spray. To give limp hair a lift, use a thickening mousse or lotion at the roots of dry or damp hair. Blow dry in sections on a low heat setting while using a brush to give added volume.

My hair is dull and lacks sheen, how can I bring shine to it?
For a great shine, squeeze half a lemon into a mug of water and pour over the head after a shampoo. This should be used as a final rinse.

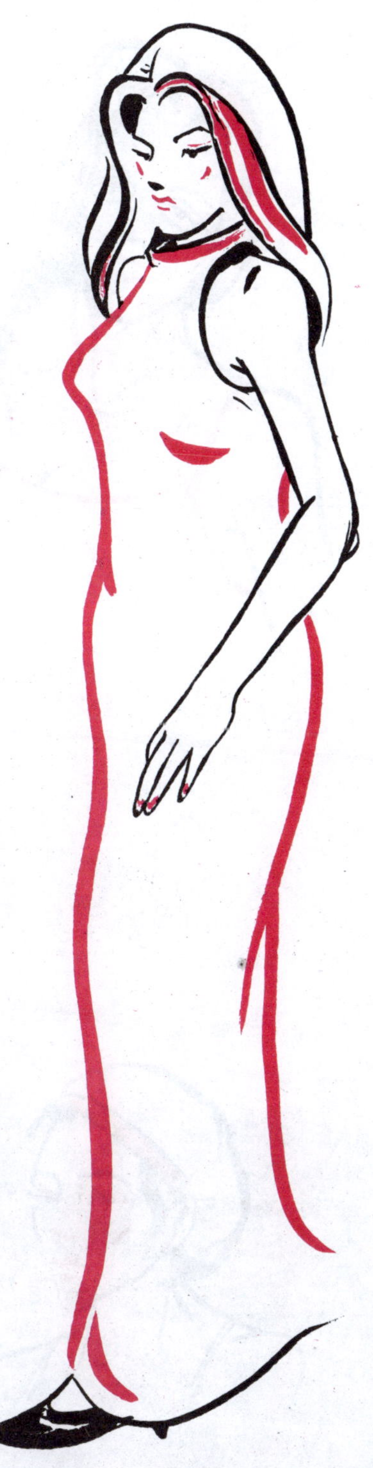

FACE SHAPES AND HAIR STYLES

It is foolish to follow fashions blindly. One has to have a basic knowledge of what suits her facial features and her figure. An outlandish style that looks good on a model may not necessarily give a flattering look to everyone.

I have a small face, what type of hairstyle will suit me?
You should stay away from long hair. Stick to short hair cuts, instead preferably above the shoulder line. This will give an illusion of length to your face.

What is the ideal hairstyle for a round face?
For a round shaped face, one should opt for a style that will cut down on the cheeks. A shoulder-length bob cut will make the face look slimmer and longer. Alternatively, one

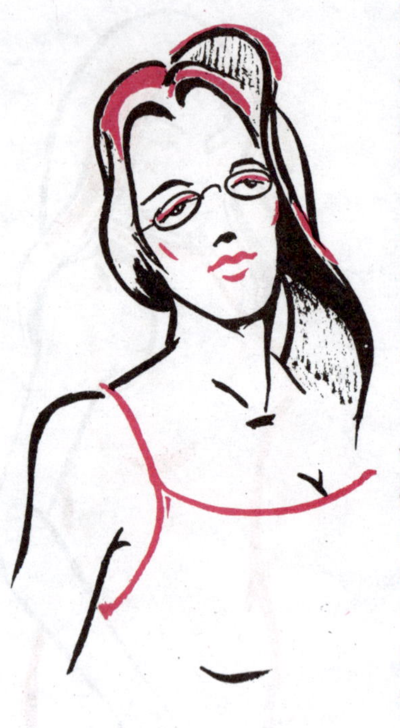

could pile the hair on top of the head, leaving a few loose tendrils to frame the face. This will add height and the face will achieve a delicate look. Avoid pulled back hair, chignons with oval shapes, heavy fringe and short hair. Tease hair to give height to the crown. Long and straight hair can also have a stunning effect on round faces.

I am disappointed with my new hairstyle. It makes my square-shaped face look more angular. What style will suit a square face?

For a suitable style, try to add as much height to the face as possible. Keep hair off the face and avoid a fringe.

Which is the most suitable hairstyle for a diamond shaped face?

For a diamond-shaped face, one should avoid a style that has volume at the cheekbone level. Hairstyles, where the sides are clipped at the back of the head, look best on this type of a face. Go in for styles that add hair volume near and under the jaw.

Which is the ideal shape of face that can take all hairstyles?

An oval-shaped face is the perfect face. It can carry off all types of styles. For a chic look, gather hair at the nape of the neck and wear it in a bun.

I want a good hairstyle that will suit my triangular, heart-shaped face.

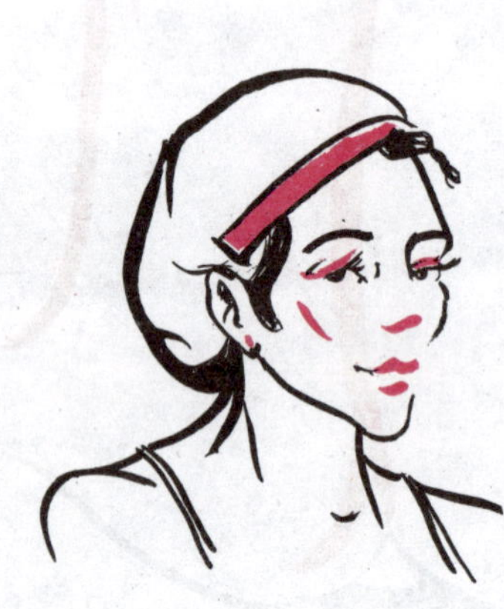

A triangular heart-shaped face has a pointed chin. One must avoid any style that enlarges the forehead, like hair that is flicked out, top hair, which is very fluffy, and pony tail. Try semi-long hair with a light and even fringe. Part hair on one side or wear the hair without a parting. Try and add volume towards the front of the head. For short hair, turn the ends inwards.

I have a triangular pear-shaped face, which hairstyle will bring out the best in me?

The triangular pear-shaped face is pointed towards the forehead. For a suitable hairstyle you must choose one which makes the forehead look larger. Wear hair in mid-length following the facial contour. Avoid all hairstyles that emphasise the chin. Also keep away from the styles that require middle parting and never wear a fringe.

Please suggest a style to suit a thin and long face.
Long or mid-length hair looks good on a thin and long face. One could also wear chignons or very short hair.

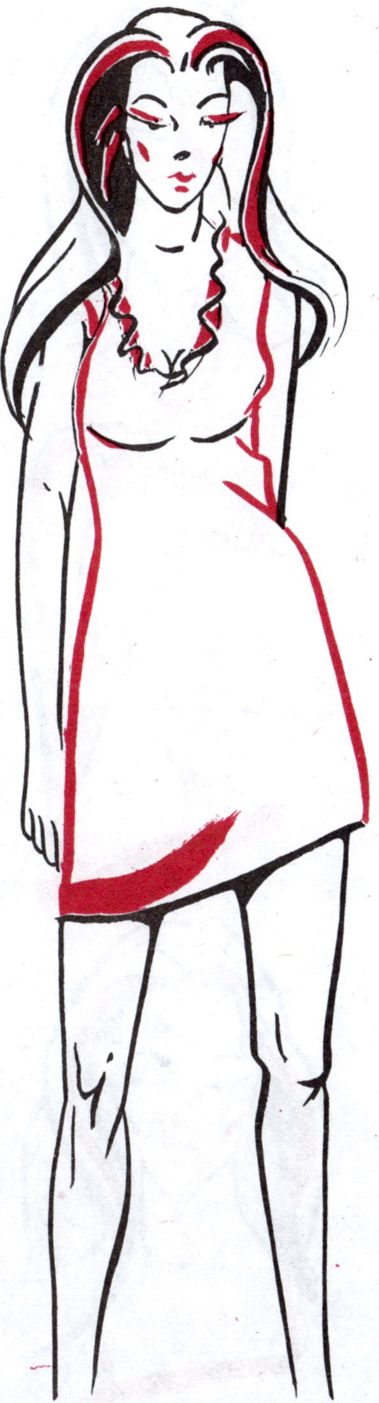

YOUR FIGURE AND HAIRSTYLE

While deciding on the hairstyle, one has to keep one's figure in mind. There are hairstyles which can give illusions of slenderness or solidity. Selecting the right kind of hairstyle can give a very flattering end result and improve the general personality.

Could you give guidance on what kinds of hairstyle looks good on different types of figures?
To decide what kind of hair looks nice on you, you must not only consider the shape of your face, but also your stature.

- If you are tall and slim: avoid a bun-like chignon, and a very short cut (page boy cut). Choose medium length styles, which will cover your neck.
- If you are small and plump: never wear long or medium long hair, it should be short and soft in style.
- If you have rather wide hips: avoid a voluminous or 'puff-ball' style. Instead select a style that is not too wide.
- If your neck is too short: short hair, which leaves the ears and the nape of the neck exposed, will look good. A chignon is suitable if you are very young.

What sort of hairdo goes with various dresses? Could you elaborate on it?
If you are wearing a cocktail or evening dress at night try a neat hair-style without dragging your hair back. That could give a severe look. No hair should fall on the shoulders.

Large collars and fur collars do not suit long or medium length hair.

Much depends on the type of occasion and the shape of the face.

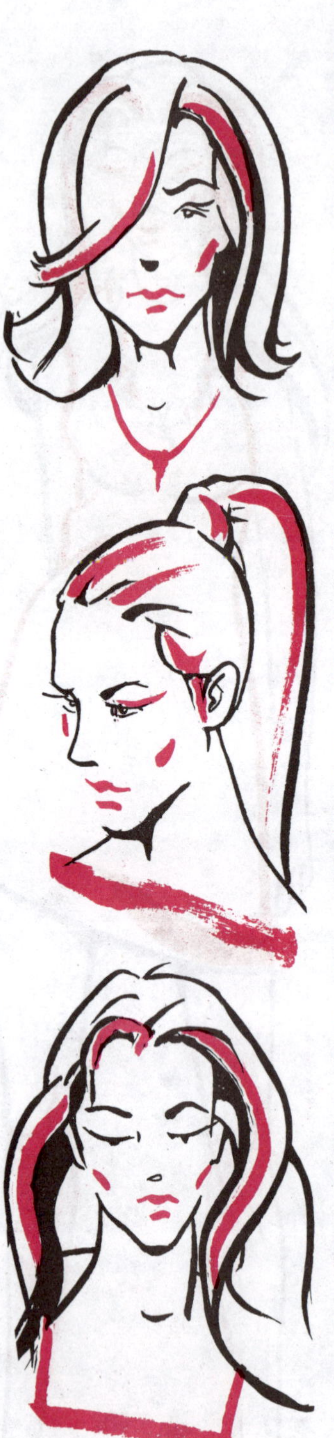

CAMOUFLAGING THE FLAWS

It is really amazing, what a good and suitable hairstyle can do to a person. It can cover up many flaws and bring out the positive traits of the person's features. It can camouflage the wide nose, the receding chin, the short stature, the drooping mouth and what not. One must bear the shortcomings in mind, while going in for a suitable hairstyle.

How can I hide my receding chin, I am very conscious about it?

To camouflage a receding chin, one should wear the hair close to the chin, over the cheeks and the forehead. This takes away the emphasis on the chin.

What can I do to make my big nose look less prominent?

You could puff your hair towards the cheeks and wear a fringe. Remember to avoid a flat hairstyle because that will highlight your nose.

I have a very large chin. Can a hairstyle reduce the bulbous look?

Definitely. You could take the attention off the chin area by wearing a suitable hairstyle. Try to style the hair towards the nape and keep it back from the temples.

Could you give ideas about hairstyles for small eyes and a heavy and strong chin?

For small eyes, you could try a fringe. To camouflage a heavy and strong chin, I would suggest a short and fluid hair style. The cut must be graduated at the nape of the neck.

I have a round face and I wear spectacles. I want to change my present hairstyle. Which style should I opt for?

While selecting a suitable hairstyle, one must keep several things in mind. The facial features like the nose, eyes, jawline, neck etc. are important factors that require consideration. Your figure, the texture and the length of the hair matter as much as the shape of your face. For a round face, the length of your hair should be up to your shoulders. To lengthen the face, the style should have a straight line and a straight parting. There should be no curls or waves to break the line of hair. It should not be cut in a ragged line. Avoid any height above the browline or width at the ear level. These are just basic guidelines and a variation could be worked out to suit your individuality.

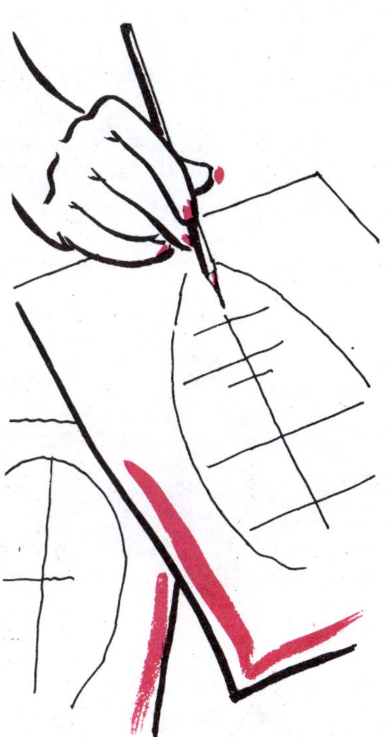

What can one do to hide a large forehead?

Remember the Sadhana cut? It was designed to hide her large forehead. You could do the same by wearing a fringe.

Any suggestions regarding a style to camouflage a low forehead?

Avoid keeping any hair on the forehead. Wear style with height and draw back the hair. High chignons look beautiful on such faces.

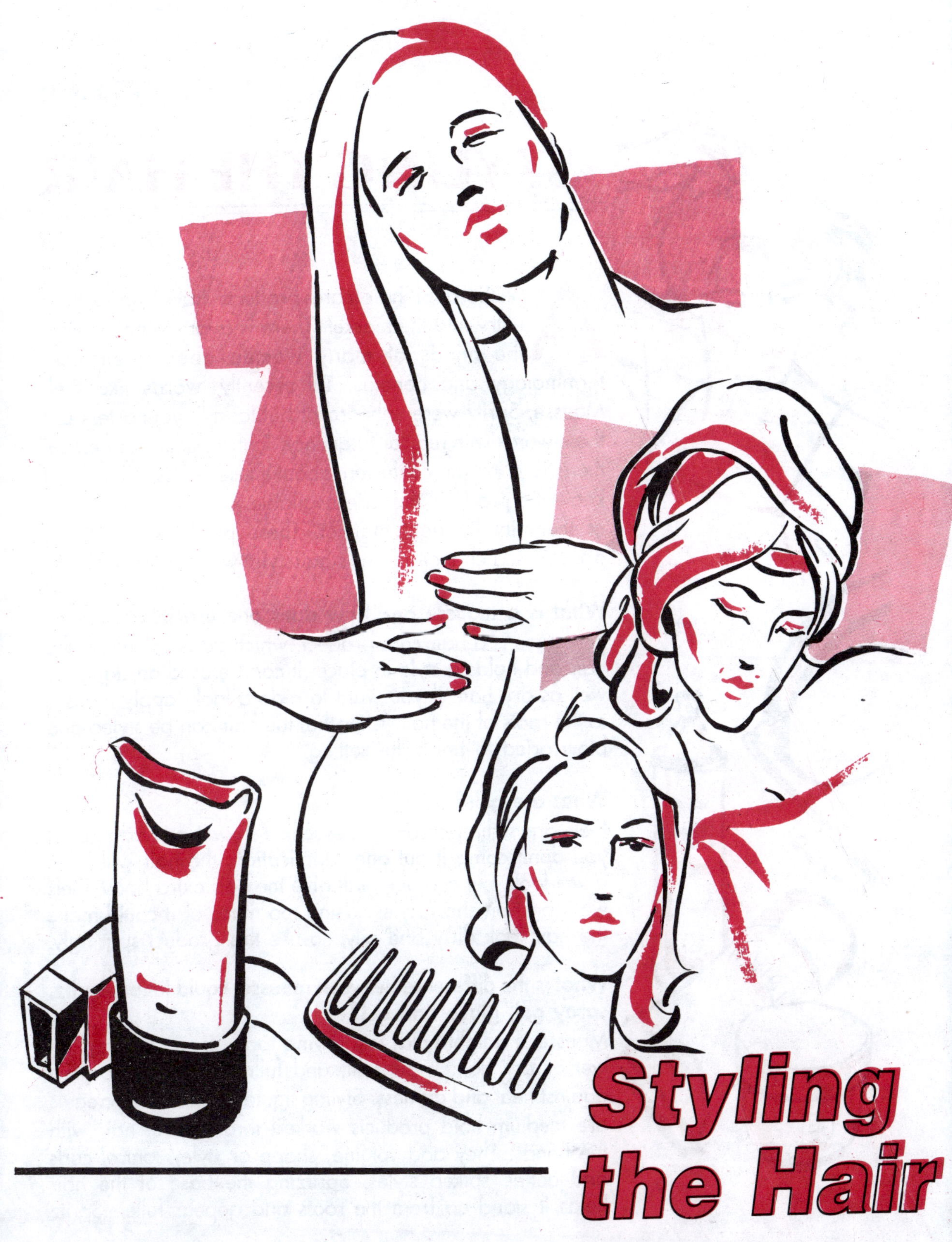

Styling the Hair

CHAPTER II

STYLING THE HAIR

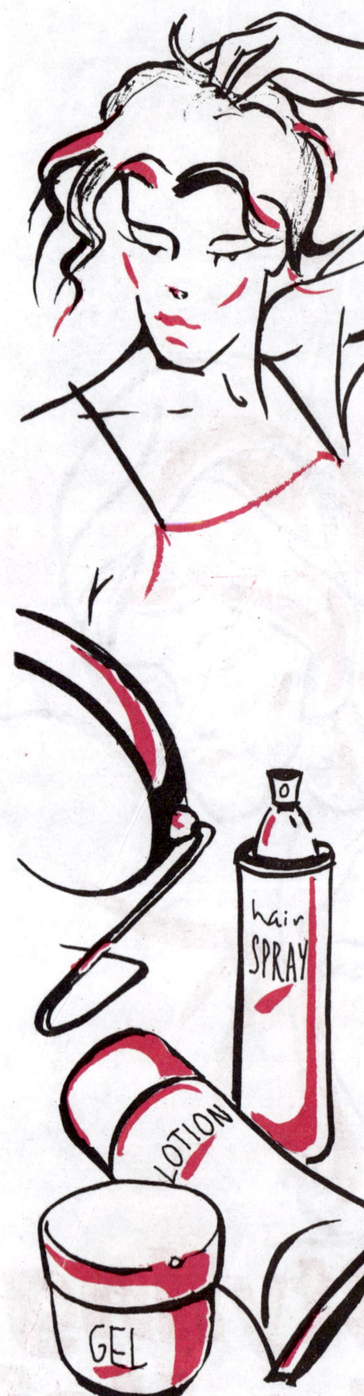

A plethora of hair care products have made their entry into the market. There is a lot of confusion in the minds of many women about their use, terminology and benefits. Till recently, words like Gel, Mousse, Spritz were unheard of but today's youngsters use these words with regular frequency. To the uninitiated person, there is a major confusion about these terms. One must know the products that are available today and make use of them in the right manner. These products can bring about a sea change in one's hairstyle, when used correctly.

What is a mousse and how does one use it?

A mousse is a hair care product, which adds volume to the hair and holds a style in place. It can be used on damp as well as dry hair. If you want to redo a look, apply mousse to the roots of the hair. After that the hair can be styled and blow dried to finish the setting.

What are gels?

Gels are setting creams. They come in wet or body gel. If you don't comb it out after application, the hair will have a wet look, but combing will give the hair extra body. Gels work best on short styles. Using too much of it could make the hair look dirty and oily, so use this product sparingly.

What is the difference between mousse, liquid lotion, spritz, spray gel, glaze and gel?

Mousse is a light hold, fast drying foam. It can be used on wet or dry hair. It adds lift and fullness and can protect against heat and dryness. Styling liquids, lotions and creams are medium hold products worked through wet hair with the hands. They add volume, shape or style, control curls and define spiked styles. Spritzing the base of the hair helps it stand up from the roots and appear fuller. Spritz and spray gels are pump sprays, which are usually used on dry or damp hair to sculpt or control it. They add body and texture to the hair. Spritzes tend to be stiffer than spray gels. Spray gels can achieve the wet look. Glazes and gels are thick liquids used on wet or dry hair. These are generally used for sculpting wet looks, for accenting particular curls or controlling thick, wavy hair.

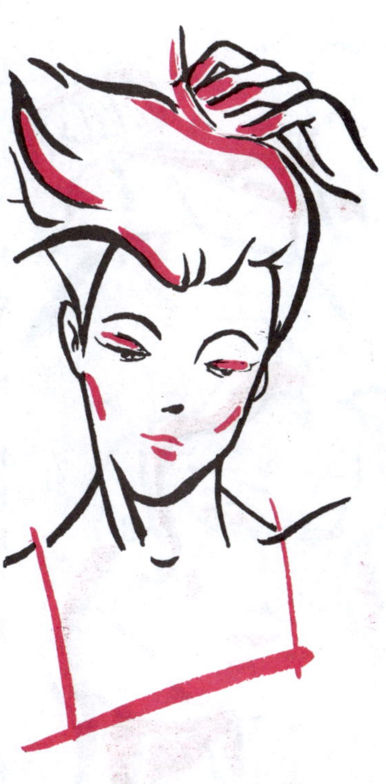

I have heard a lot about anti-frizz serum sprays. What are these?

Anti-frizz serum spray is used to defrizz hair. It is good for dry, damaged and chemically treated hair. It should be used after styling the hair.

I have very fine, thin hair but my hair needs a lift. What type of styling products should I use to give it the required lift?

Mousses work best for giving a lift to the hair. They add fullness and bounce to it. By applying mousse to the scalp, and then blow drying the hair, one can produce an effect of added fullness to the hair. After that you can use a hairspray to keep the hair in place.

Is it better to use mousse or gel to style your hair. When do you apply them, before or after using the blow drier?

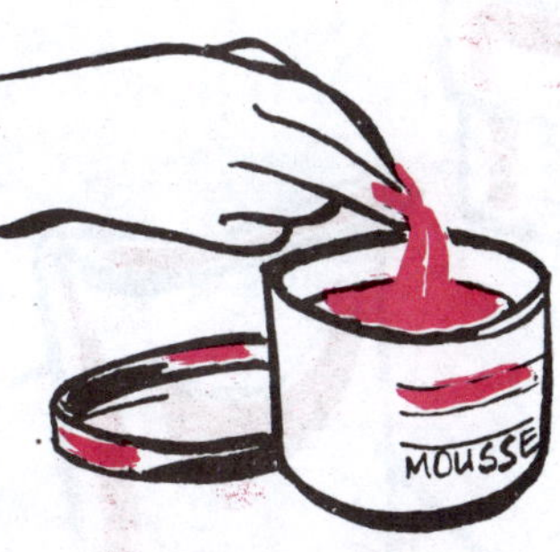

A mousse or gel should be applied to the hair before blow-drying. Most of them have an ingredient, which helps to protect the hair from the heat of a blow dryer. When applying a mousse or gel after blow drying, re-wet the hair to build extra body. However, you may not get the desired effect because the hair may get weighed down or flattened if you apply these styling aids after blow-drying. Spray gels tend to work better on fine hair, because the spray allows for a more even distribution.

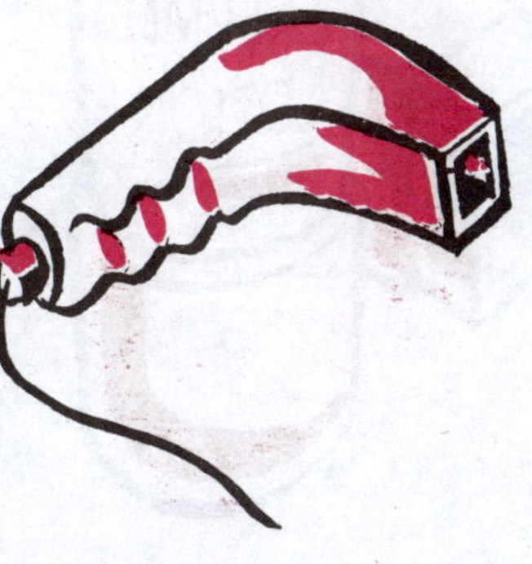

I've tried using a gel for styling my hair but it thickens up and makes my hair look dull. What can I do to hold my style and yet have my hair looking soft?

Mousse is probably the best solution. It has the lightest hold, yet is the most versatile styling agent. It adds volume when applied on wet or dry hair and fluffs it up, too. You can apply it to the sides for a slicked back look. If you apply it just to the roots, it could hold the hair away from

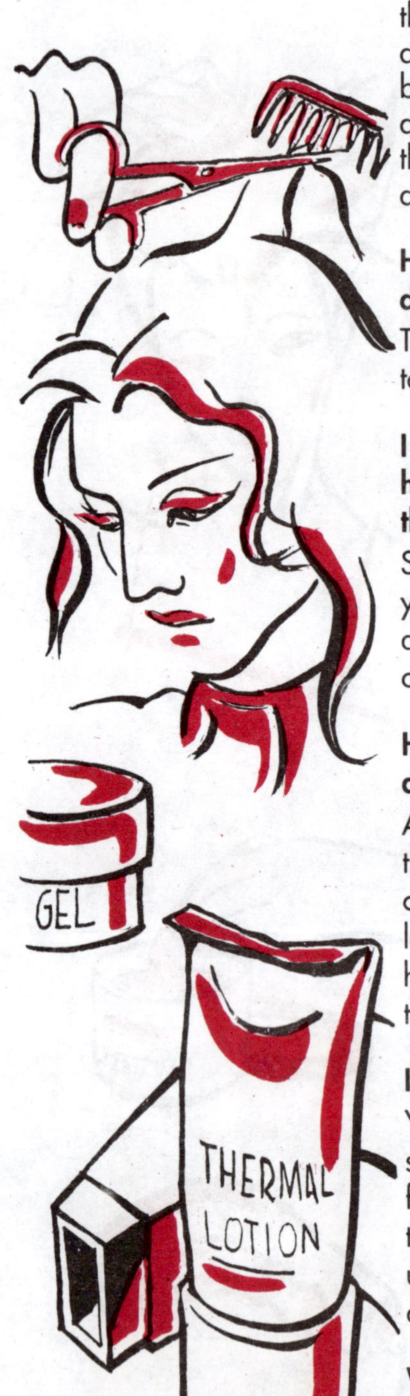

the head and make it appear fuller. Mousse is easy to use and combines the property of hold of a gel along with the benefit of making the hair feel softer. It can also work as a thermal protective shield and so can be used to prevent the damage of hair, from the heat of curling irons and blow dryers.

How can I add body to my hair without getting a perm done?

Try having your hair cut in layers and use a mousse or gel to add body to the hair.

I love to have my hair styled into a French twist but my hair doesn't hold the style. How can I style my hair into the desired style?

Sophisticated hair-dos become much easier to make when you use gels, styling sprays and mousse. They add body and hold the hair. Mousse makes hair easier to shape into chignons or French twists and provides an excellent hold.

How can I give a wavy look to my hair without getting a perm done?

A wavy look requires a curl formation where the base of the curl is directed in alternating directions. For example, one row of curls is directed to the right, the next row to the left. Styling gels hold waves that are combed into short hair. Wave clamps work well to hold the waves in place till the hair dries.

I have short hair. How can I give it an illusion of thickness?

You can create an illusion of thickness by making the hair stand out without lying flat. Brush chin-length hair away from the face with a flat brush. Apply mousse sparingly to the hair. Now, bend over and blow-dry the hair flat and up, beginning at the nape of the neck. Lastly, smooth it into a style.

What is a thermal styling lotion, and when should it be used?

A thermal lotion is a specifically formulated lotion which protects the hair from getting damaged from heat related styling gadgets like a blow dryer, curling iron and hot rollers.

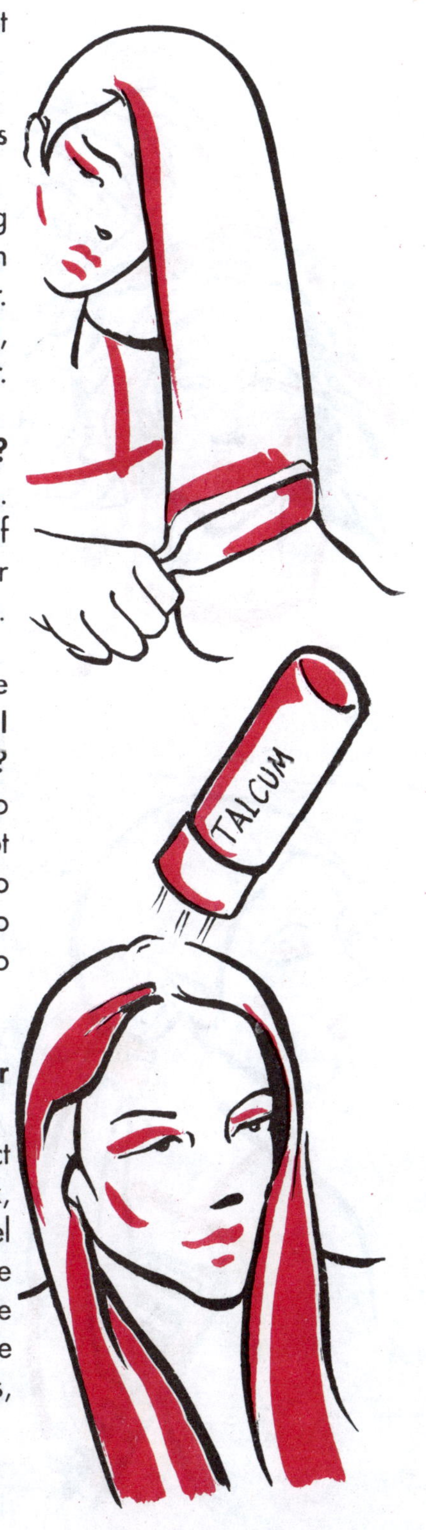

I have heard that styling products like mousse and gels dry the hair. Could you give me a tip on these?
Gels tend to have more water, making them less drying while some types of mousse may contain alcohol as an ingredient, which could have a drying effect on the hair. There are several types of mousse, which contain Panthenol, a product that imparts a healthy and shiny look to the hair.

What is the proper method of applying gel to the hair?
Apply gel first to the hands, rubbing it on palms and fingers. Then apply it to the roots of the hair from the underside. If you apply gel through to the ends, you can weight the hair down so it is safer to stick to the roots while applying it.

I face a problem while restyling my hair after I have gelled it. My hair becomes so stiff that it pulls when I brush it. What should I do to avoid the hair from breaking?
You might be using too much gel or a product, which is too strong. The problem could also be that the product is not evenly distributed through the hair. What you can do is to use a leave-in conditioner before adding gel to the hair to provide more manageability to the hair, making it easier to comb after the hair is dry.

I want to give a natural look to my hair. How do I finger sculpt or scrunch curls in my hair?
Generally, a gel, spray gel or mist-type of gel product works best for finger sculpting. To give a natural look, simply spray gel all over the head or work a regular gel evenly throughout hair. Lift curls at the base and continue lifting as the hair dries. Lifting is important because the moisture in the hair can weigh it down. What you are trying to do is to lift the curl formation closer to the roots, which achieves that 'scrunched look'.

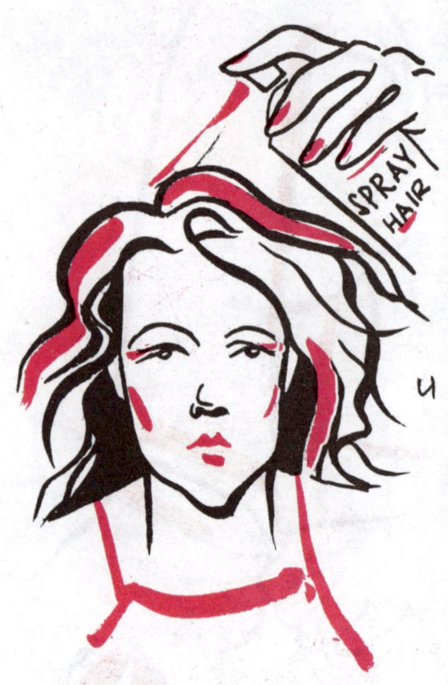

I am an advertising executive and often I have to attend social gatherings in the evening but my hair becomes limp by then. How could I give my hair an instant pick-up?

Many working women face this problem. If you have an engagement after office hours, you could pep up your limp and tired hair, with a little effort. You could simply apply talcum powder at the roots and comb it. This will give it a freshly shampooed look. If you have the time and the stamina, you could go in for an alternative method. First of all, brush through the hair. Then section front and sides, tease slightly at the roots and spritz or spray with a hairspray at the roots only. Smooth the hair into a style and then spray lightly again to hold the style. You will be surprised at the instant transformation.

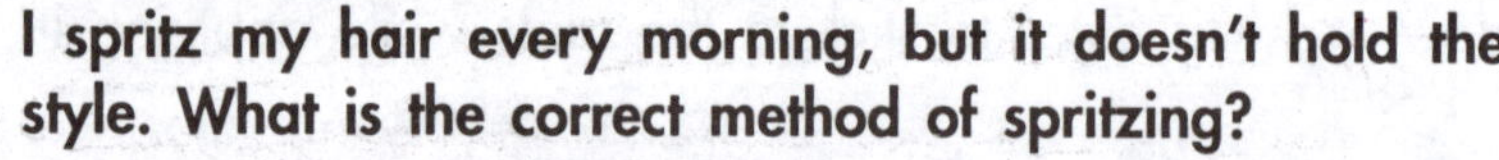

I spritz my hair every morning, but it doesn't hold the style. What is the correct method of spritzing?

You may have confused yourself over spritz and hairspray. But there is a very important difference between the two. Spritz has a holding resin like all styling support products. These add body and texture to a style. Hairsprays also have some resins, which are like 'memory' resins. They cause the hair to remember the way it was styled and to return it to that style after it has been combed or fluffed. To hold your style, use a hairspray and not a spritz.

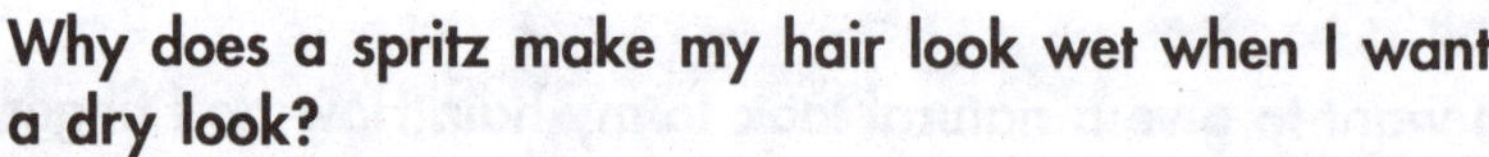

Why does a spritz make my hair look wet when I want a dry look?

A spritz or spray of any type should not make the hair look wet unless it is being used too heavily or being sprayed too near the hair. Spritz is a firm-hold and fast-drying spray that should be used sparingly.

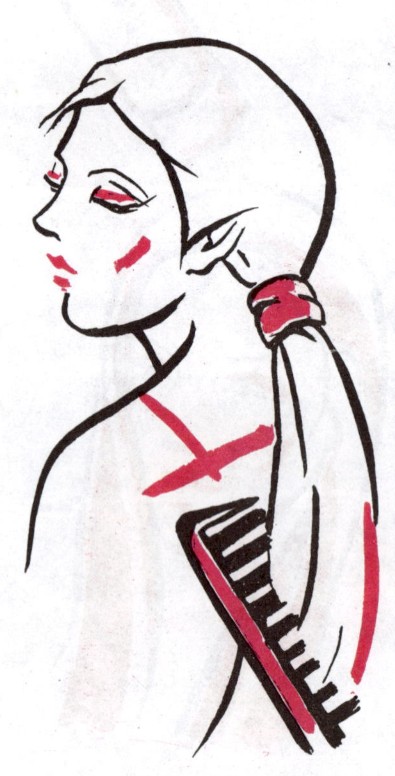

How much of a styling product should one use?

When using styling products like gels, mousses and sprays, remember to use them sparingly to avoid weighing down of the hair and causing heavy build-up. A small blob of gel is enough for short hair. You can double that amount for long hair. But apply only half the amount at first, and then apply the rest so that the product is evenly distributed throughout the hair.

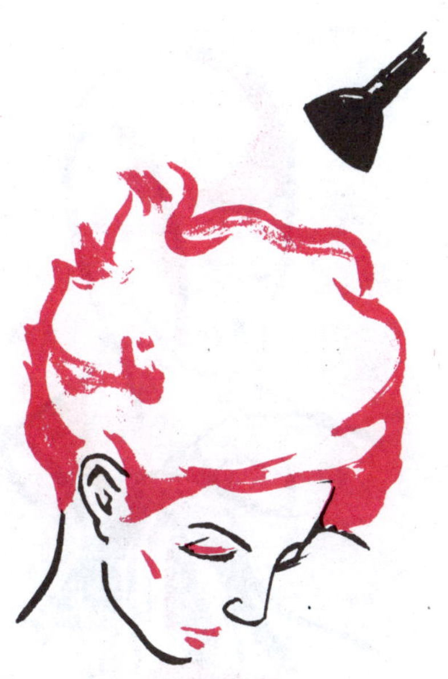

What are setting lotions, and how should they be used?
Setting lotions are medium hold products designed to be worked through wet hair with the hands. They add volume, shape and style; control curls or define spiked styles.

I love making a pony tail but the hair doesn't stay too long in that style. How can I make a perfect pony tail?
For a perfectly sleek pony tail; comb a light weighted gel through the hair from roots to ends. Secure with a covered elastic band. Wrap a small section of hair around the band to cover and secure with pins. You have the perfect pony tail you can think about.

Is it damaging to comb or brush hair that has been sprayed with hairspray?
Combing or brushing the hair after applying styling aids can break and split the hair. Wet the hair first, then comb or brush before styling. Let the hair dry. Then re-apply the styling product. Avoid overuse of styling products if you comb or brush your hair often during the day. Be sure to use a wide-tooth comb or brush with flexible ball-tipped bristles.

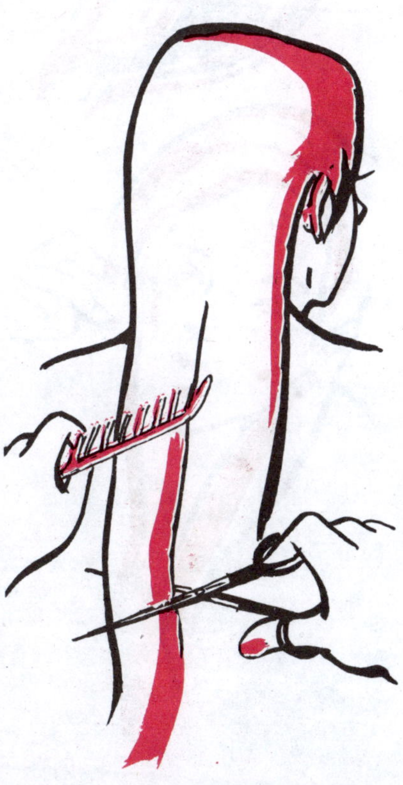

Can a hairspray cause the hair to fall out?
There are no chemicals in the hairspray, that will cause hair to fall out. If you use a strong hold hairspray to keep your style in place, it is better to shampoo it out before you brush your hair. Sometimes brushing through the sprayed hair can put a lot of stress on the hair, making it fall out.

I read in a magazine that most of the styling products leave a build up. How can that be avoided?
Most styling products are water-soluble. With proper use and regular shampooing, you can avoid a build up. One must remember to shampoo the hair regularly with a mild shampoo and moisturise it well.

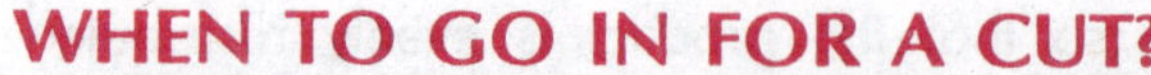

WHEN TO GO IN FOR A CUT?

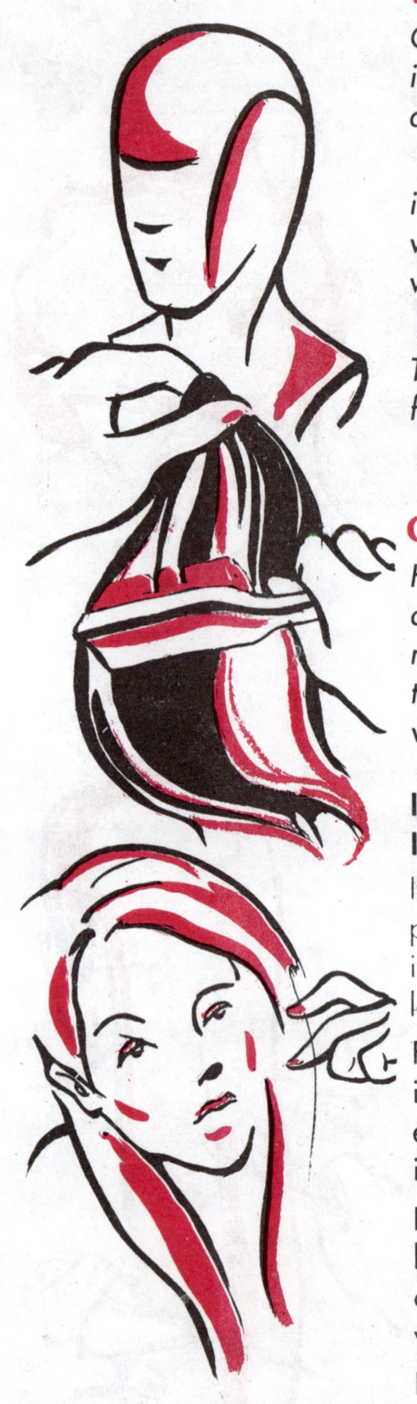

Chin length hair has to be trimmed every 6-8 weeks. This is the best style for those who don't like frequent cuts and don't have the time to style.

Medium length hair has to be cut every 6 weeks. This is mainly suitable for women who like long hair and the versatility it offers in styling. It should be conditioned every week.

Short hair with steps should be trimmed every 4 weeks. This is most suitable for the women who do not like any fussy styling and don't mind frequent trims.

CARING FOR THE HAIR PIECES

Hair pieces have been used from time immemorial, to give additional body to the natural hair. Whether it is used to make the bun or the chignon or to give additional length to the plait, hair pieces are an invaluable treasure for most women.

I am using a hair piece for the last six months. How do I look after it?

It depends on whether yours is a natural or a synthetic hair piece. You must look after a hairpiece carefully otherwise it is far better to wear natural hair instead of a piece which looks limp or badly set.

For maintaining a hairpiece made from natural hair- Brush it well to remove hairspray, dust etc. Then comb it out to the end. Pour cleaning liquid in a glass bowl and dip the piece in it for 5-6 times. Do not rub. Towel off the excess fluid.

For drying, a full or half wig, you should pin it on a headstand, comb out and set the hair according to the type of hairpiece you have. Dry out the hairpiece and comb it well.

For a hairpiece made from synthetic materials take the following steps: never wash the hairpiece in warm water, use only cold water. Brush the piece well before washing.

Use a special cleaning fluid. When washing, try not to knot the hair. Rinse under a water jet. Lay it flat and let dry.

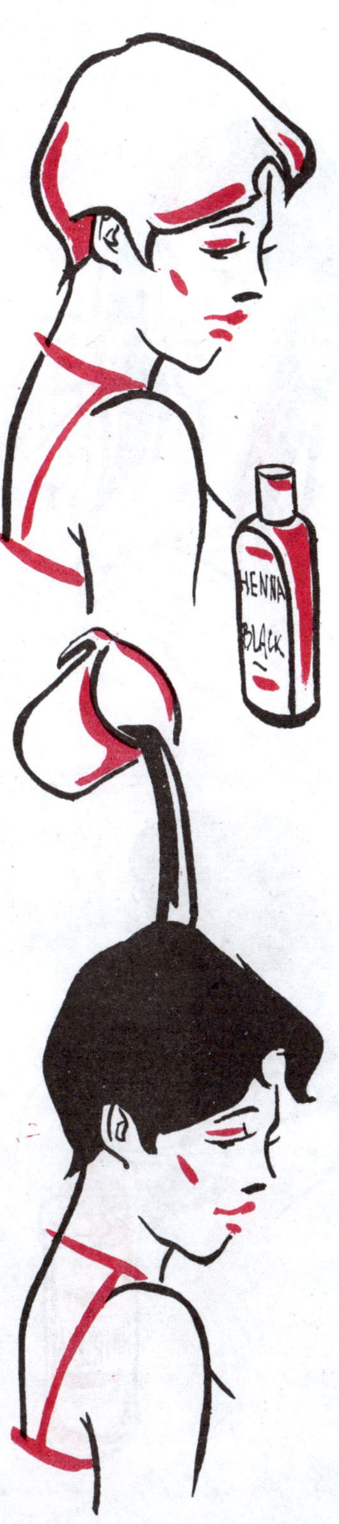

GREY HAIR

Not only do women want lovely and thick tresses; they also want to retain their youthful look by avoiding the grey that appear in their hair. What was referred to as the middle age a few decades back, is now known as the prime of youth. People are living longer and trying to preserve their youth for a longer time.

My hair is turning grey very rapidly. What can I do to retard this phenomenon?

The gradual greying of the hair with age is a physiological process. The loss of the pigment melanin in hair shafts is due to the non-functioning of the pigment producing cells called melanocytes, which are present in the hair roots. In the roots of white hair, functioning melanocytes are either less in number or are absent. Premature greying, (greying which begins before the age of 20), could be due to genetic causes. It can also be caused due to acute fever, debilitating diseases, emotional stress, nutritional deficiencies, pernicious anaemia, thyroid disorders and cardiovascular diseases. There is no treatment for retarding the process but you can use a hair colourant.

I have a very short hair cut. My hair is greying very fast. I would hate to use a hair dye and I don't like the colour henna gives to the hair. What could I do to camouflage the grey hair?

Using gel on your hair will give it a wet look and the grey hair will appear darker. Apply a medium or strong-hold gel to damp hair and then leave it to dry. Hair will continue to look damp even when it is dry. This will make the hair look darker and the grey will become unnoticeable. If you feel that the hair has begun to look dry, just spray on a little water to refresh the gel effect.

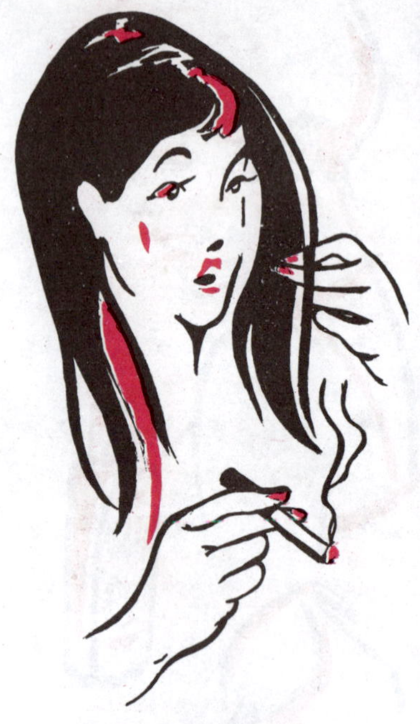

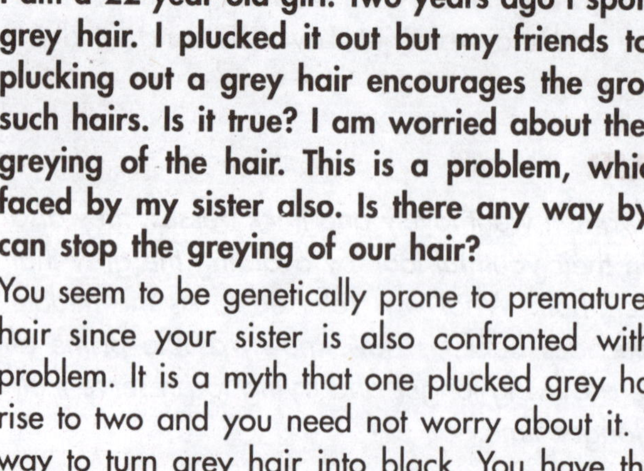

I am a 22-year-old girl. Two years ago I spotted my first grey hair. I plucked it out but my friends told me that plucking out a grey hair encourages the growth of two such hairs. Is it true? I am worried about the premature greying of the hair. This is a problem, which is being faced by my sister also. Is there any way by which we can stop the greying of our hair?

You seem to be genetically prone to premature greying of hair since your sister is also confronted with the same problem. It is a myth that one plucked grey hair will give rise to two and you need not worry about it. There is no way to turn grey hair into black. You have the option of using the natural dyes like henna or the chemical formulas, which are marketed by several companies in the country. Several foreign brands are also available these days.

I am a 40-year-old woman and have sufficient number of grey hair that require dyeing. But I am not very happy with the colour that is imparted to the hair whenever I use henna. Could you tell me how long should I keep it on my hair to achieve a black tinge?

First of all, let me begin by removing the fallacy that henna can give the hair a black tinge. Henna can only give a reddish or brownish tinge to the hair, depending on its quality, frequency of its use and the duration of time it is kept on the hair. The longer it remains on the hair, the deeper the colour. Keeping it on for 4-6 hours will get you the right depth of colour. In case you require a black tone on your hair, you will have to resort to the use other types of hair dyes or colour rinses.

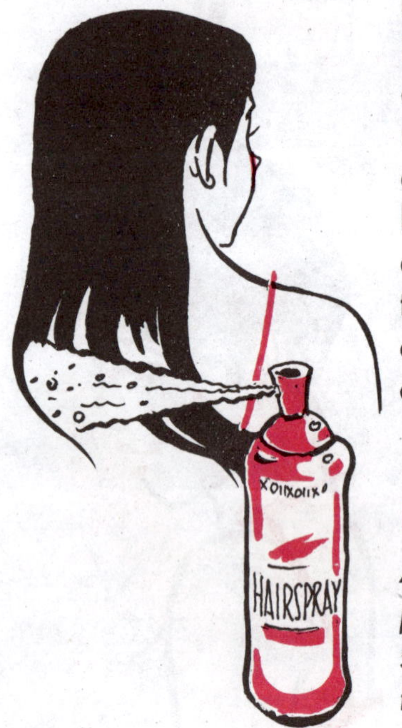

DANDRUFF AND OTHER PROBLEMS

Almost every third person I meet has some type of hair problem or the other. Dandruff, oily hair, dry hair, lice, scanty hair, falling hair etc. An effort is being made here to address some of the common queries related to hair problems.

Lately, I have been reading a lot about the effects of sun on the hair. Since we live in a country, which is hot and dry for major period of the year, how can we avoid the ill effects of sun on the hair?

Sun does a lot of damage to the hair. You can protect the hair from the direct sunlight by using a sun hat. To reduce the sun damage and to soothe the sunburst scalp, massage a mixture of 2 drops of lavender oil and 1-teaspoon of sweet almond oil into the scalp and leave it overnight.

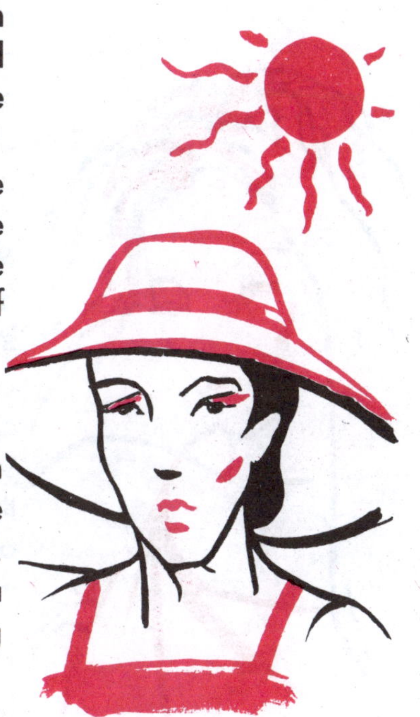

Could you explain about dandruff in detail?

Dandruff affects more than 60% people. It is a mild form of eczema in which scales of the dead skin of the scalp are shed along with the dried secretions of the sebaceous glands. Sometimes dandruff can be confused with psoriasis; a condition in which skin cells multiply abnormally fast, forming larger and thicker flakes.

Although I shampoo my hair regularly, I am besieged with the problem of dandruff. Could you suggest a remedy for my problem?

Dandruff is caused due to hormonal imbalance, bacterial or fungal infection on the scalp and poor hygiene. It could also be caused due to excessive use of hair care products and chemicals applied on the scalp or hereditary influences and emotional stress. Dandruff is difficult to get rid of because the scalp produces a new supply of flakes every three days. Medicated shampoos generally contain either sulphur, zinc selenium, tar or a combination of all these elements. You have to find one that suits you. If the dandruff does not respond to frequent shampooing, you may be suffering from seborrheic dermatitis, psoriasis or some other condition, which may require expert medical help. Hence consult a dermatologist if the problem persists.

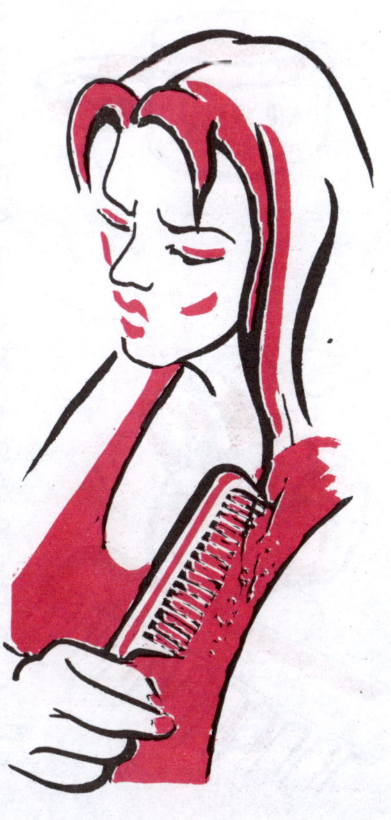

How can dandruff be controlled?

There are many ways and means of controlling dandruff. The best treatment for dandruff is to wash hair regularly with a mild shampoo. Some doctors recommend the use of anti-fungal agents for the treatment of dandruff, but this remedy is quite controversial. Dandruff is best treated with a specific dandruff shampoo. To reduce flaking, gently shampoo your hair using the pads of your fingers and try not to scratch.

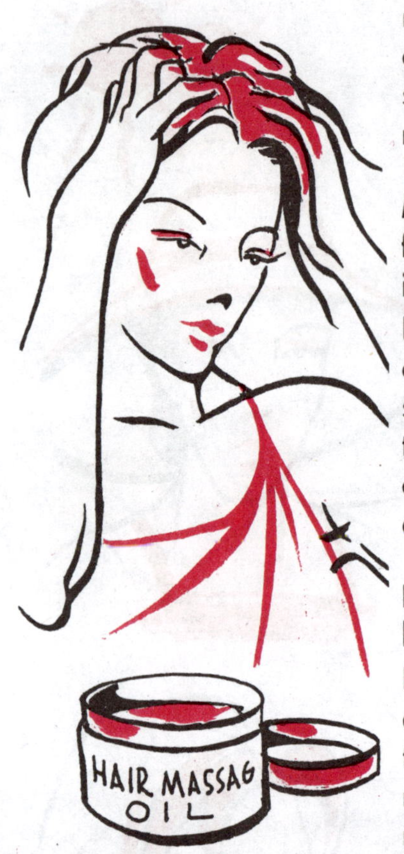

My school going daughter generally brings some lice back from the school. What can one do to prevent lice infestation in children?

Lice infestation is a very common problem among school children. Lice causes itching which leads to infection of the scalp and so action should be taken to remove the lice from the scalp, immediately. Lice are also the most common cause of swollen neck glands in children. Regular use of shampoos containing lindane can eliminate them.

I have heard that regular hair massage helps in stopping hair loss. Is it true?

Regular massage of the scalp helps in stimulating and exfoliating the scalp. The massage also helps in relaxing a tense scalp. For dry scalps, an oil massage could help by moisturising the scalp. But, it is better to avoid scalp massages if one has oily hair because the stimulation may activate the oil-producing sebaceous glands on the scalps making the hair oilier.

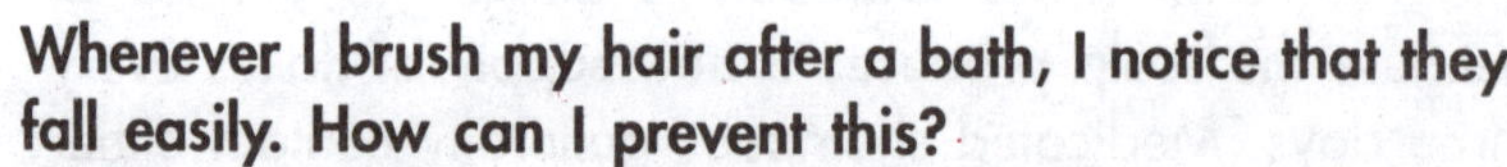

Whenever I brush my hair after a bath, I notice that they fall easily. How can I prevent this?

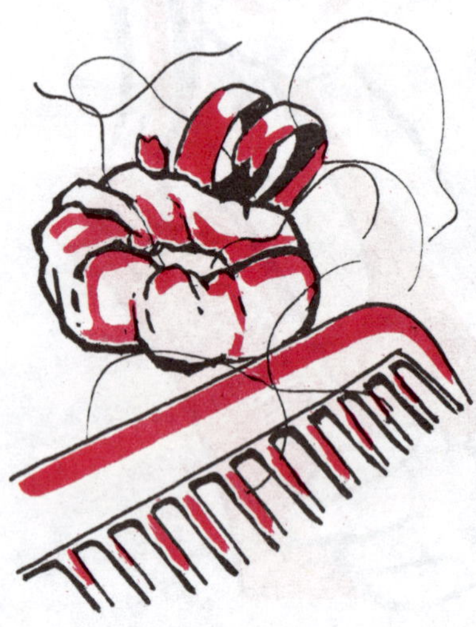

Wet hair is softer and tends to break easily, so be soft and gentle with wet hair. Avoid combing while the hair is wet. And if at all you must comb it, use a wide toothed comb or a brush with very soft and pliable bristles.

Do elastic bands also cause breaking of hair?

Elastic bands tear and break the hair. Cheap hair accessories and poor quality combs also contribute to this problem. It is best to use scrunchies or accessories, which are made out of fabric.

I have very rough and unruly hair. How can I make it softer?

Your hair type may be hereditary in nature. However, you could begin by eating a healthy and balanced diet, using a mild shampoo and conditioning your hair regularly. A regular hot oil massage may also benefit your hair.

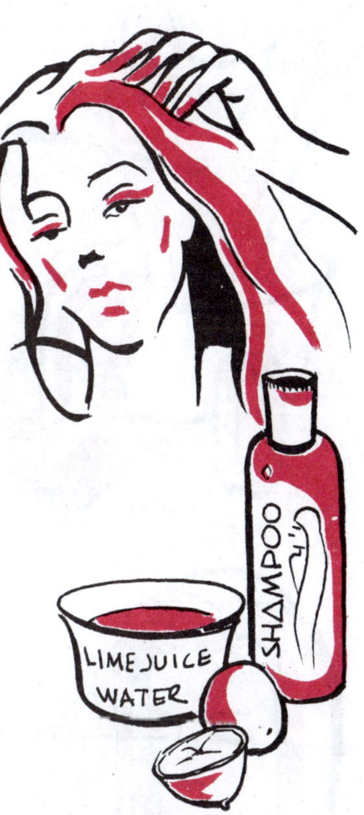

I have silky, straight hair. It turns oily within a day after the shampoo. As a result I have to shampoo every alternate day. This worries me because I have heard that frequent shampooing may spoil the hair. What can I do to reduce the greasiness?

You need not worry about shampooing your hair frequently. If your hair is greasy in nature, and you use a mild shampoo, the chances of damaging the hair are very slim. Use a shampoo, which is specially formulated for oily hair. You could rub a little limejuice diluted with water on the scalp an hour or two before washing. Do this regularly and you will notice the change.

I am a 39-year-old woman. Although I have done everything to prevent hair loss, I have been losing a lot of hair for the past six months. I use coconut oil regularly and have also been taking vitamin B Complex but this has not stopped the falling of hair. Could you suggest some treatment to prevent the hair loss?

The major factors for hair loss in females are the hormonal changes after childbirth, certain endocrinal tumours, birth control pills or ovarian problems. The hair loss also could be the result of hereditary factors. Ageing causes a diminished production of the female hormones and the hair follicles become weak and sluggish. Some of these hair follicles no longer produce hair. Anaemia and dandruff or fungal infection of the scalp could also cause hair loss. I would suggest that you check your haemoglobin count and take some iron supplements if the same is on the lower side. A diet, which is rich in proteins and vitamins, will also help in checking the hair loss.

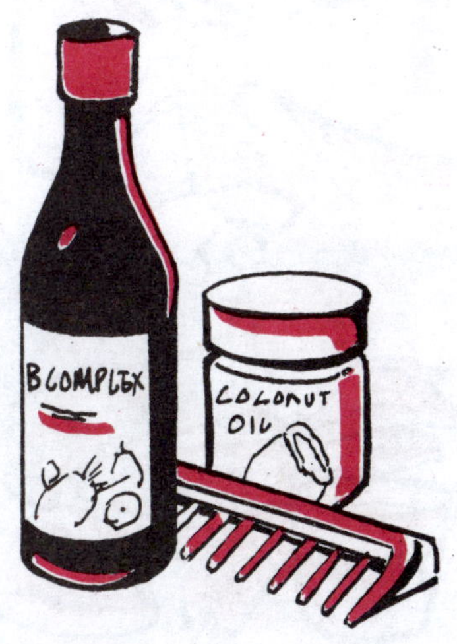

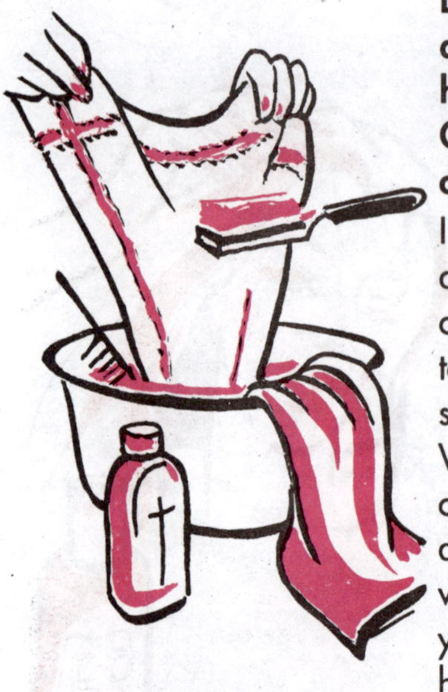

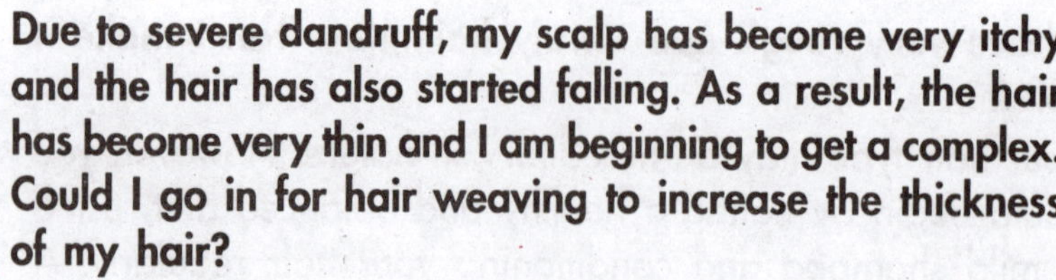

Due to severe dandruff, my scalp has become very itchy and the hair has also started falling. As a result, the hair has become very thin and I am beginning to get a complex. Could I go in for hair weaving to increase the thickness of my hair?

I do not think there is reason to despair. There are many anti-dandruff products in the market, which you could try out. There are two types of dandruff. Dry dandruff is easy to control while oily dandruff can cause itching and the scales mix with sebum which then become difficult to remove. Wash your hair with a good anti dandruff shampoo twice or thrice a week. Sanitize combs, brushes, pillow covers and towels which have been used by you. You could also visit a good dermatologist. However, if you have made up your mind about hair weaving, here is some information to help you. Hair weaving is quite a safe method. You can use the services of a trained and reputed hairdresser who is expert in this method.

I am an 18-year-old college student. I suffer from dandruff and falling hair. I never oil my hair but I wash it once a week. Is there a specific diet that strengthens the hair and enhance hair growth?

As mentioned earlier, dandruff is of two types, the powdery type, which is caused due to very dry scalp. This problem could be inherited and can occur when the hair is exposed to chemical treatments like perming, colouring etc. The greasy type of dandruff is caused by the overactive sebaceous glands in the scalp. Both these conditions can lead to hair fall. Stress, dietary factors and drugs can also aggravate dandruff. You can treat the powdery dandruff with a warm oil and lemon juice massage while the oily and flaky dandruff requires frequent shampooing to keep the scalp clean. Try using shampoos, which contain ketaconazole.

High protein diets with vitamin B, vitamin A and D and betacarotene are also vital for good and healthy hair. Your diet must contain lots of green vegetables, carrots, fish, liver, yoghurt, cottage cheese and pulses.

Hereditary factors also determine the length and thickness of hair.

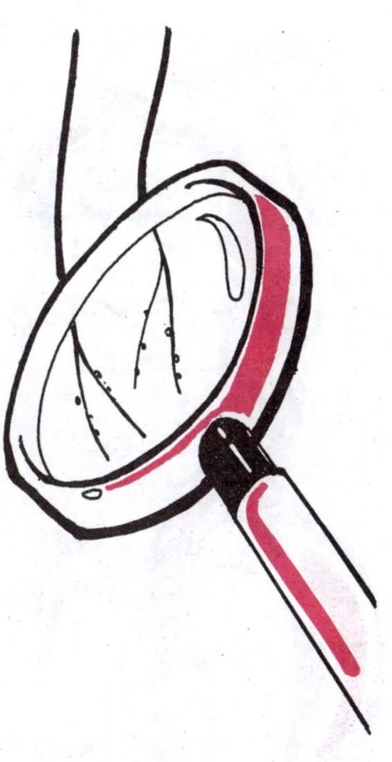

During the monsoon my hair becomes very matty and lank. How can I prevent this and bring back the bounce and shine to it?

The humidity in the air during the monsoon causes the hair to lose its shine, body and bounce. Since humidity causes perspiration, the hair tends to swell and become matty. You need to shampoo your hair more frequently. It is quite safe to shampoo frequently if you use a mild herbal shampoo. Use very little shampoo and rinse your hair well to get rid of all soapy residues.

My hair does not itch but I have noticed some flakes in it. Could it be dandruff?

I think it is a case of dry scalp. Maybe you are using too much of shampoo or shampooing your hair too often. You will benefit by massaging the scalp with your fingertips while the hair is damp. If the dryness persists, use a dry scalp treatment shampoo.

Why does the hair split?

The hair splitting is due to a slight bio-chemical imbalance (lack of certain fatty acids). This reveals itself under a microscope as a tiny mushroom set like a parasite on each hair. In spring this capillary phenomenon is normal and goes away without special treatment. You should not brush your hair too hard, use too many chemical based products or use the blow dryer.

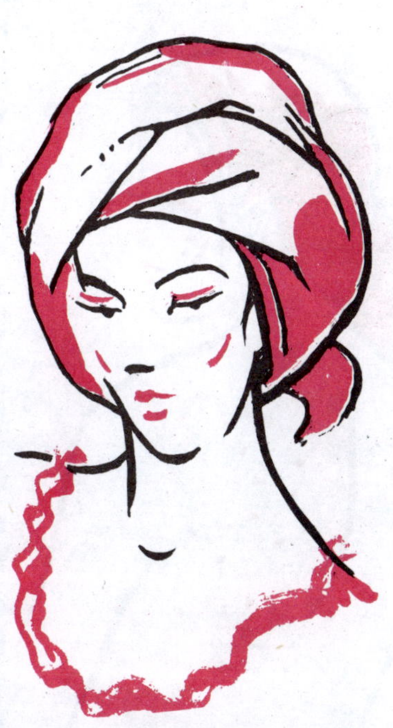

I have split ends which make the hair look untended,what should I do?

Get your hair trimmed every four to six weeks. Hair appears healthier after the dry split ends are trimmed off regularly.

What is the hot turban therapy?

Hot turban therapy is the process of steaming the hair with a bath towel dipped in hot water. Massage hot oil into the scalp and keep it overnight. An hour or so before you go

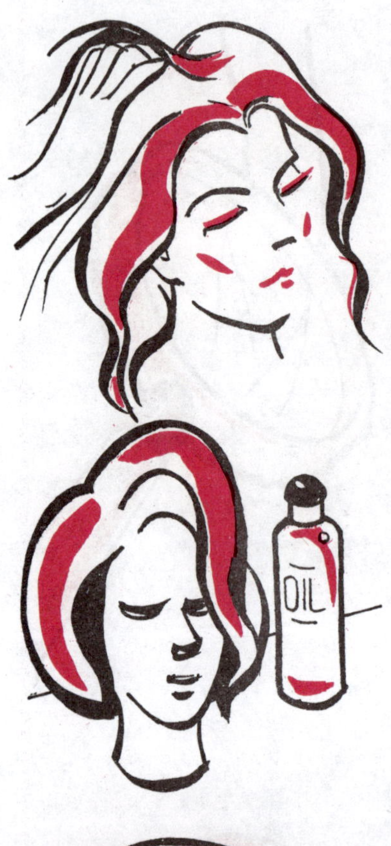

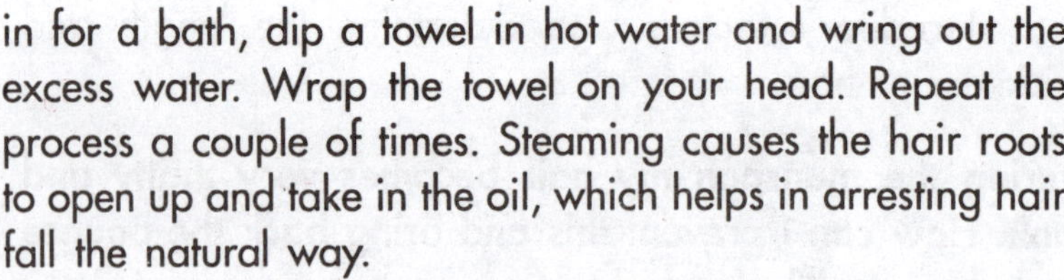

in for a bath, dip a towel in hot water and wring out the excess water. Wrap the towel on your head. Repeat the process a couple of times. Steaming causes the hair roots to open up and take in the oil, which helps in arresting hair fall the natural way.

We were transferred to Jodhpur recently. Ever since we have come here, I have been losing a lot of hair. The hair has become rough and unmanageable and I have also been suffering from dandruff. The environment has a high dust factor. Could it be due to this?

Since there is a lot of dust around, you will have to shampoo your hair more frequently. Since that may cause drying of the scalp, you need to replenish the moisture and the oil by hot oil massage. Lightly massage the scalp with your fingertips and steam for about 5 minutes. You could also give it the hot towel treatment or the turban therapy. This will make your hair softer and manageable. Keep the oil overnight and wash it off in the morning. Don't keep the oil on the hair for long, as the oil may attract more dust.

I have very fine hair. I use false hair along with my real hair. I am worried because someone told me that using false hair would cause hair loss. Is it advisable to continue with the false hair?

There is no harm in using false hair. Some people have finely textured hair and resort to the use of false hair. As long as you can keep the hairpiece clean and tidy, there should not be any affect due to its use. Take adequate care to keep your own hair clean and well nourished. Give it a weekly oil massage and eat a protein rich diet to keep your hair in good health.

Due to dandruff, I have been suffering from pimples on my back, neck and face. Please suggest a remedy for this. Although I have tried oiling the hair and keep my combs scrupulously clean, I have been suffering from falling hair. What could I do to control the problem?

There are a number of anti dandruff shampoos available in the market. All are equally good and you could choose one according to your hair type. Avoid any hair oil, hair cream or anything greasy on your hair. Apply calamine lotion on pimples and eat foods rich in vitamin B, iron and carotene. Foods such as whole-wheat cereals, vegetables, fruits, yeast and marmite are good for the hair. While bathing, wash the hair separately and do not allow the water from the hair to drip on your body and face to control pimples.

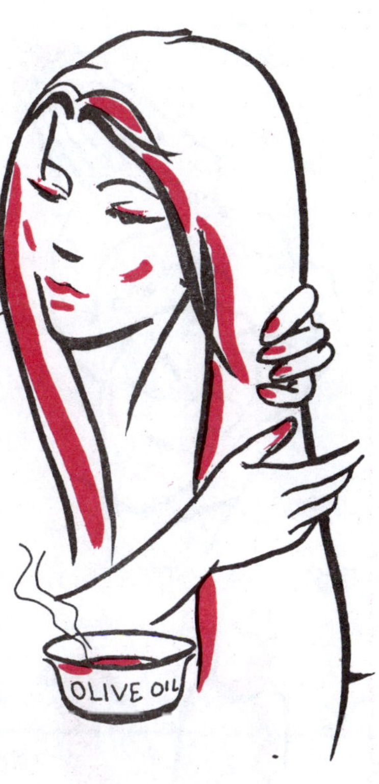

I have very dry hair, which is cut in steps. The problem is that I want to leave it open but it becomes fluffy and unmanageable after a few minutes. I apply hair oil 3-4 times a day and shampoo the hair every day. I also condition the hair once a week. Is it all right to continue with these methods?

Yours is a case of overkill. One need not resort to every trick in the trade in order to take care of the hair. The hair only needs thoroughly cleansing and a good conditioning treatment. Use a mild protein enriched shampoo and conditioner every day. Dirt can also make the hair unmanageable and dry. Massage your hair with warm olive oil at night three times a week to improve the blood circulation to your scalp. This will make your hair soft and glossy.

My hair has split ends and these have stunted the hair growth. I have to trim them off, very often. I want to grow my hair to a good length. Does olive oil help in curing split ends and increasing hair growth?

A massage with warm olive oil twice a week at night will help in improving the condition of your hair. It will take a few months for this treatment to have effect. The length of the hair depends on hereditary factors. Since you have to trim frequently because of split ends, they cannot grow to their maximum length. Once the problem of split ends is taken care of, your hair will begin to grow. You should also take a protein rich diet because hair needs a lot of proteins to grow long and healthy.

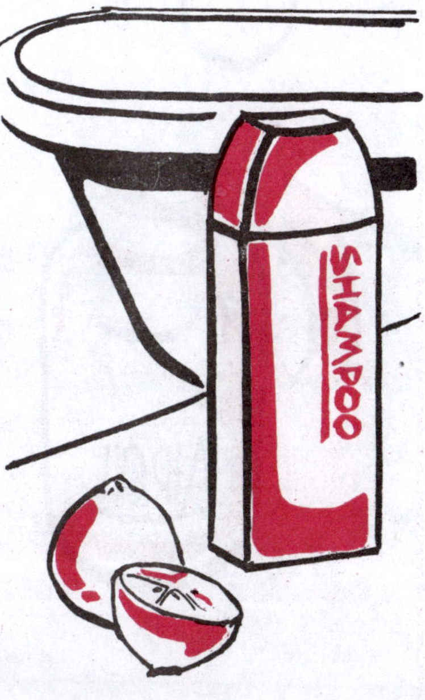

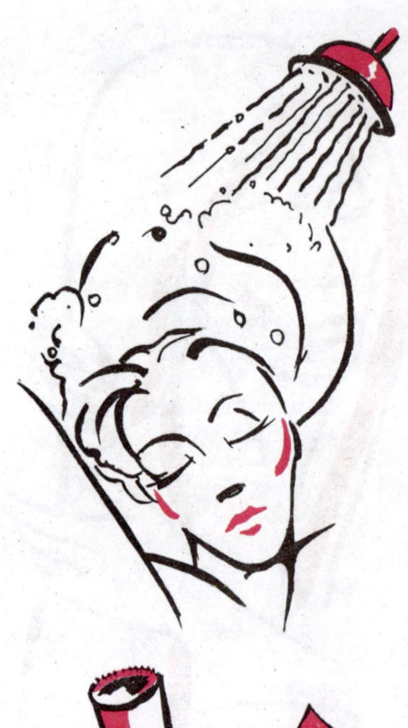

I had very good hair when I was a child, but I have been steadily losing hair ever since I became a teenager. My hair is dull and lifeless and I have an itching problem, too. I have experimented with several hair care products, both herbal and others, but there has been no benefit. Could you suggest some means of making the hair healthy?

A clean and healthy scalp does not itch. Wash your hair with a medicated shampoo three times a week. If you have a greasy scalp, use a lemon shampoo or add fresh lime juice to the last rinse. As a precaution, clean your combs and brushes, pillow covers and towels, everyday. You could be suffering from dandruff or some scalp infection so you should meet a dermatologist.

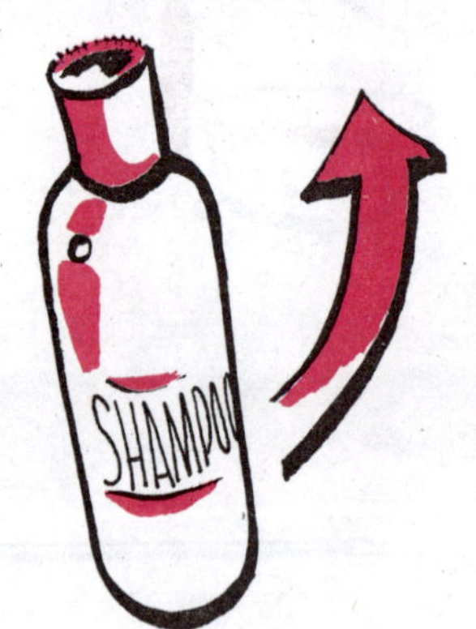

Should the hair be oiled each time it needs a shampoo? My mother insists that I oil my hair and keep it overnight before I shampoo it the next morning.

It is not essential to use oil each time you need to shampoo your hair. Oily hair requires more shampoo, which in turn robs the scalp of its natural essential oils. You could oil your hair once a week or a fortnight and that will take care of the conditioning part. After shampooing your hair, use your fingers to comb out the tangles. Brush later, with a wide toothed comb.

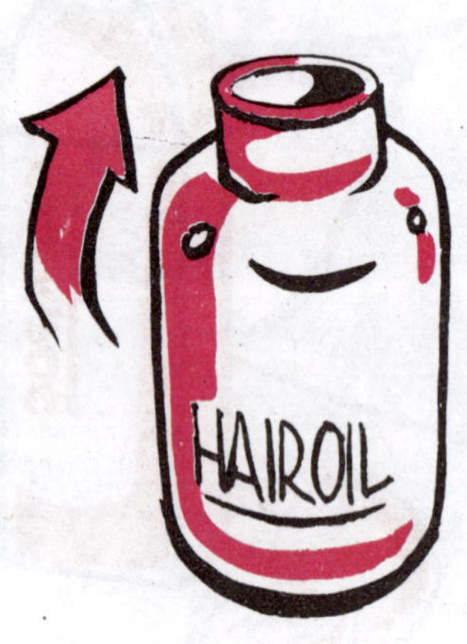

I have very straight and long hair. I want to try out different styles to look different. Can I perm my hair at home? What is the procedure for the same?

Some people would be very happy with straight and long hair. Perming is not a good solution. Some treatments, which need special expertise, should be left to the experts only. In permanent waving, strong chemicals are used which require proper training and experience. Most important are the precautions because a mistake could be quite damaging for the hair. You can easily fashion your hair into different styles with a shoulder length, straight hair because this type of hair is more pliable than a curly type. In fact shoulder length is ideal for the hair.

I have a problem of dry and brittle hair. What could I do to prevent it from splitting?

It is essential for you to replenish and moisturise your hair. A good conditioner helps in softening dry hair. Use only a mild shampoo as harsh shampoos can rob the hair of the essential oils. These can cause excessive dryness of the scalp, which in turn produces dandruff. After shampooing the hair, keep your damp hair in a towel for about 15 minutes. Use your fingers to comb the hair in gentle massage like movements. This will help in activating the oil glands in your scalp. Brush gently. An oil massage followed by a steamy, hot turban therapy on the hair, done every fortnight, will also help in getting rid of the dryness.

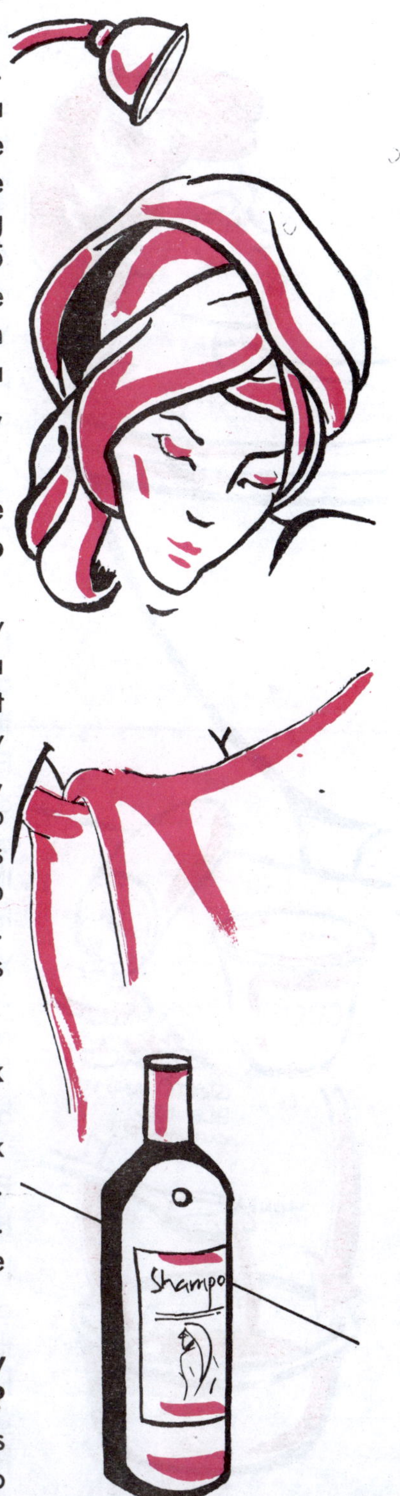

My job requires me to travel widely and this causes the hair to get dirty and limp within no time. Is it all right to shampoo every day?

Although a daily shampoo is not recommended for dry hair, if you have oily or greasy hair, you could use a shampoo every day. Do take care to choose the right shampoo otherwise your hair could turn into a very dry and brittle one. Baby shampoos are normally quite mild, you should take care to choose a shampoo according to your hair type. If your hair is not very dirty and feels sweaty, just rinse it out with plain water. After a wash, keep your hair in a towel, tied like a turban, for about 15 minutes. After that, just finger massage the hair in gentle movements to release the sebum. Brush it gently.

I have very thin and limp hair. How can I make it look fuller?

Thin and limp hair has a tendency to fall flat and look dead. Choose a shampoo, which is meant for limp hair. Use your fingers to comb your hair while it is still wet. When the hair is dry, bend forwards and comb it in reverse direction. This will make it look fluffier and fuller.

I have very oily hair. It turns oily within a day of my shampooing it. What can I do to control the greasy look?

Your scalp has a tendency to secrete excess oil, which is making the hair look lank and greasy. Take special care to

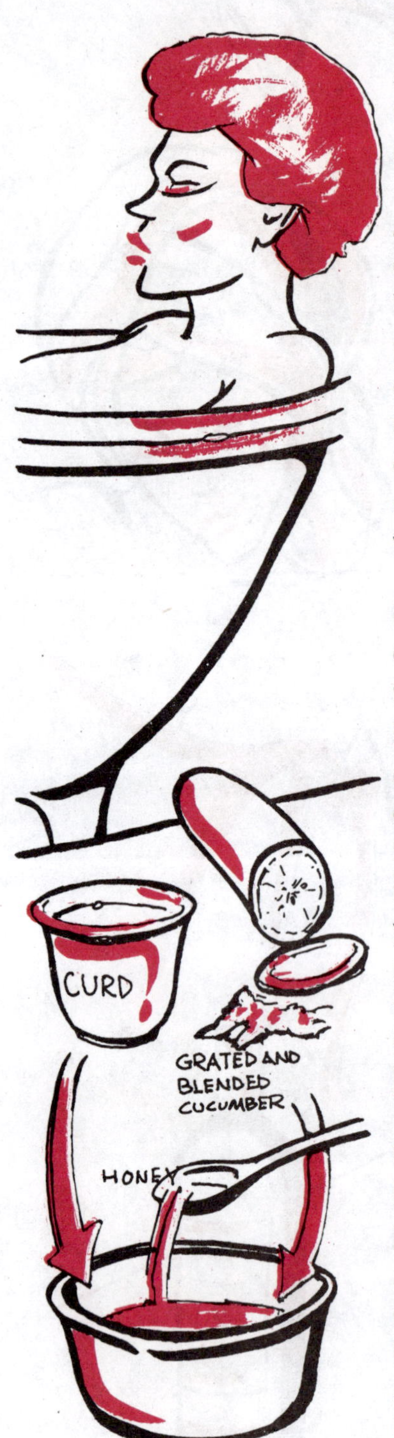

keep the scalp scrupulously clean. Using a special shampoo formulated for oily hair is essential. Do not scrub the scalp or comb it very often, as these actions will activate the sebaceous glands to secrete more oil. You may be required to shampoo your hair frequently so use one, which is very mild and does not cause harm to the hair.

After an outing my scalp feels hot and dry. How can I combat the ill effects caused by the harshness of the sun?

You can use a cup of curd, 1-teaspoon of honey and a piece of grated and blended cucumber. Blend these together and apply to dry hair, leave it on for 10 minutes and then use a shampoo. This will help you combat the drying effects of the sun. Also remember to treat your hair gently. Don't rub it vigorously after a shampoo, instead, blot it gently with a towel.

I am a 43-year-old woman. Could you please guide me on hair care at my age and also tell me a simple style that would suit my age?

Forties is the time when a woman begins to notice the changes in her skin and hair. It is the time to take care of oneself. Problems like dry hair and scalp get intensified at this age. You could start by using a shampoo especially formulated for dry hair and take care of its nourishment. If you have abused your hair over the years, it is bound to show up now. You should be careful about taking a protein rich diet, which will keep your hair in a healthy shape. As for the style, with age, softer and face-framing styles look better than the severe, pulled back hairstyles.

Ever since I lost a lot of hair, I have wanted to go in for hair transplant. What exactly is hair transplant?

Hair transplantation is the surgical procedure of transferring a patient's own living hair from a part of his scalp where the growth is denser to the part where it is thin. Healthy hair roots are taken from the occipital region (back of the scalp) and planted on to the frontal region. It is quite a harmless method and a successful one, too.

Please give some basic guidelines for hair care.

1. Never treat the hair harshly.
2. Avoid using dyes. Use henna as a conditioner as well as a colouring agent.
3. Take a calcium supplement if you don't take at least 2 glasses of milk everyday.
4. Add iron and minerals in a natural form in the diet.
5. Include proteins like eggs and nuts as well as pulses in your diet.
6. Take a lot of fresh fruits and vegetables.
7. Trim your hair once in 7 weeks to avoid split ends.
8. Give it a good oil massage once a week.
9. Use a mild shampoo and rinse it out well.
10. Avoid all types of chemical treatments, perms and hair dryers.

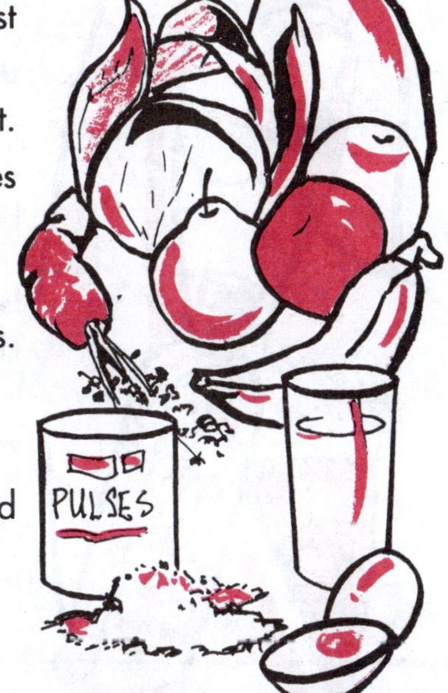

SHAMPOO FACTS

There are hundreds of brands of shampoo available in the market and each one claims to be the best. Under such circumstances, it is easy for people to get confused and keep changing their shampoos. Some of the myths propagated by the companies that manufacture shampoos have been dispelled in this chapter.

Is there a shampoo, which can make my hair grow faster?

No shampoo can make the hair grow. They can add fullness and keep the scalp clean and healthy.

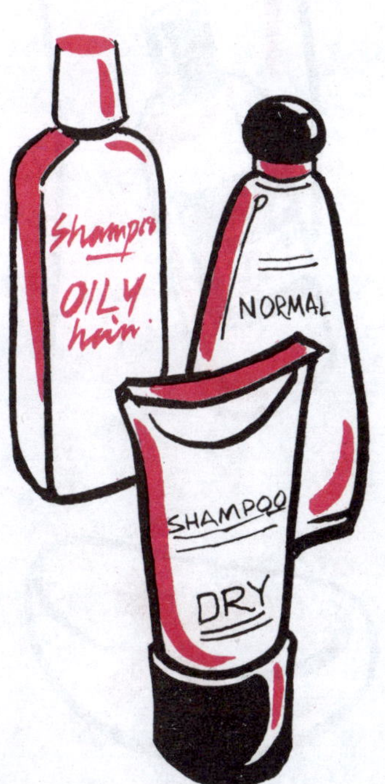

Can shampoo be used everyday?

Although it is not advisable to shampoo the hair everyday, there are a few shampoos available in the market, which are mild and have a slightly acid pH level that the hair likes. It is important to choose a shampoo according to your hair type (oily, dry, normal etc.)

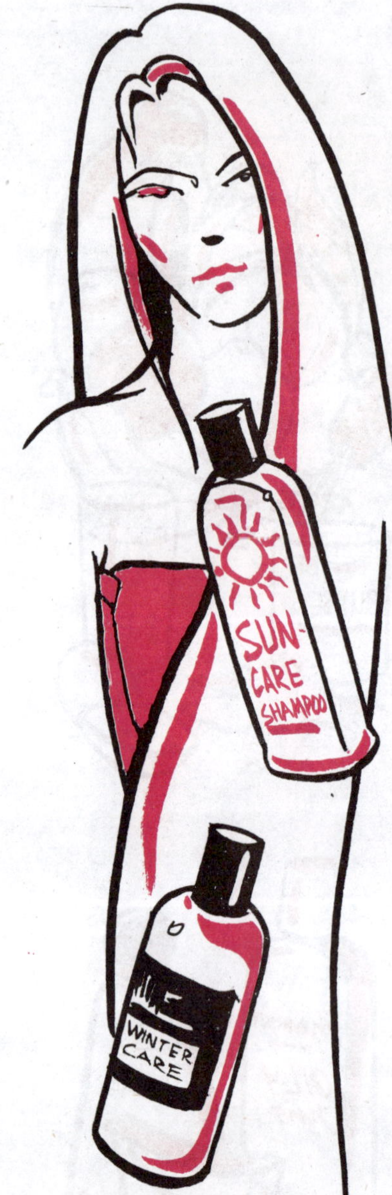

If the shampoo is left on the scalp for 2-3 minutes, does it clean the hair better?

Shampoos are designed to attract dirt and lift it off the hair. Shampoo does not absorb the dirt and so leaving it on for a longer time will not have any cleansing effect.

Will frequent shampooing make my hair oilier?

Frequent shampooing cannot make your hair oilier but if you massage your scalp for longer time, the scalp could become oilier.

Is it better to use the same brand of shampoo or keep changing it after some time?

It is all right to use the same shampoo regularly as long as you are using the right kind of shampoo meant for your hair. However, weather changes may prompt the need to change the brand. In dry winter air, you may need a moisturising shampoo while summer may call for a volume-building shampoo that keeps the hair looking fuller.

My friend insists that a bar soap especially made for washing the hair is better than a shampoo. Is it true?

No. A bar soap is too alkaline and could strip the hair from its natural colour and leave a fatty residue.

I have been using a mousse and gel to give body to my hair. I feel that my shampoo is not getting rid of the build up. What should I do?

Use a gentle, deep cleansing shampoo routinely, once or twice a week. Depending on the extent of the build up, use a shampoo of the right type. A shampoo, which contains more detergent, is designed to lightly strip the hair. It usually has a higher pH level, too. Use as needed and follow up with a hair conditioner.

What is the pH factor?

The term 'pH' refers to the balance between acid and alkaline, which must be measured with the presence of water, because dry substances do not have a 'pH'. The pH level can range from 0-14 with 7 being neutral (water). Anything under 7 is acid and anything above 7 is alkaline. Human hair likes a mildly acidic pH level. Although hair has no pH, the scalp and the natural oils, which coat the cuticle of the hair, do have a pH between 4.5 and 5.5. Shampoos that claim to be pH-balanced usually range from, 4.5-6.5. Basically, a pH-balanced shampoo is gentle and not harsh.

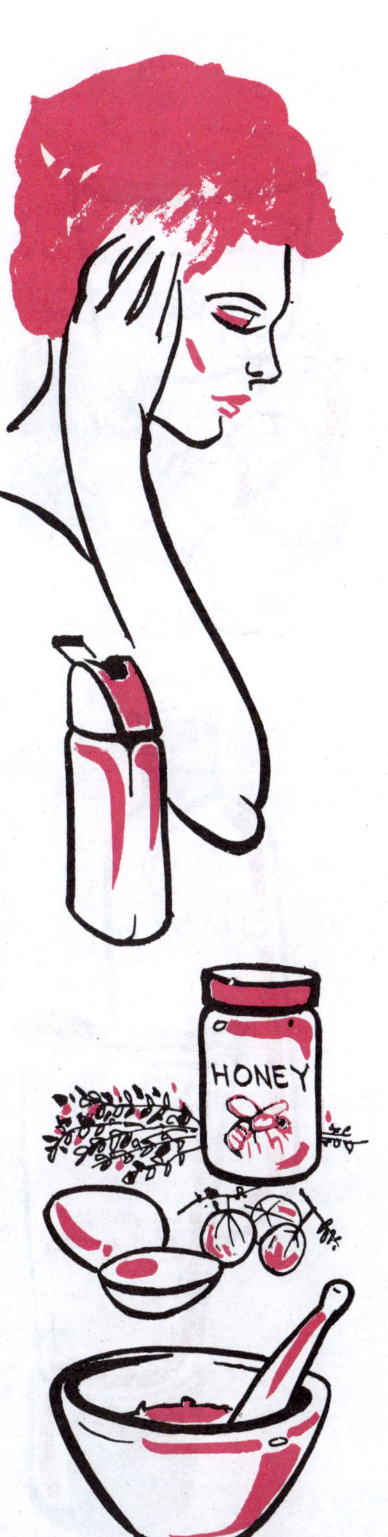

What is the ingredient that one should look for in a shampoo?
Sodium laureth sulfate. This is a surfactant, which adds cleansing properties to the shampoo. Most shampoos contain this element. Avoid heavy conditioning shampoos, which could add to the build up problem.

I have heard that rusty water turns your hair into a reddish one. Is this true?
Yes. Chemicals in the water can discolour porous hair resulting in orange or brownish stains.

What makes a body building shampoo work?
A body building shampoo cleanses without leaving any residual conditioner on hair. It has a rinse-clean factor to make the hair feel fuller by leaving the hair cuticles slightly ruffled.

How can one stimulate the scalp?
To stimulate circulation to the scalp use a rubber scalp massager while shampooing. It promotes healthy hair growth. One can also use the fingertips for massage like movements in order to stimulate the circulation.

How effective is the claim made by certain shampoos that they add body to the hair?
Such shampoos cleanse the hair without leaving any residual conditioner on the hair. They have a rinse clean factor, which makes the hair feel fuller as the cuticles get slightly ruffled by their action.

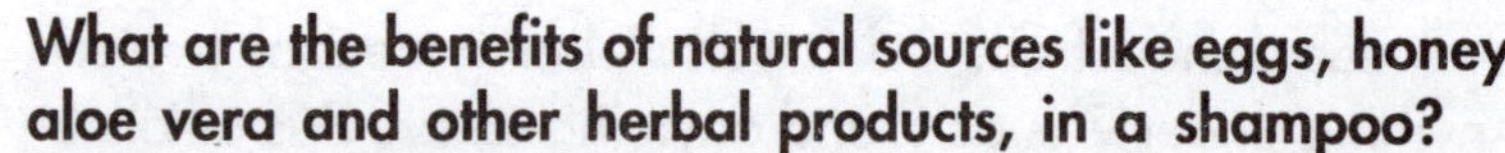

What are the benefits of natural sources like eggs, honey, aloe vera and other herbal products, in a shampoo?

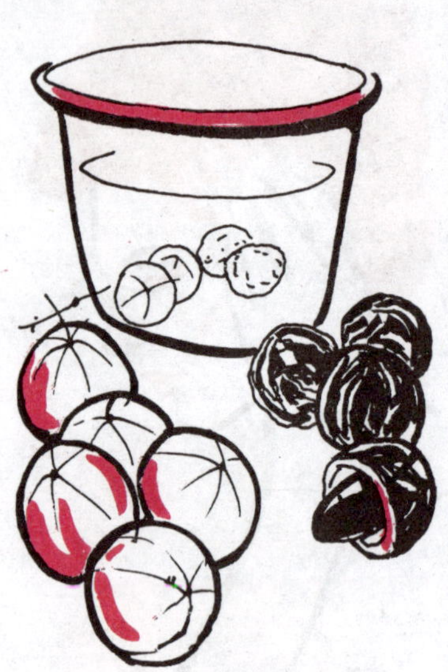

Some natural herbs have cooling properties while some rejuvenate the hair roots. Eggs add proteins and conditioning agents to the shampoo. The extracts from plants and vegetables benefit the hair as they moisturise the scalp and keep it cool without doing any damage to it. Herbs like spearmint act as an antiseptic and help in cleaning an oily scalp. Camomile is believed to lighten the hair. Comfrey and rosemary aid in cleansing while henna acts as a conditioner. 'Amla' strengthens the hair roots and 'reetha' and 'shikakai' are very good cleansing agents.

I have a sensitive scalp and am allergic to detergents. What kind of shampoo can I use?

You must look for a shampoo with natural ingredients such as 'reetha', 'shikakai' and 'amla'. There are many good herbal shampoos available in the market. Or you can make your own shampoo by soaking these ingredients in water overnight. In the morning, boil it for a few minutes, strain and let it cool. Wash your hair with the concoction.

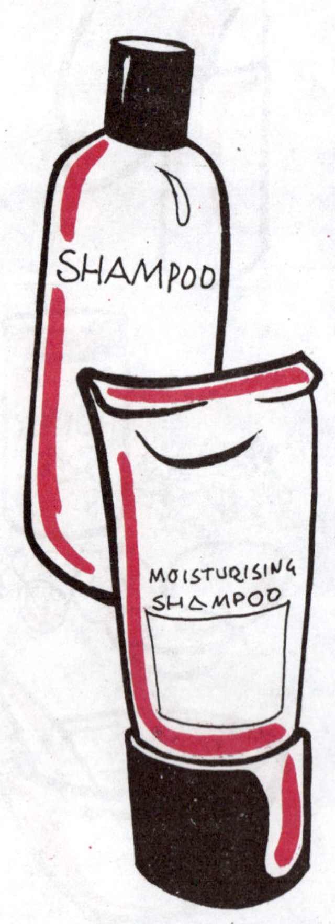

What kind of shampoo should be used for hair, which has been colour treated?

Shampoos that are designed to control colour loss are lower in pH, ranging from 2.5 to 4. This enables the cuticle of the hair to close, thus enabling the hair to retain its colour.

I have very dry hair. What kind of shampoo would suit my hair?

For dry hair, you must choose a shampoo, which has a conditioner. This will help in cleaning as well as conditioning the scalp. A moisturising shampoo has a rinse-out conditioner mixed in it which prevent the loss of moisture by closing the cuticles and it helps fight dryness caused by blow-dryers, curling irons, heat rollers and sun.

I have heard that salt water damages the hair. I love bathing in the sea. What can I do to prevent the damage?

Salt water does a lot of damage to the hair. When salt water dries on the hair, it creates a high-saline solution, which can cause mineral deposits to build up; resulting in hair that is weighted down and cannot grow. Hair should be washed or rinsed as soon as you get out of the salt water.

You can oil your hair before bathing in the sea and protect it with a tight waterproof cap.

I do not feel clean until I can feel my hair squeak, after a shampoo. Does it mean the hair is really clean or is it my imagination?

Squeaky-clean indicates that the oils have been removed from the hair. However, it may also indicate a raised hair cuticle. Rely on a thorough rinsing rather than the squeaky clean feeling.

What is the right way to rinse the hair after a shampoo. Should one use warm water or cold one?

A cool water rinse helps in closing the hair cuticles which makes the hair feel smoother. Hot water stimulates oil production. So if your hair is dry, you may want to use warm water. If your hair tends to get oily very soon, cool or tepid water rinse is recommended. The temperature of water should be determined by what you want to achieve.

The weather also dictates the type of water you want to use. You definitely can't use cold water for rinsing when the weather is cold and vice versa.

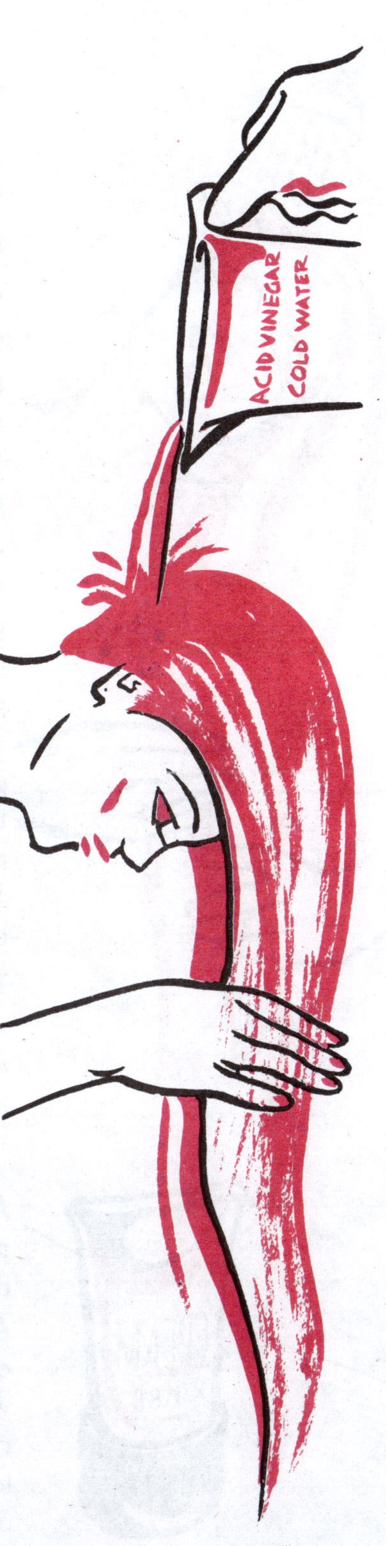

Will rinsing the hair with cold water or vinegar after shampooing make the hair shine?

Cold water and acid vinegar rinse helps in closing the hair cuticle, making the hair appear shiny.

How long should one rinse the hair after a shampoo in order to be sure of leaving no residue?

The average time required to rinse out the shampoo, is about 60-90 seconds. You can make out that the shampoo has left your hair, just by the feel of the hair. Hair should not feel like it is coated. It is best to rinse with the water flowing in the direction of the cuticle and not against it. If you hold your head back and allow the water to flow from the forehead towards the back of the head.

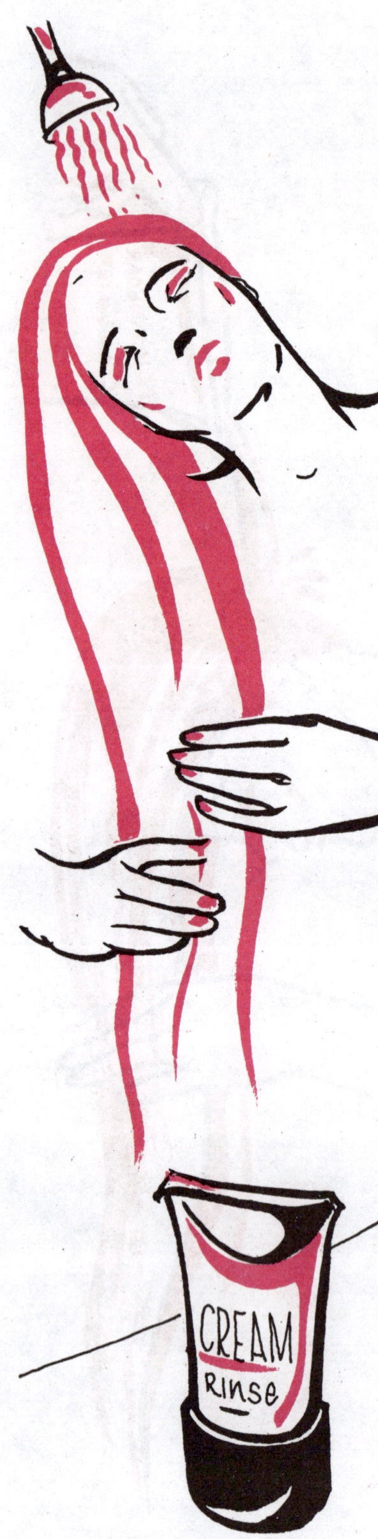

HAIR CONDITIONERS

It is not enough to style the hair and keep it clean. There is a need for conditioning the hair, which cannot be ignored. Without condition, one can never expect a good quality of hair. Conditioning has to be done regularly and made a part of the beauty ritual.

What is a conditioner and how does it help the hair? What are the different types of conditioners available these days?

Conditioners, as the name denotes, help in putting the hair in a good condition. They could be the deep penetrating types, which penetrate the cortex for longer lasting results and should be used only occasionally for extremely damaged hair. They actually open the cuticle to let moisture or protein get into the cortex, which is the middle part of a hair and gives strength to the hair. There are two basic types of deep penetrating treatments: moisturising and protein supplementation. The moisturising treatment consists of putting moisture in the hair, softening it and adding bounce to it. Protein treatment rebuilds strength in hair and adds protein to the cortex in order to bring back the lost elasticity. This treatment is generally given before a perm or a hair colouring in order to get the hair back to a good shape.

The other types of conditioners are the rinse-out conditioners, which are to be applied for a certain span of time and then rinsed out like a shampoo. The leave-in conditioners are light conditioners, which are left on the hair. They do not flatten the hair or weight it down.

A friend of mine told me that a cream rinse is better than a conditioner. What are the advantages of using a cream rinse?

A cream rinse detangles and doesn't penetrate like a conditioner does. It works instantly but it must be rinsed out well or it can leave a residue, making the hair look dull. A conditioner, on the other hand, imparts moisture or protein to strengthen the hair. Deep penetrating conditioners can actually penetrate the cortex also.

There are so many types of conditioners in the market. What is the difference between the ingredients contained in them?

The difference mainly lies in the formulation of the moisturiser, proteins, herbs and silicones in these conditioners.

I have observed that many of the conditioners and styling aids contain alcohol in varying degree. Doesn't the alcohol have a drying effect on the hair?

The kind of alcohol found in some shampoos and conditioners is cetyl or stearyl alcohol. This type of alcohol actually helps in conditioning the hair and making it softer. Isopropyl alcohol, which is found in the hair spray and many styling aids, is usually called 'SD-40' alcohol. It is this ingredient that makes hairspray dry quickly. Generally, there is not enough SD-40 alcohol in any professional beauty product to cause harm to the hair. However, over a period of time, styling aids can build up and sap the moisture in the hair.

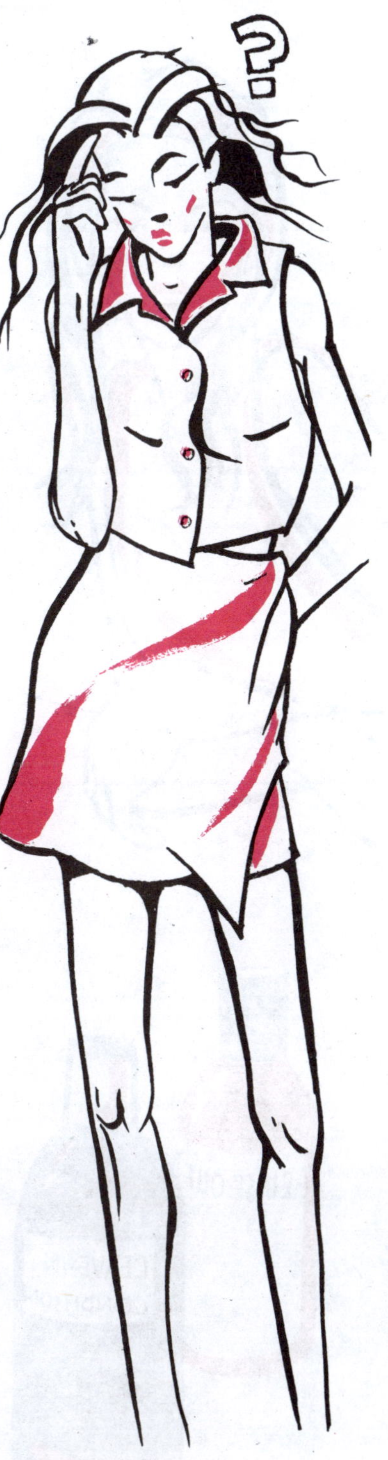

My hair is badly damaged due to abuse during my younger age. Will it help if I leave on the conditioner on my hair, longer than indicated in the directions?

Conditioners usually take a certain amount of time to penetrate the hair. After that time, there is no added benefit in leaving it on the hair. Leaving a conditioner for a longer period can actually do more harm than good as it dries out the hair. Follow the directions on the package instead of trying out new stunts.

Why is it that the hair feels greasier after the use of some conditioners?

The weight of the conditioner and its capacity to rinse out without any residue, rather than the amount used, contribute to that greasy feeling. Choose a light weight conditioner and use it as per the directions given on the package. That should take care of the greasiness in your hair.

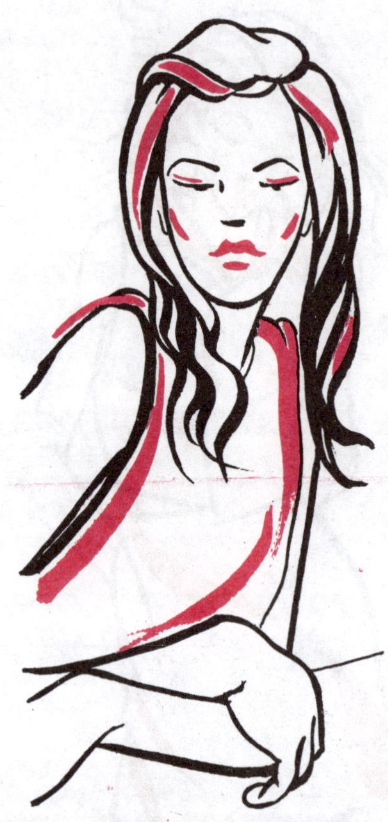

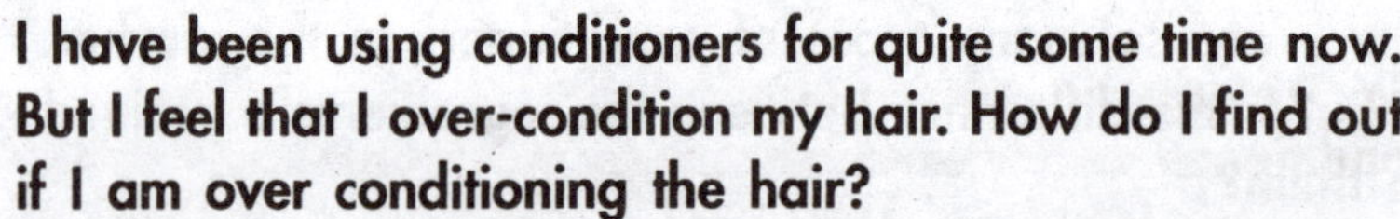

I have been using conditioners for quite some time now. But I feel that I over-condition my hair. How do I find out if I am over conditioning the hair?

An over conditioned hair become very limp. Hair that is over proteined is brittle and hard. If you have been using too much conditioner or conditioning your hair too often, it could lead to the above conditions. Rinse out with a good, mild shampoo.

On his trip abroad, my brother brought me a leave-in conditioner and a rinse out one. I am confused about the two types of conditioners that are available these days. What is the difference between a leave-in conditioner and a rinse-out conditioner?

A rinse-out conditioner does a permanent conditioning by filling in the cuticle or snags in the hair and making it stronger. But a leave-in conditioner is made to maintain the hair on a daily basis. The leave-in conditioner makes it easier to comb the hair, which in turn reduces the friction, prevents breakage and adds sheen to the hair before drying. Leave-in conditioner also protect from additional moisture loss. Another type of leave-in conditioner, a perm rejuvenator, adds elasticity to the hair in order to encourage the curl formation and adds bounce, too. Moisturisers in the formula give the hair a healthy look.

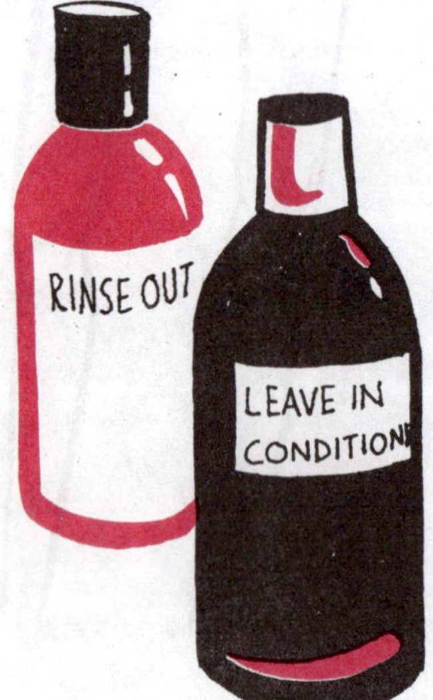

Can a leave-in conditioner be used on all types of hair?

Yes. It can be used on fine, thin hair to condition without weighing down the hair. On coarse, thick and rough hair, the conditioning agents soften and make the hair easier to manage.

I have fine hair. Should I avoid conditioners that weight down my hair and make it look flat?

Conditioners, which were available in the past, seemed to plaster down the hair on the head. But the recent ones are much lighter in formula. A leave-in conditioner may actually work better for you than a rinse out conditioner because it is formulated to be lighter on the hair. Avoid conditioners, which have a waxy ingredient in them.

My beautician recommended that I use an instant conditioner just after shampooing my hair. What is the reason for this?

An instant conditioner smoothes the cuticle, making the hair easier to comb. A smooth cuticle makes the hair shine and look vibrant.

I bought a moisturising shampoo for my hair. Is it necessary for me to use a conditioner after using the shampoo?

Yes. There is very little benefit of the rinse out type of conditioner if you are using a shampoo with a moisturiser since the formulae in both the products are almost similar. But using a leave-in conditioner will definitely improve your hair.

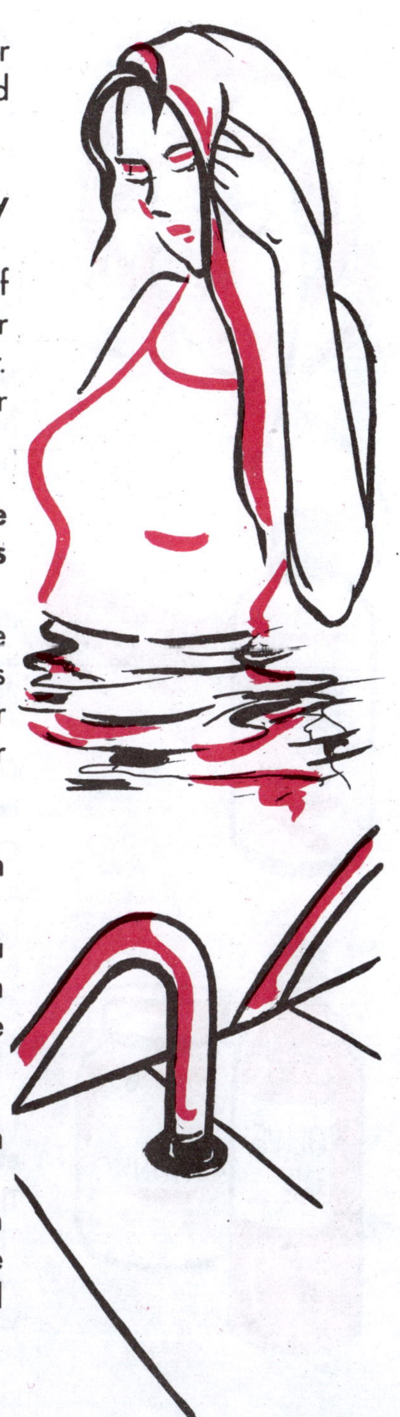

I am a regular swimmer. I have heard that the chlorine content in the swimming pool water harms the hair. Is this true?

Yes, the chlorine in the water can harm the hair. Chlorine causes oxidation and oxidation by-products cause dryness and lightening of the hair. You must rinse your hair immediately after a swim and condition it before going for a swim, in order to combat the effects of the chlorine.

I am tired of my flat hair. Is there any method by which I can bring back a little bounce to it?

You could prevent your hair from flattening by using a shampoo and conditioner in the morning. Your hair can pick up scalp and body oils from your pillow if you have shampooed and conditioned your hair at night.

Recently, I came across an article in a magazine, which talked about a scalp 'facial'. What is this treatment?

A scalp facial is a detoxifying treatment, which is undertaken in some beauty parlours. It essentially consists of a massage of the scalp, steaming and then applying essential oils and moisturisers. It is similar to the facial done on the face.

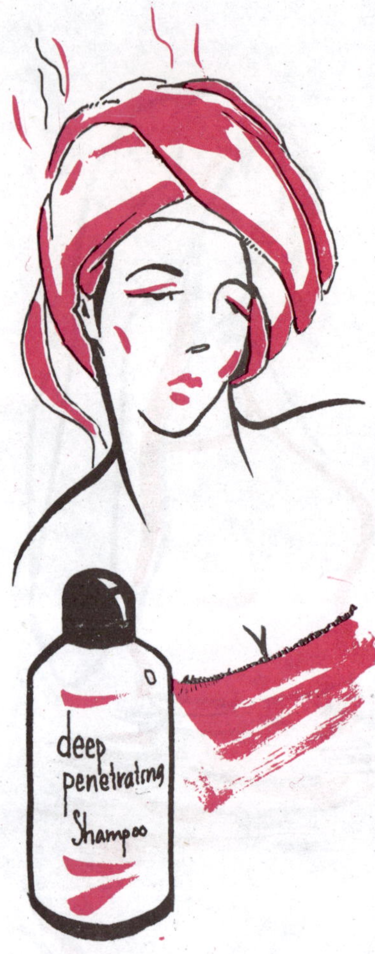

I bought a deep penetrating conditioner, recently while on my trip abroad. The instructions ask the user to wrap the hair after using the product. What is the benefit of this procedure?

Just as we oil our hair and give it the hot towel treatment to make the pores of the scalp absorb the oil better, keeping the head warm helps in opening the cuticle layer and allows the conditioner to penetrate more effectively. You could even wrap your head with a hot towel or a plastic wrap. One can also use a shower cap, which covers the scalp completely.

My friend uses mayonnaise and olive oil on her hair. Her hair is really thick and shiny. How do these two things help the hair?

Mayonnaise and olive oil moisturise and add sheen, making brittle hair more manageable. Olive oil does the same thing. However, these are very heavy for most types of hair so they are difficult to rinse out and leave a heavy residue on the scalp. For best results, it is good to use the conditioners that are available in the market, which are lighter in nature.

Can I use a hair rinse or a lemon rinse instead of a conditioner? Is vinegar as effective as any other rinse?

On fine hair, a lemon or vinegar rinse leaves hair with less tangles but it could be too acidic for some fragile type of hair. Commercially available rinses offer the proper acid balance without the softening effect of a conditioner. Conditioners work best on rough and coarse hair that needs to be softened and is difficult to manage.

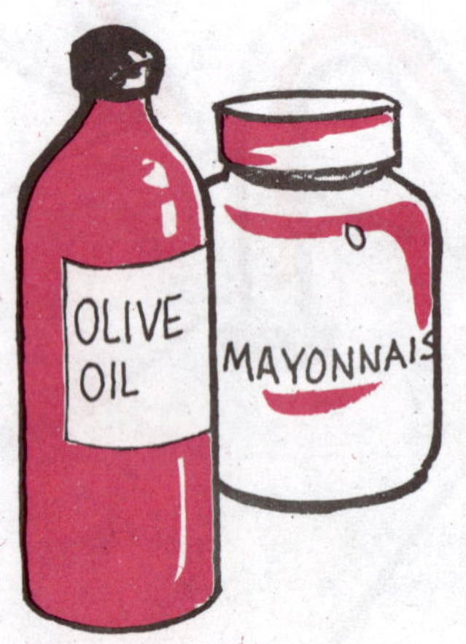

I live in a place where the water is hard. What is the effect of hard water on the hair?

The minerals contained in hard water are calcium and iron. These bond to the hair's protein making it dry and dull. You will have to take extra care to moisturise and condition your hair.

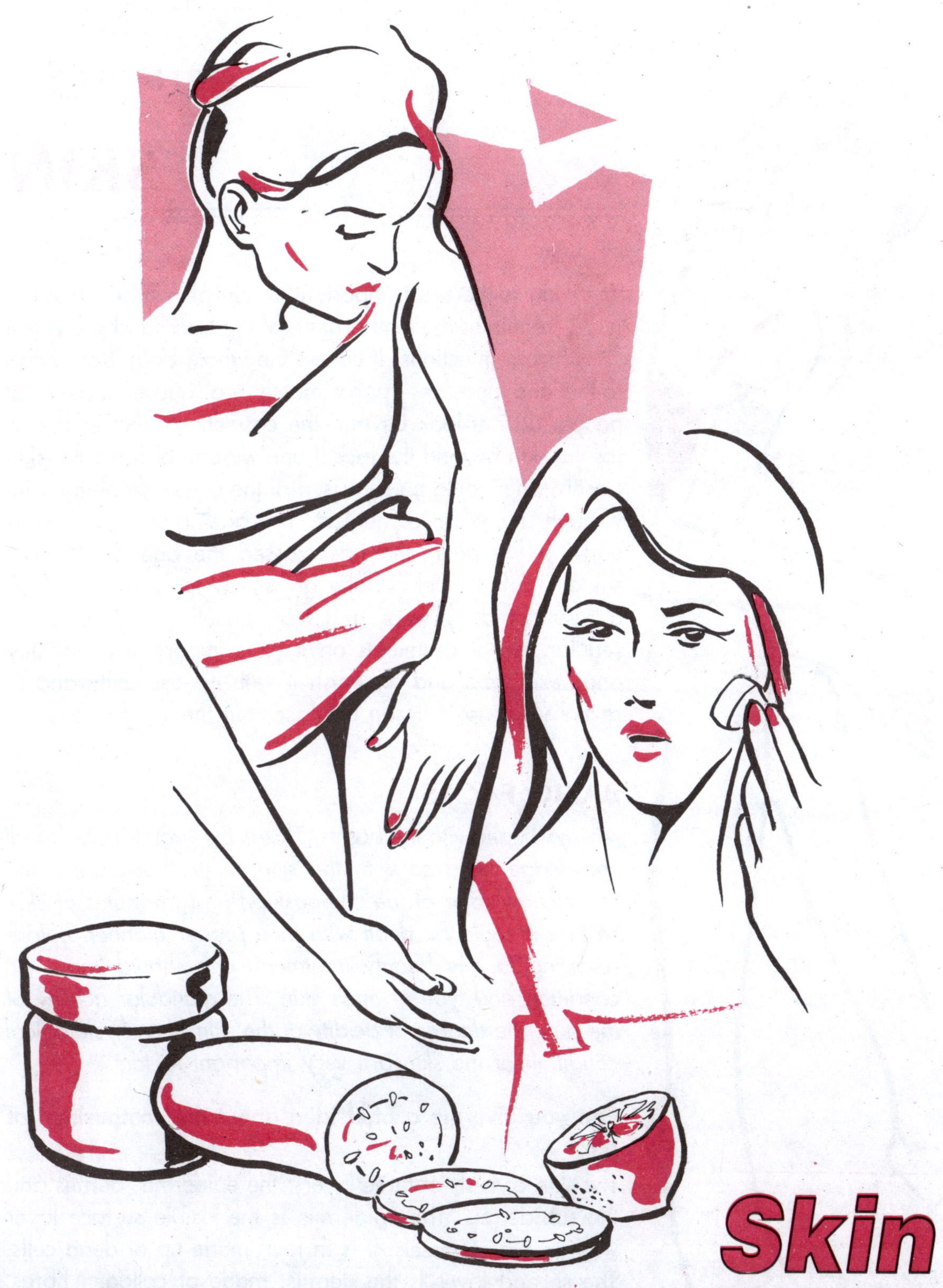

Skin

CHAPTER III

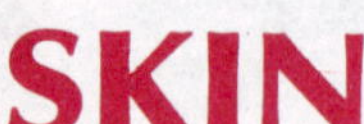

SKIN

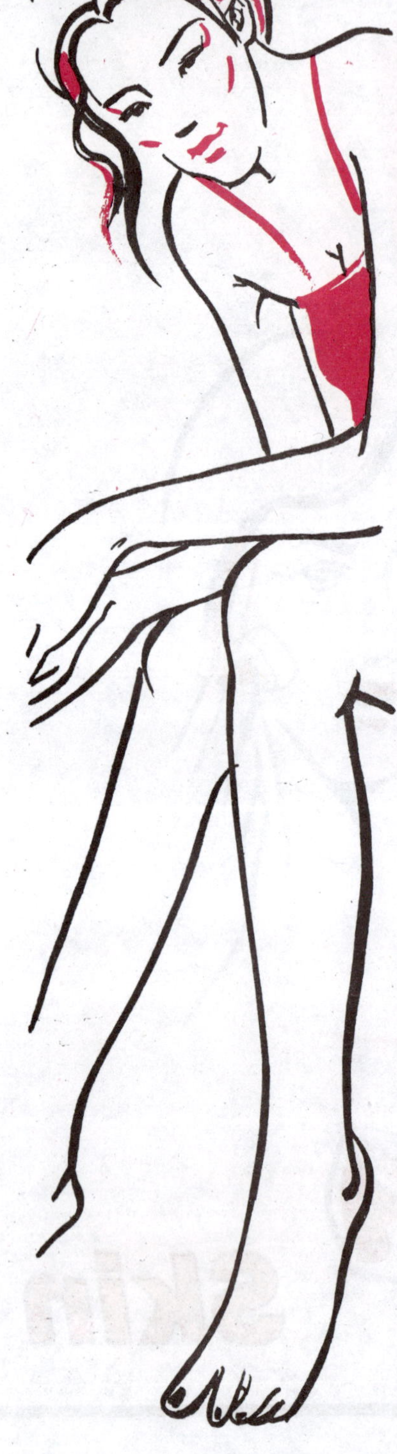

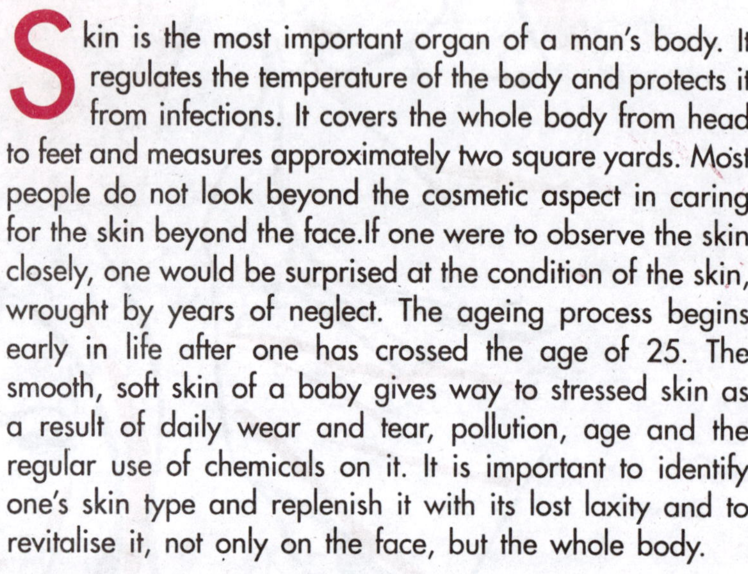

Skin is the most important organ of a man's body. It regulates the temperature of the body and protects it from infections. It covers the whole body from head to feet and measures approximately two square yards. Most people do not look beyond the cosmetic aspect in caring for the skin beyond the face.If one were to observe the skin closely, one would be surprised at the condition of the skin, wrought by years of neglect. The ageing process begins early in life after one has crossed the age of 25. The smooth, soft skin of a baby gives way to stressed skin as a result of daily wear and tear, pollution, age and the regular use of chemicals on it. It is important to identify one's skin type and replenish it with its lost laxity and to revitalise it, not only on the face, but the whole body.

BASIC FACTS

Always begin with the basics. This is the ground rule for all knowledge. And so with the skin. One should have the basic knowledge of the composition and attributes of skin so that it could be dealt with in a proper manner. Before resorting to any beauty treatment, one should know the condition and type of one's skin. The glandular activity of the skin, the degree of acidity of the skin, the physiological condition of the skin are very important factors.

Can you give me a brief idea about the composition of skin?

The skin consists of three layers: the epidermis, dermis and the sub-dermis. The epidermis is the visible surface layer with no blood vessels. It is in fact, made up of dead cells. The second layer is the dermis, made of collagen fibres, which lends elasticity to the skin. This layer has sebaceous glands, which secrete oil, and sweat glands, which regulate the body temperature. This layer acts as a cushion between the surface skin and the muscles below. The skin is a tissue which covers the whole body. It functions through pores, which are the exit channels, and if the skin is not cleaned properly they become clogged and form whiteheads or blackheads. It is the sebaceous glands, which cause oily, dry or normal skin.

The sub-dermis is the bottom most layer of the skin. It has fat cells, which make the skin supple.

Most women are worried about the skin being oily or dry. It is the sebaceous glands, which are responsible for the oiliness or dryness of the skin.

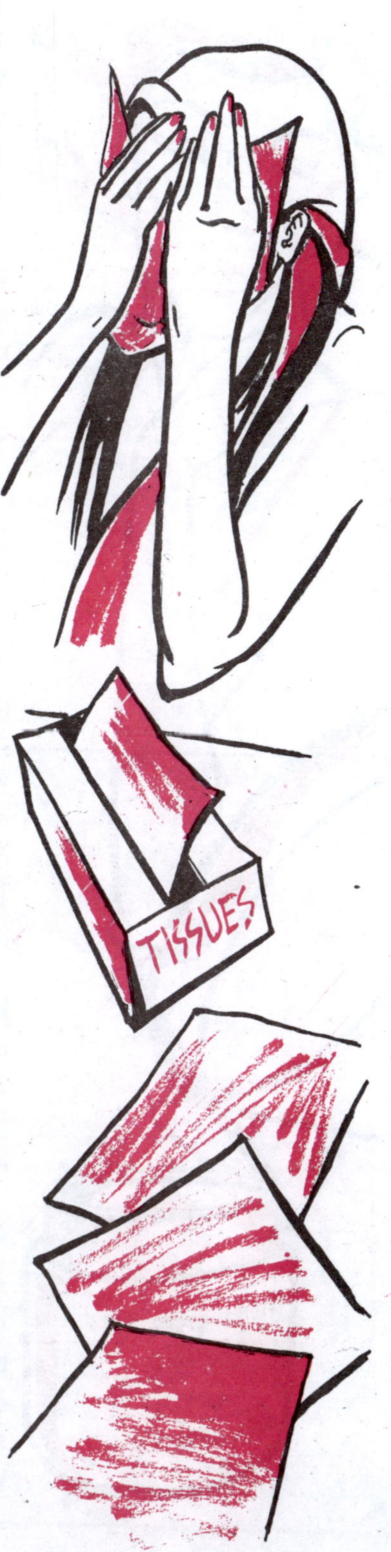

What are the different types of skin and how can I identify my skin type?

There are three types of skin: the oily, normal and dry skin. To know your skin type, perform this test. Place a dry tissue on your face and press it against your face when you get up early in the morning. If the tissue is stained you have an oily skin, if there is a T-shaped stain in the centre panel, then yours is a combination skin. And if there is no oily patch you have a dry skin.

What are the attributes of a normal skin?

You are a very lucky person if you have a normal skin. It is a healthy skin, which has no blemishes. Since the sebaceous glands are working at the optimum level, there is no secretion of excess or less sebum. It remains velvety, smooth and supple. There are no enlarged pores or flaky dead cells. There is a healthy glow and soft texture to it.

How does one care for a normal skin?

A normal skin hardly needs any care. Remember the key words are cleansing, nourishing and toning. The skin needs to be cleansed twice daily, in the morning and before going to bed. For nourishment, any cream can be used and for toning you can use an astringent or skin tonic. Don't forget to use a moisturiser during the day to retain the moisture of the skin.

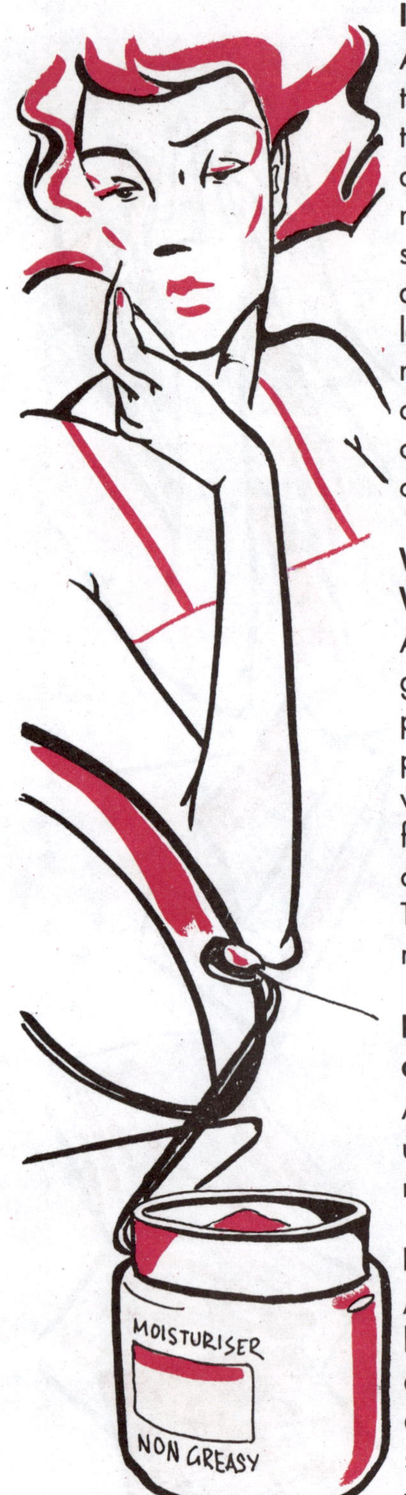

I feel I have a dry type of skin. How can I look after it?

A dry skin is flaky and dull in appearance, especially around the eyes and the cheeks. Fine lines appear very soon when the skin is dry. It also has a tendency towards, flakiness, dry patches and sore skin in cold weather. A dry skin needs a lot of care. The oil glands of a dry skin do not supply enough lubricants to the skin so the skin becomes dehydrated. For a dry skin, it is imperative that you use a lot of nourishment and moisturise it adequately. It is best not to use too much of soap on the face as that will compound the problem. At night, use a rich-nourishing cream before retiring to bed. And keep the skin scrupulously clean with a mild cleansing cream or lotion.

What are the main identification traits of an oily skin? What is the proper method of caring for such skin?

An oily skin looks shiny, thick and dull. The sebaceous glands of an oily skin produce more oil than required. The pores are enlarged and the oily skin is more prone to problems like acne and blackheads. One needs to keep it very clean so that excess oil is not formed. Use a mild toner for toning. Toning will improve the circulation and the texture of the skin. Keep away from greasy creams and moisturisers. There many specially formulated lotions and non-greasy moisturisers, available for the oily skin.

I have heard about the combination skin. What exactly is a combination skin?

Actually, most of us have a combination type of skin. It usually has a T-shaped panel of oiliness down the forehead, nose and chin. The rest of the face is dry.

How does one care for the combination skin?

A combination skin requires special care since you will have to combine two different types of care for the two different zones. One for the oily T-zone and another for the dry areas. Cleanse the oily part with an astringent or a strong skin tonic and the cheeks should be treated as you would treat a dry skin. Lubricating and nourishing are the main requirements of the dry zone. Apply a good moisturiser during the day time and a rich nourishing cream during the night. The oily T-zone should not be put under the heavy creams, as that will only aggravate the oiliness. For that area, just a mild, oil free moisturiser is fine.

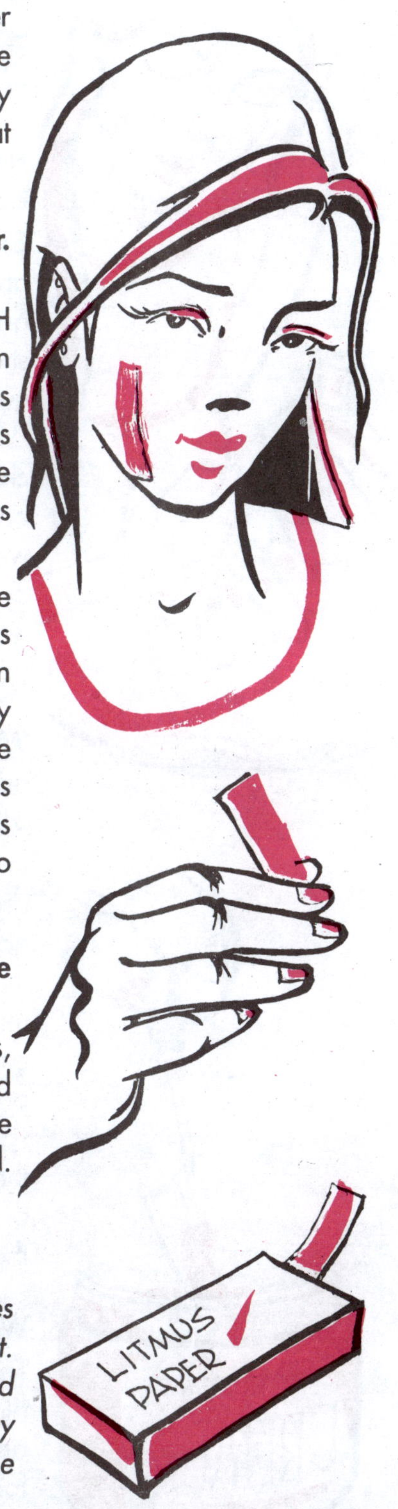

In the recent years I have heard a lot about the pH factor. How can I get to know the pH level of my skin?

The degree of acidity of your skin is known as the pH factor. To determine pH is to ascertain the hydrogen potentials. The hydrogen particle, when in excess, causes alkalinity. When the hydrogen particle is deficient, it causes acidity. The pH factor is neutral when at 7. When the figure is under 7 then it is acidic and when it is above 7 it is alkaline.

To find out whether your skin is acidic or alkaline, take a litmus paper and apply it to the face (an hour after it has been washed). Keep it there for a few minutes and then remove it. If the paper has remained blue, you lack acidity and your skin is a breeding ground for infection. If the paper has turned to a rose-lilac, the acidity level is satisfactory. If the paper has become pink-red, your skin is too acidic and it is delicate, sensitive as well as likely to age prematurely.

What are the general types of skin problems that one faces?

The general types of skin problems are acne, blackheads, pigmentation, freckles, dark circles under the eyes and enlarged pores. Of these acne troubles most young people and the dark circles are common among the middle aged.

SKIN CARE

Once we discover the type of skin we have, it becomes much easier to deal with it and the problems related to it. Skin care is a science by itself. It requires a lot of time and perseverance to deal with it. The ritualistic processes may be scorned by some but they cannot be neglected if one wants a healthy and glowing skin.

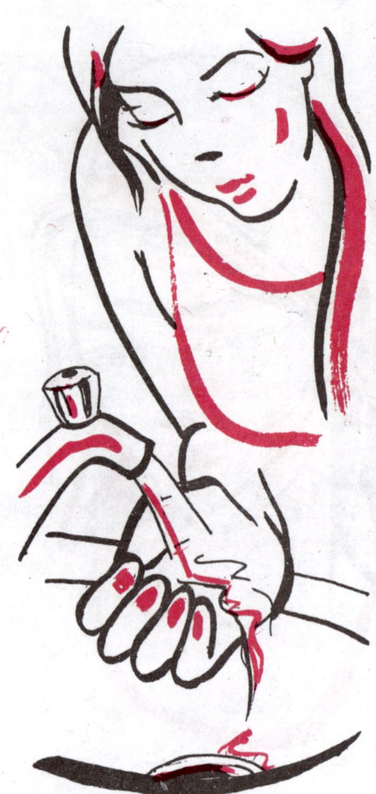

What are the essential steps towards skin care?

The essential steps towards skin care are: cleansing, toning, nourishing and rejuvenating.

How important is the daily ritual of cleansing? How can I cleanse my skin effectively?

Cleansing is a very vital part of beauty and skin care. We are living in a very polluted environment, today. The dust, grime and impurities in the atmosphere play havoc with the skin. It is, therefore, extremely important to clean the skin, every night. An oily skin requires more cleaning than a dry skin because the open pores, on the oily skin become clogged with dirt and oil. If you do not want to use the branded products available in the market, do the cleaning with home-based products. Take 2-teaspoons of cold milk, apply it on the face and wipe away with a moist cotton wool. For oily skin, add a little water to the milk. Follow it up with a toner.

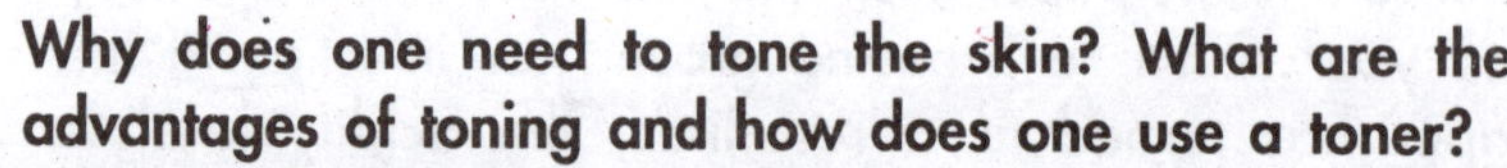

Why does one need to tone the skin? What are the advantages of toning and how does one use a toner?

All types of skins need a freshener or a toner. Toners come in alcoholic and non-alcoholic forms. The alcoholic ones are meant for the oily skins whereas the non-alcoholics are good for the dry skin. Toning helps to clear away all residues that have been left by a cleanser. It also tones up the facial muscles besides stimulating blood circulation. It restores the pH balance, which might have got disturbed during the process of cleansing. The best way to tone the skin is to splash a lot of cold water on the face. This helps in closing the pores, which might have opened up during the process of cleansing. After that one can apply a toner suitable to the skin type.

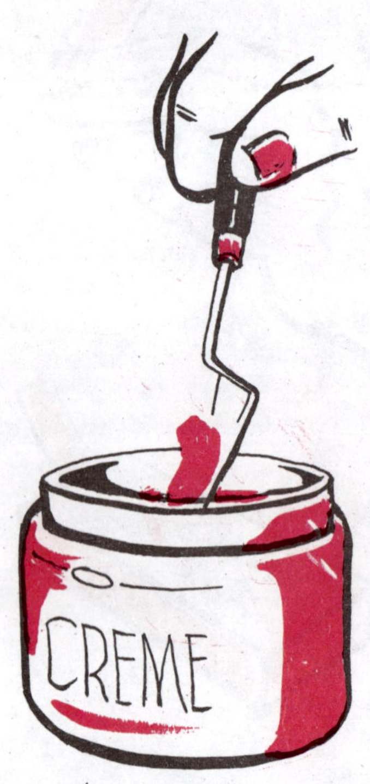

What is the function of a moisturiser?

The moisturiser functions as a shield on the skin. It forms a film over the skin's surface, holding in the natural moisture and providing a base for the make-up. The make-up stays for a longer time if a good moisturiser has been applied as a base. A moisturiser forms a barrier between the skin and the environment. Most people think that there is no need for moisturising an oily skin. This is a wrong concept. All kinds of skin require moisturising. An oil free or light moisturiser is needed for the oily skin whereas a rich, oil-based one is a must for the dry skin. One must, however, remember to remove the moisturiser at night.

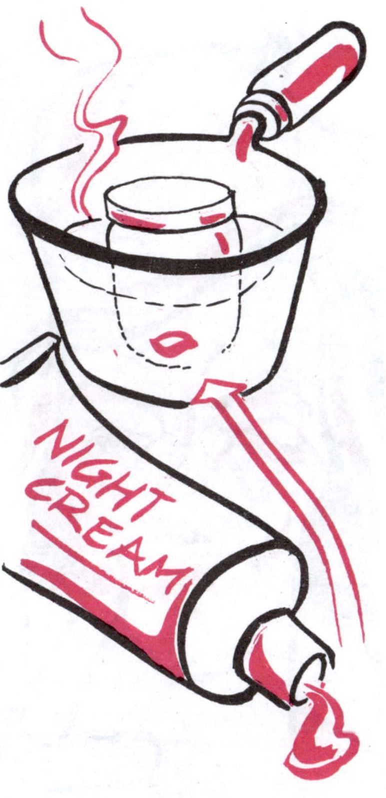

What is the proper method of taking out a moisturising cream from the container? My cream always gets spoilt.

The right way of taking out moisturising cream from its container is to use a spatula. Although you feel your fingers are clean, they are capable of transferring bacteria to the container.

What is the right way of applying the night creams so as to make them more effective?

To make night cream more effective, place one application in a sealed jar and leave in a sink of hot water for a few minutes. Apply it on the face with gentle, upward strokes. The cream is absorbed by the pores more rapidly because of its warm state.

Why do we need a face pack?

A face pack or mask cleanses, revitalises, stimulates and exfoliates the skin. It also functions as a deep pore cleanser. A good mask helps to free clogged pores, loosens the blackheads, removes dirt and recharges the cells. There are several types of face masks available in the market. Some need to be washed away while some are peeled off.

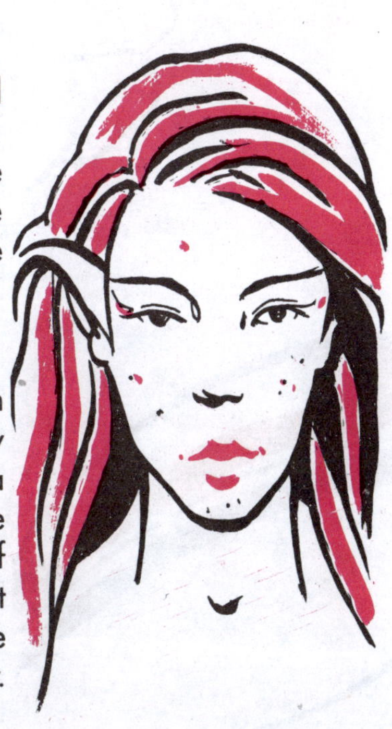

What is an exfoliating face mask?

The exfoliating mask is designed to remove dead cells from the surface of the skin and to encourage the growth of new cells. It helps in increasing blood circulation and brings a glow to the skin. A good home-made face scrub is made from a mixture of wheat husk or chokker, a few drops of milk and rose water. Apply it on the face. When it is almost dry, rub off the scrub by using circular strokes. Regular use of the scrub also discourages the growth of facial hair. Wash off the face with cold water.

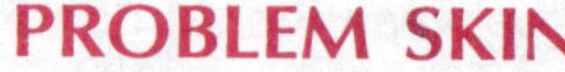

PROBLEM SKIN

Meet any girl who is in her teens and she will complain about the acnes and blackheads that plague her. To her, they are the biggest misery of her life. Not only the teenagers but even the middle aged women and the older ones also have various complaints about their skin. The flood of international creams and lotions that have made an entry into the Indian market has not helped those who do not know the solutions to their problems. Trying out each product with a hope that it will wave a magic wand, and bring about a glowing complexion, is not possible. So, here we bring you the solutions to most skin problems. Identify the one you are facing and then take the remedial measures.

I have a lot of pimples on my face. All efforts to get rid of them have failed. Could you people explain a little about the causes for pimples?

Acne, commonly known as pimples, is a variety of skin eruptions ranging from whiteheads and blackheads to solid red bumps and pustules. The pimples result because the sebaceous glands, the oil glands in the skin which are connected to hair follicles, secrete an oily material which normally softens and lubricates the skin. But these do not become active till puberty. Under the influence of hormones released at puberty, these glands burst into activity, excreting the oil up through the follicle on to the skin surface and causing the face, especially the nose, to become shiny. This problem is more or less normal during adolescence. Acne is caused when the outlet of the gland gets plugged with a lump of oil and dead cells. Bacteria acts upon it and further aggravates the process. The free fatty acids and other substances produced by these bacteria cause irritation to the surrounding skin.

What are blackheads?

Blackheads are nothing but clogged pores. They generally appear on an oily skin. On combination skin, they appear on the nose. Unclean skin is a breeding ground for blackheads. They are a mixture of dead cells of the skin, oil and bacteria. When they come into contact with the atmospheric oxygen, a chemical reaction takes place and the mixture darkens to form blackheads.

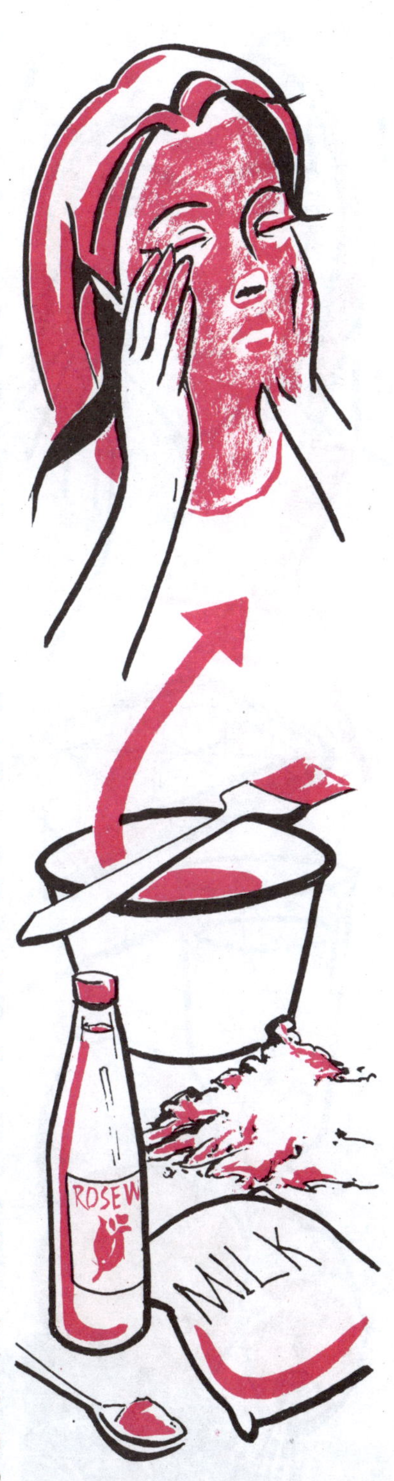

What is a whitehead?

If the plug formed by the clogged pore on an oily skin does not push to the surface but remains just below the skin, it appears as a tiny, rounded, whitish elevation. This is called a 'whitehead'. Both blackheads and whiteheads may remain in the skin for a long time and generally seen in mild cases of acne.

I have been told that only teenagers get acne. Is this true?

No, it isn't. Acne can be experienced in childhood and later during the adult years. It is, however, more common between the years 13-18. Almost 80% of teenagers have acne.

I have an oily skin. Due to this I have pimples. When these pimples dry up, they form a dark spot on the skin. I have several small holes on my skin. What could be the cause?

The black spots are scars that are left behind by the pimples after they have dried. To lighten them, use chokker, mixed with rosewater, raw turmeric and milk. Apply it on the face and neck region and scrub it off till the flakes fall off the face, using circular movements of the fingers. The small holes on your skin are the open, enlarged pores. Splash ice cold water on your face three times a day. Eat a lot of fruits and vegetables. Avoid fried foods, sweets and aerated foods.

I have tiny dots on my nose. When I squeeze them, a scale like substance comes out of them. Could they be whiteheads?

The spots mentioned by you are definitely, whiteheads. These are quite common in teenagers. You must try to keep your skin totally clean. Avoid using any oily products on the face. Cleanse the face with a face wash and avoid using soap. Apply an astringent lotion to give it a toning. Also

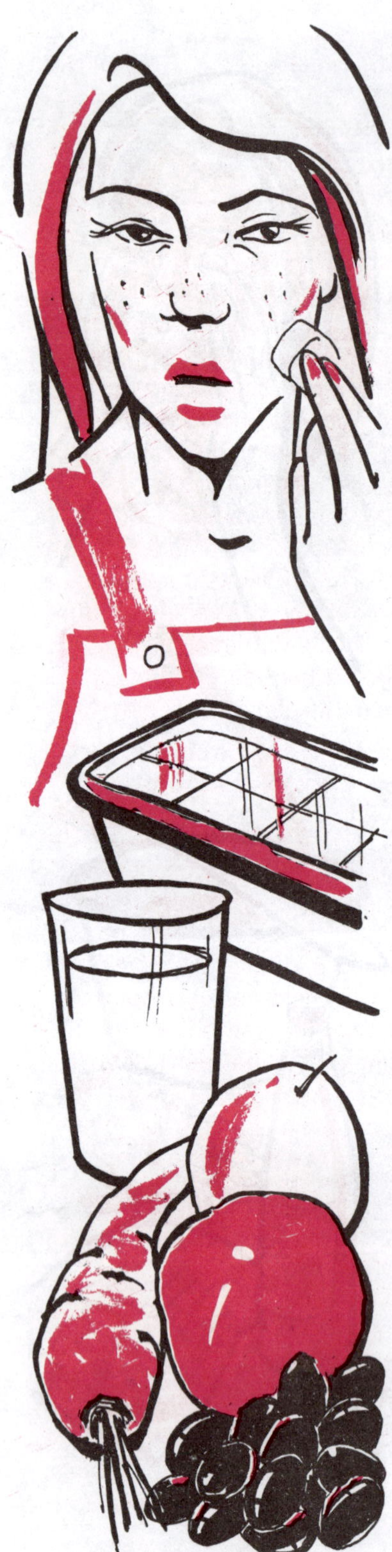

remember not to use any rich nourishing cream or oily moisturiser on the face. You will benefit from a weekly face pack and a thorough scrub.

Recently, I have noticed some black spots on the nose. I have been using a face pack of honey and curd twice a week. Could it be due to this?

What you have mentioned leads to a conclusion that you have blackheads on the face. You must avoid the face pack that you are currently using because curd may be causing the greasiness. The tiny skin pores on your nose are clogged with dirt and grime. They need a thorough cleansing treatment. Get the blackheads removed by an expert and do not attempt it yourself. Wash your face at least thrice a day with a medicated soap or with a face wash. Steam the face for five minutes every week and then splash the face with cold water to block the pores. Tone it with a good skin toner. Following this regime will help you in getting rid of the blackheads.

I am a thirty five-year-old woman and have a very sensitive skin, which has oily patches. I have recently developed black spots around my chin, cheek and nose. What could I do to counteract these?

Your skin needs a three pronged treatment. Firstly, make sure that your skin is scrupulously clean and to do so you have to wash your face several times a day with a good medicated soap. This will help in checking the flow of oil on the surface of your skin. Secondly, you could steam your face to open the pores of your skin and remove the dust and grime. Splash your face with cold water or rub a cube of ice on your face to close the open pores. What I suspect is that you have a lot of blackheads on the oily T-zone of your face. Get it removed by an expert.

Thirdly, you must include a lot of fresh fruits and vegetables in your diet. Added to that a daily intake of about 8-10 glasses of water will make a lot of difference to your skin condition.

I have a fair complexion and a lot of freckles on the face especially on the nose and cheeks. Can these be checked? I have been advised to use a melalite ointment.

Freckles are generally a genetic problem. They are your body's protection against the exposure to sun. Melalite cream, with hydroquinone as an ingredient, helps dissolve the melanin pigment. Since this pigment appears from the basal layer of the skin, more and more of melanin cells will keep appearing in the form of freckles. There is no permanent cure but you can take precautions so that there is no darkening effect. To do so, avoid being exposed to sunlight by carrying an umbrella or wearing a sun-hat. Also use a sunscreen with a high SPF (Sun Protecting Factor) of above 30.

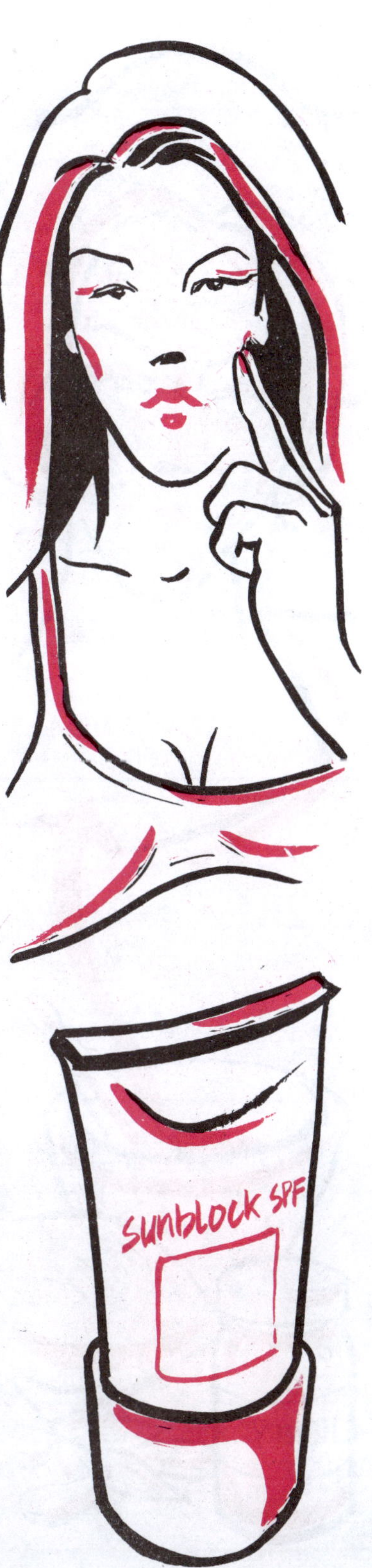

I am an 18-year-old college student. Of late, I have noticed a lot of tiny dots on my chin, which make the area look darker than the rest of the face. On squeezing them, a white scaly object emerges. How could I control this problem?

The tiny dots on your chin are a collection of sebum in the open pores because of the presence of an oily zone there. Apply an erythromycin lotion on this area, at bedtime. Also use a face pack with Multani mitti, twice a week. Follow it up with splash of cold water. Wash your face with a medicated soap, several times a day.

I am a 20-year-old girl with a medium complexion. My skin has recently become very dark although I am using a sunscreen with a SPF of 30. I have a healthy, outdoor life and want to keep my tan to a low degree. What can I do about it?

A tan is basically a protective mechanism adopted by the skin, whereby the melanin pigment from the basal layer comes to the surface in order to absorb the ultraviolet rays of the sun. As long as the exposure to these rays continues, it will be difficult to get rid of your tan. Sunblocks do not prevent tanning; they simply delay the process. You should try to prevent direct sunlight by using a parasol and keeping indoors during the peak of the day.

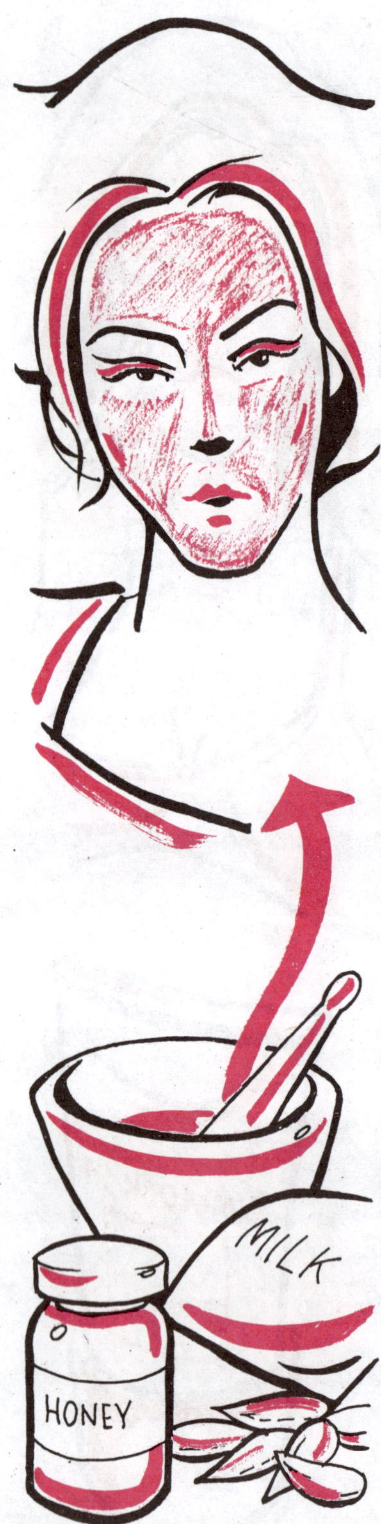

I am a 19-year-old girl from Bhutan. I have many freckles on my face. They have recently increased in number. I want to know if I can get rid of them.

You should discontinue the use of any oily cream and apply a moisturiser with a sunscreen to stop the freckles from multiplying. You could try applying sour buttermilk on your face, at night. But freckles are one problem, which generally don't go away. Since they are your skin's protection against the harsh rays of the sun, it is better not to try to get rid of them.

I have a freckled face, which has become the bane of my life. Please help!

Freckles are common with people who are sensitive to sunlight. It is your armour of protection against the harmful ultraviolet rays. Just a short time in the sun can cause the freckles to appear and the dark sun spots also make their appearance. Freckles are caused by a combination of melanin producing cells and sun exposure. Cream containing more than 5% alpha hydroxy acids can be used to exfoliate dead skin cells where pigments build up. However, to repair the skin fully, try a lightening cream. You could also use a cream, which normalises the levels of melanin in the skin and encourages the production of new collagen fibre. For this, you have to consult your family doctor.

I have a very dry skin. I have been advised to use a starch, gramflour and rose water face pack. Will it help?

In fact, this pack will make your skin still drier. A cream based pack is more suitable for your skin. Mix milk and honey and almonds to make a paste. Apply this paste to your face for 15 minutes. Rinse off with tepid water. Apart from this mask, use a good moisturiser during the daytime to keep the skin well-nourished.

I am a 24-year-old woman. There is a rash on my nose, which refuses to go away. What can I do about it?

The rash on your nose could be due to a very oily zone of combination skin type. In this case, excess oil and sticky dead skin cells, forming blackheads and whiteheads appear as raised, granular rash and clog the pores. Try a facial scrub, at least twice a week. Wash your face several times a day with a medicated soap. Steam your nose or get it cleaned by a beautician every month. The other reason could be Rosacea, which displays a reddish rash on the cheeks, too. In this case, you must avoid all types of hot and spicy food as well coffee and exposure to extreme climate.

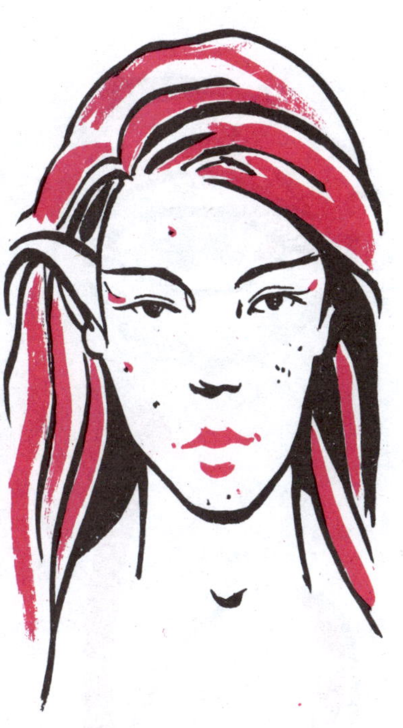

I have been suffering from pimples for quite some time, now. I keep my face absolutely clean and try drinking a lot of water but there has been no improvement in the condition. Please help!

Acne is caused by the over production of oil by the sebaceous glands. That is when the skin appears shiny. Acne is hormone-related and could be genetic in nature. You should wash your face several times a day with a medicated soap preferably a neem-based one to take off the surface oiliness. Use a mud pack at least twice a week to draw out the inner oils and toxins. Avoid creamy and oily products and don't squeeze out the pimples. Also eat a balanced and healthy diet. Stress could also aggravate the problem so try to keep stress at the minimum.

I was suffering from acne a few months ago. On the advice of a friend I began using an acne cream which has made the skin very dark and dry. When I stopped using the cream, the acne resurfaced. What can I do?

The acne cream might have suppressed the acne without getting rid of the basic problem. Acne is caused because of the overactive oil glands on the skin. You must stop using the acne medication and try to keep your skin free of oil traces by repeated washing with a medicated soap and water. Also maintain a healthy diet and keep away from all types of oil based cosmetics. The black marks can be treated with a skin lightening cream with a sandalwood base; glycolic peels to lift off the top scarred layers of the skin or by dermabrasion.

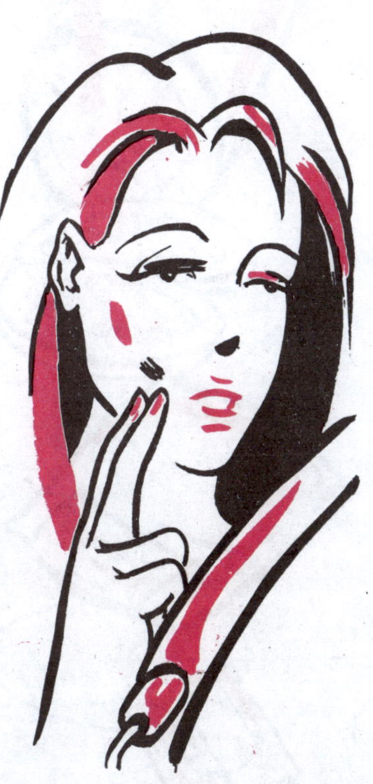

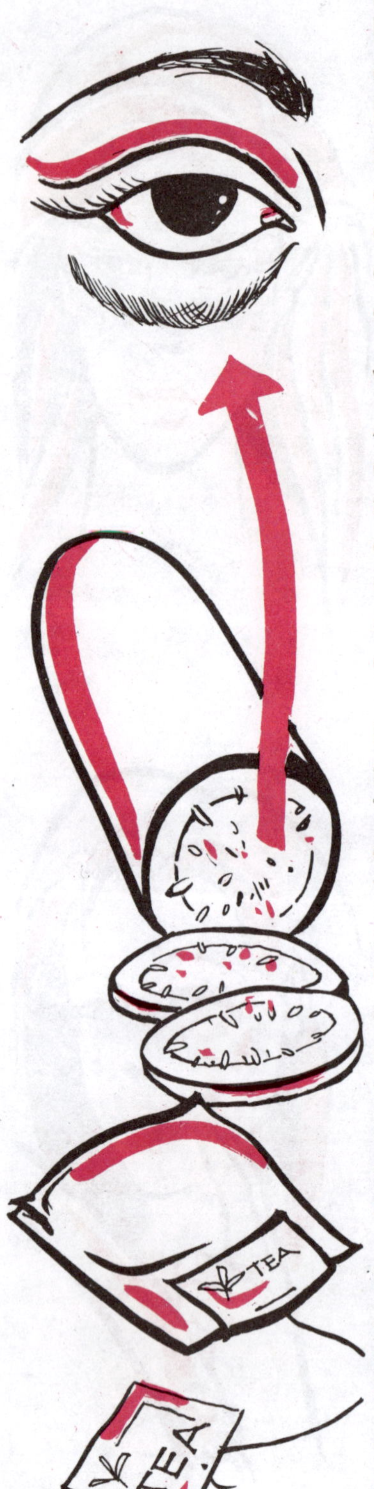

I have heavy dark circles under the eyes. This makes me look older than my age. How do I get rid of the dark circles?

Dark circles under the eyes appear due to various reasons such as eye strain, faulty reading habits, inadequate sleep, digestive problems etc. Keep chilled cucumber slices on the eyes for about ten minutes, every day to bring relief to tired eyes. Placing used tea bags will also help. A good healthy diet and adequate sleep are a must for you.

What is the benefit of using of a face scrub?

A face scrub or an exfoliating mask is designed to remove dead cells from the surface of the skin and to encourage the growth of new cells. It helps in increasing the blood circulation and brings a nice glow to the skin. It is to be used once a week only. You must apply a very thin film of moisturiser after using a facial scrub so as prevent any dryness.

I have a fair complexion but my forehead, area around the eyes and lips as well as the neck appear quite pale. This makes me look sickly. How can I achieve a uniform complexion?

The patchiness of complexion could be due to photosensitivity, fungal infection, vitamin and iron deficiencies or drug induced. Treat the cause. You could use a cosmetic camouflage for the meantime. Use a cover stick, which is a shade darker than your normal skin tone. Touch up all the pale spots. Cover this with a thin coat of foundation and then use a loose powder. If your skin is normal or dry and you are above 25, your could use almond oil to massage your face.

I am a 24-year-old woman with a two-year-old daughter. After the child's birth, I developed dark skin around the eyes and upper lips. What is the remedy?

This dark pigmentation problem is a common one and is called melasma or chloasma. It is also called the 'mask of pregnancy' because of its typical distribution over the face.

This problem usually fades away after the delivery but since it is persisting in your case, you could protect these areas from sunlight by using a sunblock with a high SPF (sun protection factor). Don't use any strong soaps, cleansers or highly pigmented cosmetics. Also try a pigment fading cream on the face. The good old lemon juice works very well in most cases. Apply the diluted juice of half a lemon on the patchy parts twice a day and rub gently.

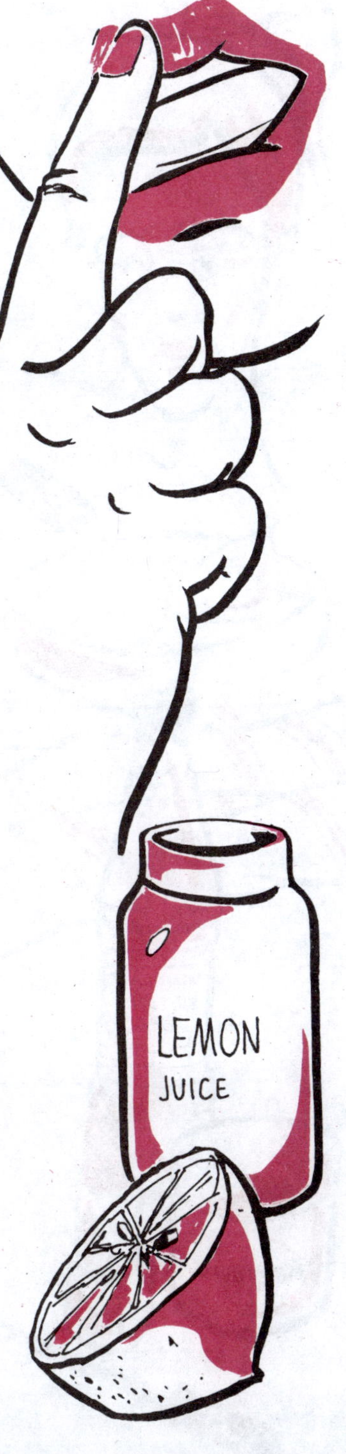

I am a 20-year-old girl. Sometime back I scratched my skin with the fingernails and since then those patches have developed into scars. Please help!

For scars, which are not very deep, use glycolic acid peels, chemical peels, laser treatment or dermabrasion. For deep scars, a new method called 'Zyderm Collagen Implant' is available. A fine needle is used to inject collagen (total human protein), directly into the depressed areas. The implant fills the depression, thus raising the skin to the level of the surrounding tissue. This, however, requires expert handling and could be a little expensive. In the meantime, you could use cosmetic cover-up techniques to camouflage the patches.

I have a problem of pigmentation around my lips. What is the cause of this problem and how do I get rid of it?

Pigmentation problems occur during major hormonal changes such as adolescence and pregnancy. Stress, prolonged exposure to sunlight and menstruation problems also aggravate it. I suggest that you combine a steroid cream with one containing 2% hydroquinone and apply this to your blemishes. The condition should improve within three months of regular treatment. Otherwise consult a dermatologist.

I am an 18-year-old girl. I suffer from the discolouration of my neck and back. I feel very conscious because of this affliction. Could you please suggest a remedy?

You are suffering from a pigmentation problem, which could be hereditary in nature. The patches darken during

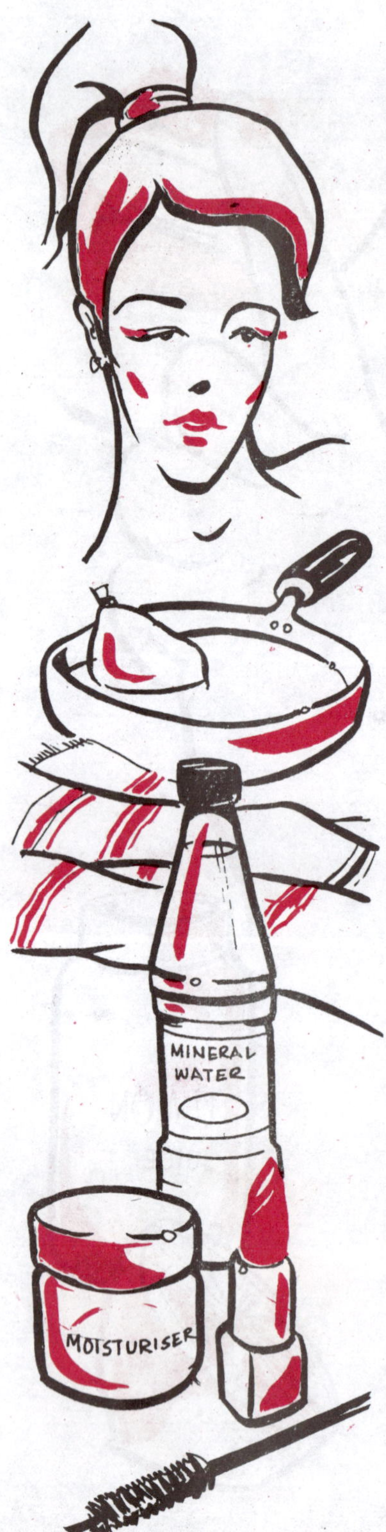

menstruation, under exposure to sun and if you are under stress. They can be lightened but it is difficult to get rid of them. Avoid exposure to direct sunlight as far as possible. Once a month, bleach the affected areas. Also, massage a cream containing 2% hydroquinone into the skin. Do this regularly for about 3 months and see if there is any improvement in the condition.

My skin looks rough because of the enlarged pores. What can I do to solve this problem?

Oily skin usually tends to cause open pores. Wash your skin several times a day with a medicated neem soap. Use a clay pack to draw out the deeper oils and eat fresh fruits and vegetables. Drink plenty of water and apply a gel containing 2.5% benzoyl peroxide on any areas that tend to break out into acne. Use only oil-free products on the face.

GLOWING COMPLEXION

Who wouldn't like to possess a thousand-watt smile and a glowing complexion? It is the secret desire of every woman walking on this earth. But a glowing complexion is not one, which is easily available for a price or sold on the cosmetics counter of the shops. A good, balanced diet, relaxed mind, healthy body, all go hand in hand with a beautiful complexion. One has to work towards all these elements to bring about the desired result.

I have a hectic social life, which gives me a tired look. I want to look good when I go out. Could you suggest a regimen for a glowing face and fresh looks?

Follow these steps for a refreshed look that will attract envious glances from the other women.

- Clean your face carefully and pin your hair back neatly.
- Fill a large pan with cold water and place some ice cubes tied in a piece of clean cloth in it.
- Dip your face into the icy water for about 20 seconds.

- Lightly pat dry the skin with a clean towel.
- Spray your face with mineral water
- Apply a light moisturiser to the face
- Now apply your usual make up.

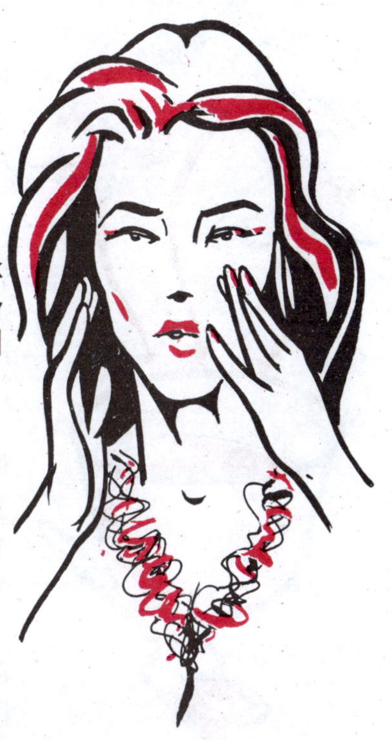

How does a facial massage help?

A facial massage keeps the muscles of the face and neck firm, it forestalls the appearance of wrinkles and ugly concentrations of fat. It stimulates the circulation of blood and induces complete relaxation of the face.

When should one massage the face?

The best time is at night before going to bed. Your features will feel more relaxed when you get up the following morning and your day time makeover will also look better.

What are basic movements of facial massage?

The basic movements are the relaxing movement, which are slow and soothing. There are the stroking movements and vibrations. Then there are the tonic movements, which are rapid and energetic. These are the kneading, pressing and percussion movements.

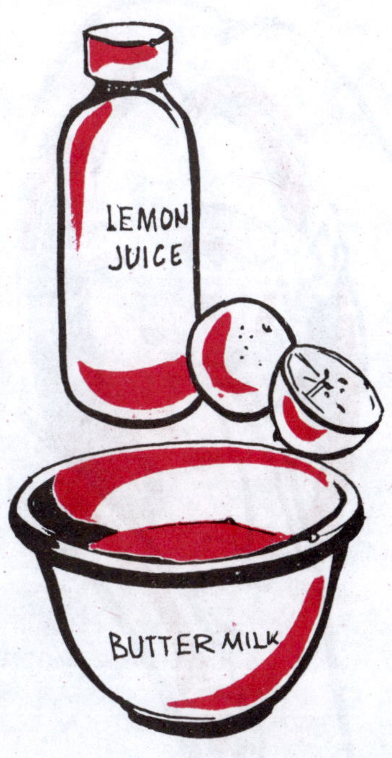

I am a college going girl. I have a very dark complexion and I feel very conscious about it. Is there any method by which I can lighten my complexion?

There are many kinds of whitening creams in the market but one must be very careful in using them. The best is to use some herbal product or a home remedy. You can try buttermilk or lemon juice, which are natural whiteners. Apply them thrice a day for a few weeks and see if it works. You should not be conscious about the dark complexion, what matters is the overall personality of a person. There are several dark complexioned ladies who are beautiful personalities and have attained fame. Try to get over your complex and concentrate on developing some positive traits to stand out in a crowd.

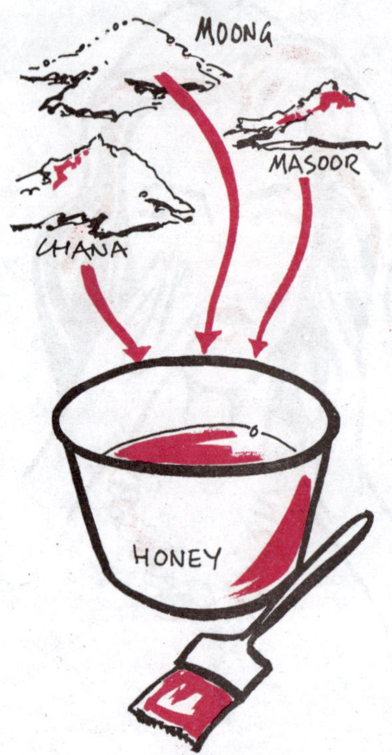

I have always envied the glow on my friend's face. How can I get a glow on my face, which looks, rather dull and tired?

A glow on the face cannot be achieved by cosmetics alone. A lot of it has to do with the state of mind and the physical condition. If you are a stressed person, no matter what you do cosmetically, the glow will be difficult to achieve. However, you can try this method. Every night, massage your face with olive oil or almond oil. Apply a little oil with the fingertips all over your face and neck in firm, rotating motion. Wipe oil off with moist cotton wool.

Please give a recipe for a home made facial scrub.

To make a scrub at home, grind small quantities of 'chana', 'moong' and 'masoor' dals in equal proportions and mix with milk, curd or honey. Apply the scrub on the face and let dry. After 15 minutes, scrub out with moist hands. Another great scrub is the orange peel one. Just mix dried and powdered orange peel with water and apply.

How can I rejuvenate my skin. It looks pale and dull.

To rejuvenate a tired skin, apply papaya pulp. To get a glow, apply fresh orange juice on the face.

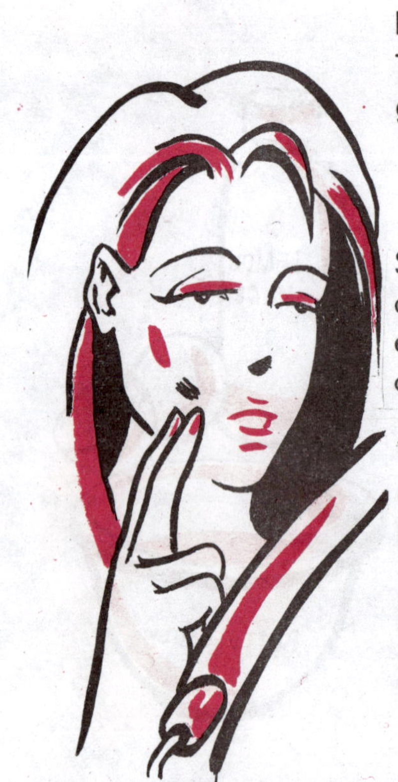

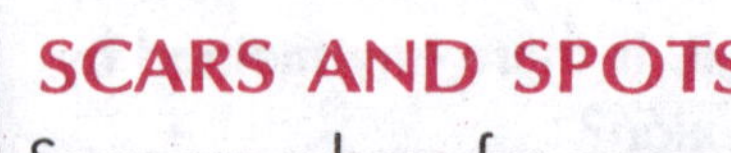

SCARS AND SPOTS

Scars are a bane for anyone aspiring to be beautiful. There are many types of scars, some of which can be removed easily while others are not easily removed and may require cosmetic surgery.

What is the difference between a glycolic acid peel and a chemical peel? Will these peels work to remove the acne scars?

Exfoliating the top layers of the skin with the help of certain acids is called 'skin peeling'. These can be either chemical or fruit peels. Chemical peels contain certain acids such as trichloroacetic acid and the 'fruit peels' contain alphahydroxy acids such as glycolic acid (or sugarcane extract). The peeling action depends on the strength of the acids as well as the sensitivity of the skin upon which they act. They help in removing scars, fine lines and lightening blemishes.

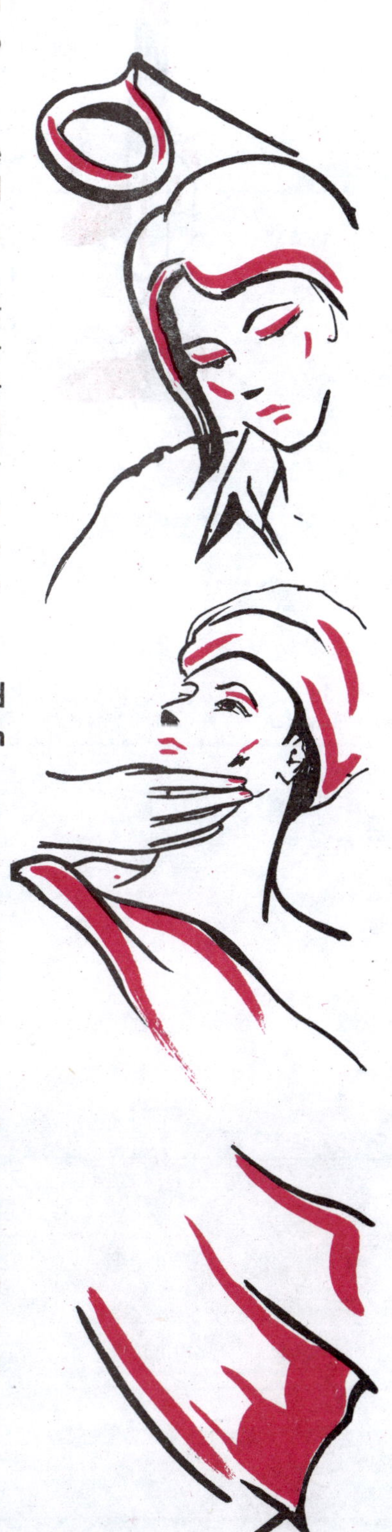

I have some dark spots at the side of my nose. There are some blackheads and enlarged pores on the nose and cheeks. Application of astringent makes my skin very dry. What should I do to get over the problem?

You seem to have an oily as well as sensitive skin and it should be treated accordingly. The first step is to keep it clean and free from skin-clogging substances. So, make it a point to wash your face with any medicated soap and cold water at least three times a day. Apply skin toner instead of using astringent, which can be strong for a sensitive skin. Using a water-based moisturiser should be good for you. You should drink the juice of a lemon thrice a day and eat a lot of citrus fruits.

I have an ugly scar on my cheek. Although I have tried various products to erase it, none has worked. Will skin peeling help me?

It all depends on the scar. Is it a deep one or a superficial one; is it recent or an old one? There are various treatments like dermabrasion or laser to remove scars or acne pits. A dermatologist or a plastic surgeon should do these treatments. You should consult a skin specialist before you attempt anything.

I have recently got tanned and my face as well as the hands have become very dark. What should I do to save my complexion from turning too dark?

Your daily activities might be keeping you outdoors for a long duration. You must protect your skin when you are under direct sunlight by using a sunscreen lotion on the exposed parts of your body such as the face, neck, arms and hands. You can also try a whitening cream for improving your complexion.

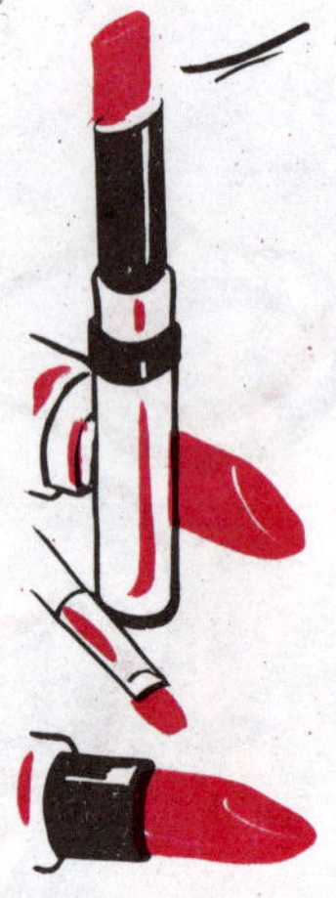

I have a fair complexion but my lips are quite dark. I want my lips to look rosy and healthy. How can I give them a normal colour?

There is no such thing as a normal colour for the lips. The colour may differ from one person to another. You could, however, massage your lips with buttermilk twice a day and apply a lip-salve at bedtime. Use only light shades of lipstick, because the lips can get pigmented due to dark coloured lipsticks.

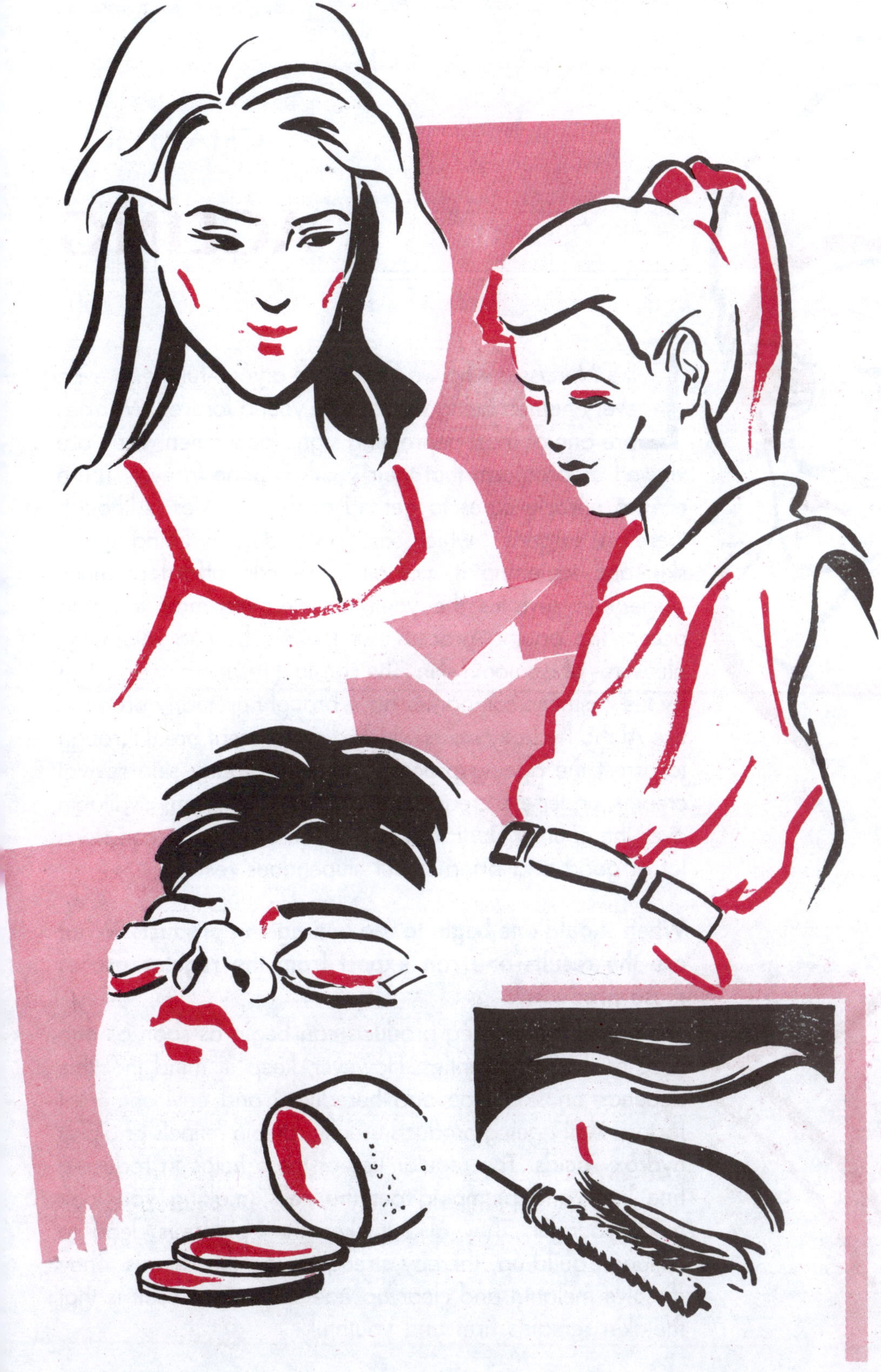

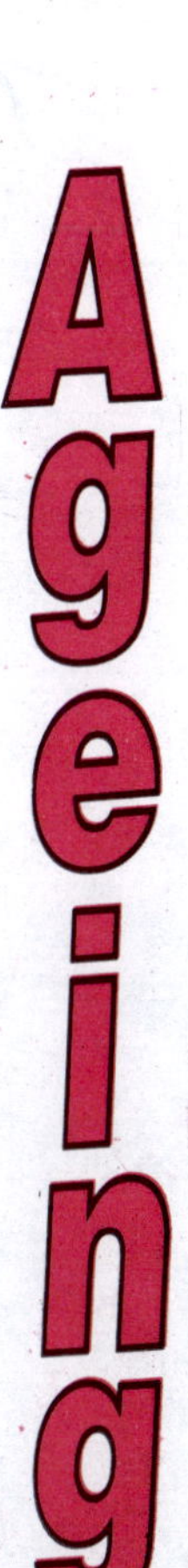
Ageing

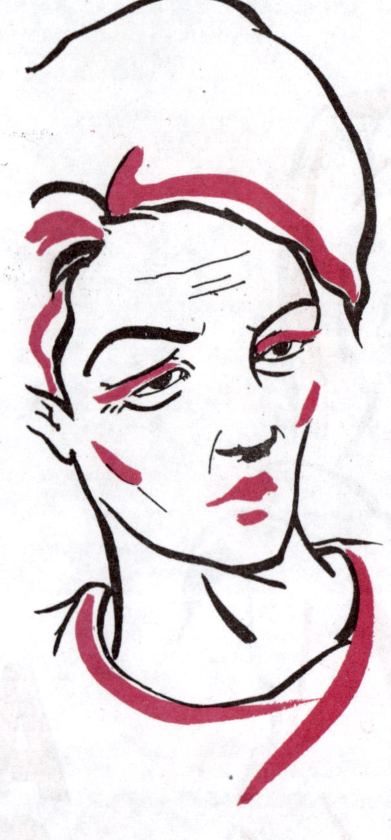

CHAPTER IV

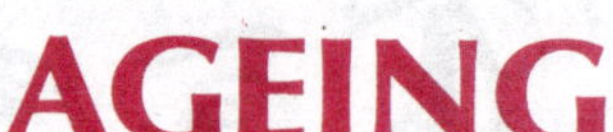

AGEING

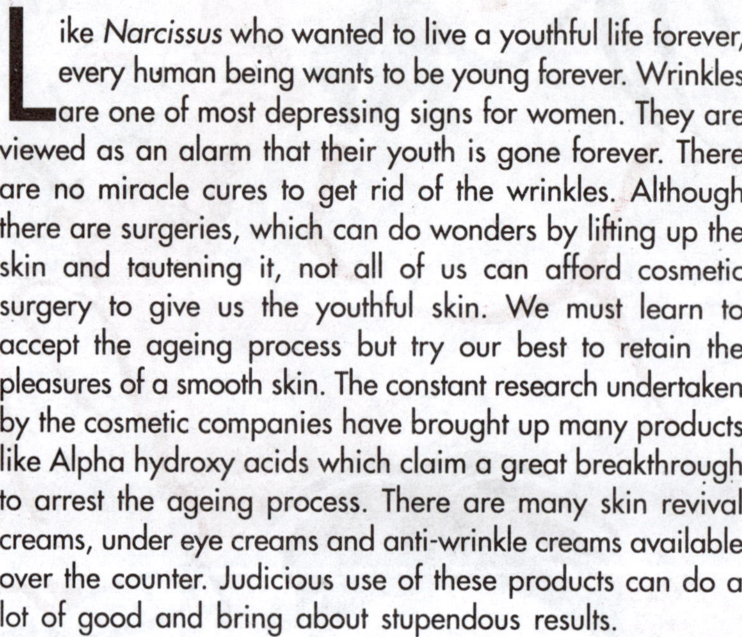

Like *Narcissus* who wanted to live a youthful life forever, every human being wants to be young forever. Wrinkles are one of most depressing signs for women. They are viewed as an alarm that their youth is gone forever. There are no miracle cures to get rid of the wrinkles. Although there are surgeries, which can do wonders by lifting up the skin and tautening it, not all of us can afford cosmetic surgery to give us the youthful skin. We must learn to accept the ageing process but try our best to retain the pleasures of a smooth skin. The constant research undertaken by the cosmetic companies have brought up many products like Alpha hydroxy acids which claim a great breakthrough to arrest the ageing process. There are many skin revival creams, under eye creams and anti-wrinkle creams available over the counter. Judicious use of these products can do a lot of good and bring about stupendous results.

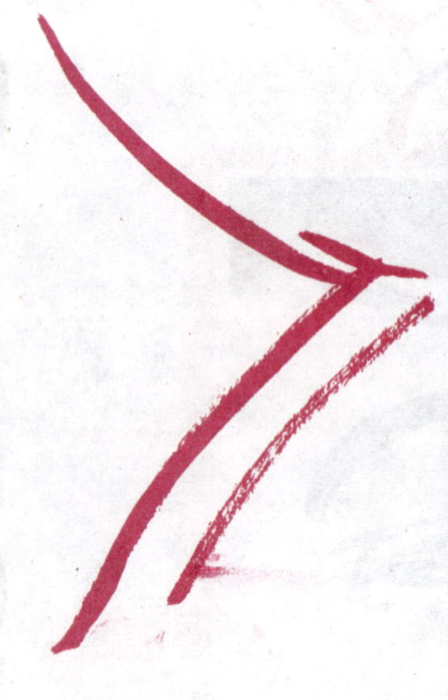

When should one begin to use anti-ageing products. What are the results one can expect from the regular use of these products?

The use of anti-ageing products can begin as soon as one reaches the late twenties. However, keep in mind that this depends on skin type and hereditary and environmental factors. Anti-ageing products usually contain retinols or alpha hydroxy acids. The regular use of these helps in reducing fine lines and plumping out the cells, making you look much younger. They also thicken the epidermis, lead to collagen build-up, thereby strengthening the dermis. They dissolve melanin and clear up age spots. The result is that the skin remains firm and youthful.

How can one retain the youthful looks? I envy women who are past their prime and yet manage to look young.

To prevent the visible signs of ageing, remember the following rules—

- Get enough sleep
- Exercise regularly
- Eat plenty of fresh fruits and vegetables daily
- Drink at least eight to ten glasses of water every day
- Stick to a good skin care routine
- Don't smoke
- Always wear a sunscreen when outdoors
- Take some time to relax, a stressed skin looks tired and haggard
- Practice meditation

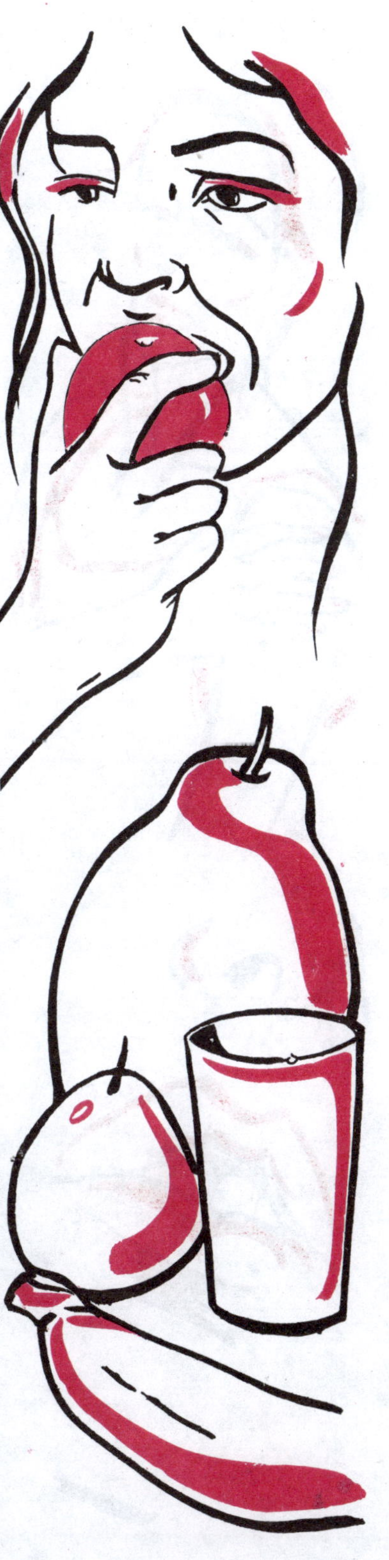

I have heard that vitamins E, C and beta carotene can work wonders as anti-ageing agents. Is that true?

There are some findings, which indicate that, these vitamins can have a retarding effect on the process of ageing. By influencing the factors responsible for the deterioration of the cells, these can slow down the ageing process. The main factor associated with the ageing process is free radicals. Antioxidants like vitamins E, C and beta-carotene react with free radicals and provide protection from their harmful effects. Free radical damage can result in sagging skin and muscles losing their firmness. Although all the antioxidants are necessary for the repair and appearance of the skin, hair, nails, teeth and gums, vitamin E is particularly important. Besides blocking free radical action, it promotes skin elasticity and boosts the circulation, giving skin a nice glow. Dermatologists have long been recommending creams and lotions, which contain Vitamin E, for minimising scars and wrinkles. Vitamin E bars the overgrowth of collagen, which forms a scar.

How does the pollution of the environment effect the skin?

Pollution is one of the major destructive elements of the world. It harms the skin in a big way. When the free radicals

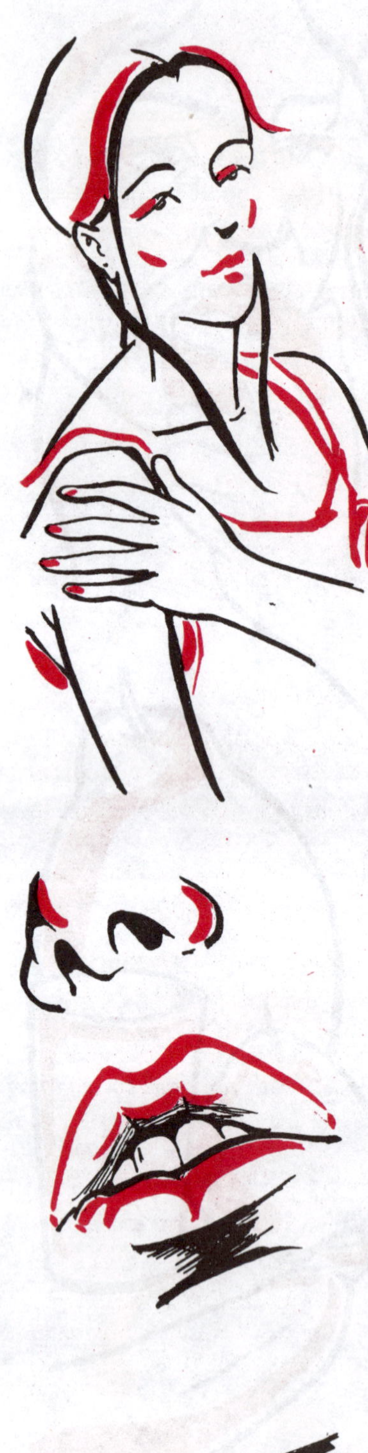

formed due to pollution, react with the skin, they harm the collagen and elasticity of the dermis thus causing sagging and ageing of the skin. They can also cause cancer and other diseases.

In the recent months I have been hearing a lot about free radicals. What are these and how do they cause damage to the skin?

Free radicals are produced by the metabolic processes of our body, like breathing, digestion etc. They are highly reactive molecules, which destroy bacteria, parasites and harmful cells, and also attack normal, healthy cells in the body. They can damage the cells and contribute to conditions ranging from skin damage to cancer. Normal metabolic processes produce some free radicals but their number goes up when the body is exposed to things like cigarette smoke, toxic chemicals or a diet high in animal fats. They can also be produced by tissue injuries from infection, toxins, reduced blood flow, excessive exercise and radiation or extreme cold and heat.

What is the function of antioxidants in counteracting the effect of free radicals?

Antioxidants like vitamin A, C and E and many other substances in plant food neutralise and fight the free radicals. They provide protection from the harmful effects of the free radicals.

I have been using cold cream and vaseline on my lips because they remain dry. Yet, I am not able to make them soft and supple. Could you suggest a remedy for the dryness?

Lack of moisture and the deficiency of vitamin B group are sometimes the cause of dry lips. A dry cold or a dry hot weather can also dehydrate the lips. Any medication, excess tea or coffee can also dry the skin. Drink plenty of water and fruit juices. Your body might be deficient in the essential vitamins and salts. So, include a lot of green leafy vegetables and fruits in your diet. To relieve the excess dryness, use a lip-salve at night. Fresh cream is one of the best emollients available in the natural form.

BLEMISHES AND DARK CIRCLES

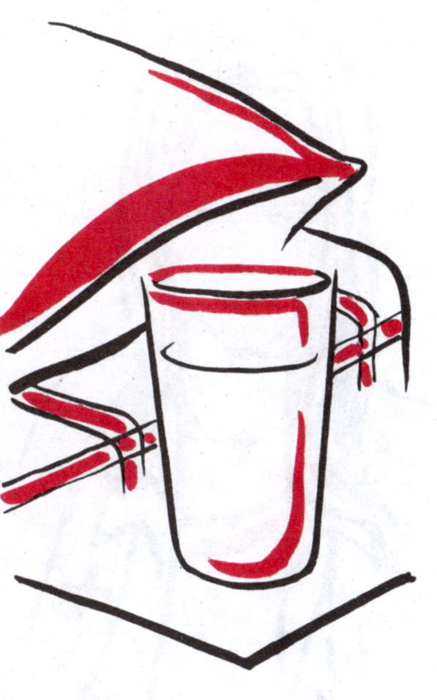

All women hate blemishes on their skin. They dream of a perfect, peaches and roses complexion where there is no place for the dark circles and spots. But not everyone is lucky enough to be born with a beautiful skin or complexion. A lot of care and love has to go into maintaining the skin to its optimum level.

I have dark circles around the eyes. Is there any permanent cure for dark rings around the eyes?

Dark circles under the eyes are due to various factors. Lack of sufficient iron in the diet, acute fatigue or eye strain, insomnia and late nights are some of them. Try to relax before going to sleep by doing some yoga. A glass of hot milk at bedtime also induces sound sleep. For eye strain, consult an eye specialist. Meanwhile, you can disguise the dark rings by applying a pale, light textured foundation cream with a soft, moistened make-up sponge. Pat a little loose powder to give a matt surface.

I have bags under my eyes. How do I get rid of them?

To get rid of the bags under your eyes, dip two wads of cotton wool, either in chilled cucumber juice, witch hazel or rose water. Keep aside. Wash and dry a small sized potato. Grate it and put over the eye lid. Apply the wool over the eye-lids. Lie down and relax for 15-20 minutes. Gently wash off the grated potato with tap water. Pat dry and apply a little baby oil.

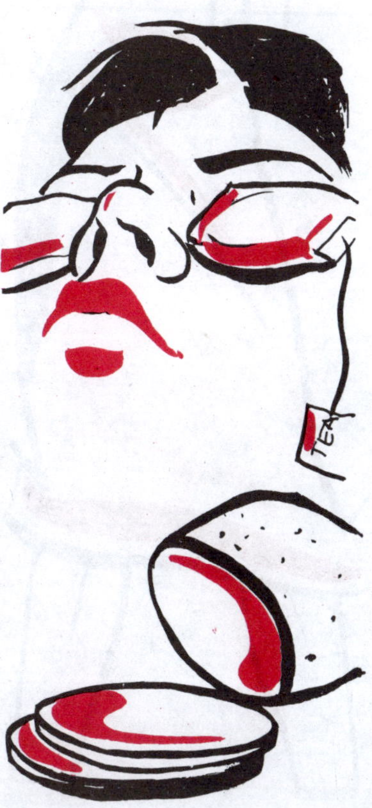

Please suggest a way by which I can get rid of the puffiness around my eyes.

Puffiness is generally due to accumulation of excess fluids. To get rid of the puffiness around the eyes, place chilled used tea bags on the closed eyelids and keep them in place for about ten minutes. The caffeine in the tea works like a diuretic to help rid the eyelids of excess fluid and the puffiness vanishes in no time. Alternatively, you could place two slices of potatoes on the eyes and relax for 10 minutes.

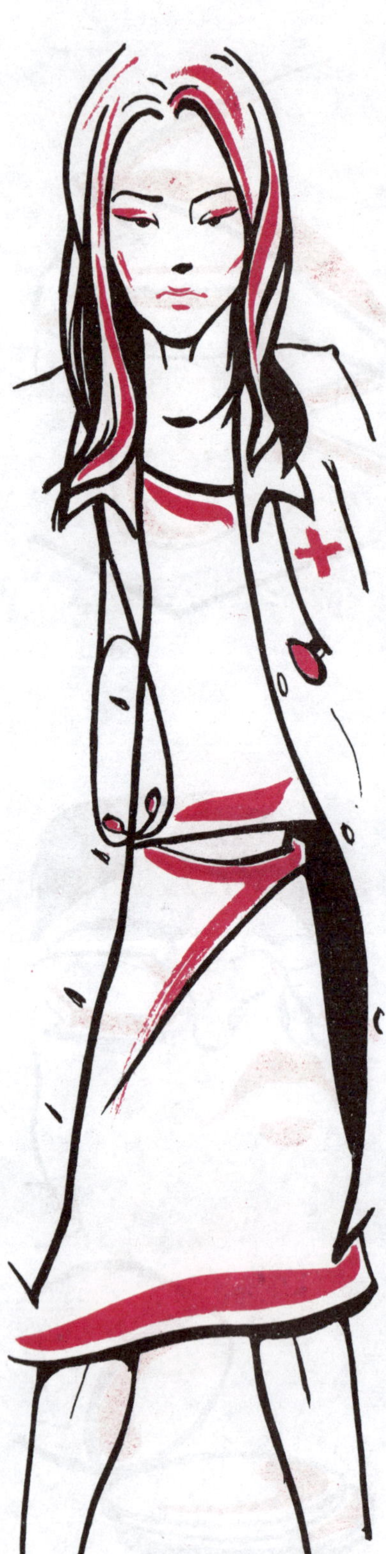

How can I camouflage the dark circles around my eyes?

Dark circles around the eyes are caused by iron deficiency in the diet, lack of sleep and stress. Try to get rid of the causes before you begin to try out cosmetics. Try to begin by eating an iron rich diet to take care of the body's iron requirements. Get adequate sleep and banish stress from your life. To camouflage the dark circles, you can use a little foundation, which has been blended with eye-cream. Apply this under the eyes and blend it properly so that it doesn't stand out. If you have bags under the eyes, blend a little dark brown pencil under the eyes to divert attention from the puffiness.

I have a low haemoglobin count. Because of this, I've developed dark rings around the eyes. What sort of diet will help me raise my haemoglobin level?

This is a question, which should actually be addressed to your doctor. However, I can suggest that you supplement your diet with iron rich food. Squeezing lime juice over any vegetable makes the body absorb the iron in them. Alfa-alfa sprouts are a very rich source of iron. They help in increasing the haemoglobin levels. These protein rich sprouts are low in calories and can be taken as salads or as juice. The alfa-alfa juice should be taken with tomato juice and a dash of lime juice. Drinking half a glass of this mixture daily will definitely raise your haemoglobin and erase the dark rings around your eyes.

I am a girl of 21 years. I have a wheatish complexion. There are some blemishes on my forehead, cheeks and chin. I want to improve my complexion. Please suggest some natural home remedy.

The best home remedy is sour buttermilk, which should be applied on the face. You will have to be patient since this takes a long time to make a difference. If you are in a hurry, you can use the whiteners available in the market.

The skin on my chin and upper lip has turned dark. My friend suggested that I use a bleach but I am not sure about it. What can I do to lighten the area around my lips?

When a dry skin is exposed to direct sun, it becomes dark and tanned. Use a sun screen or lotion and a revitalising cream at night. Don't use a bleach as suggested by your friend as it is likely to have a drying effect on your dry skin. You should also take food rich in vitamin B such as raw carrots, cabbage, tomatoes, cucumber, salad and seasonal fruits.

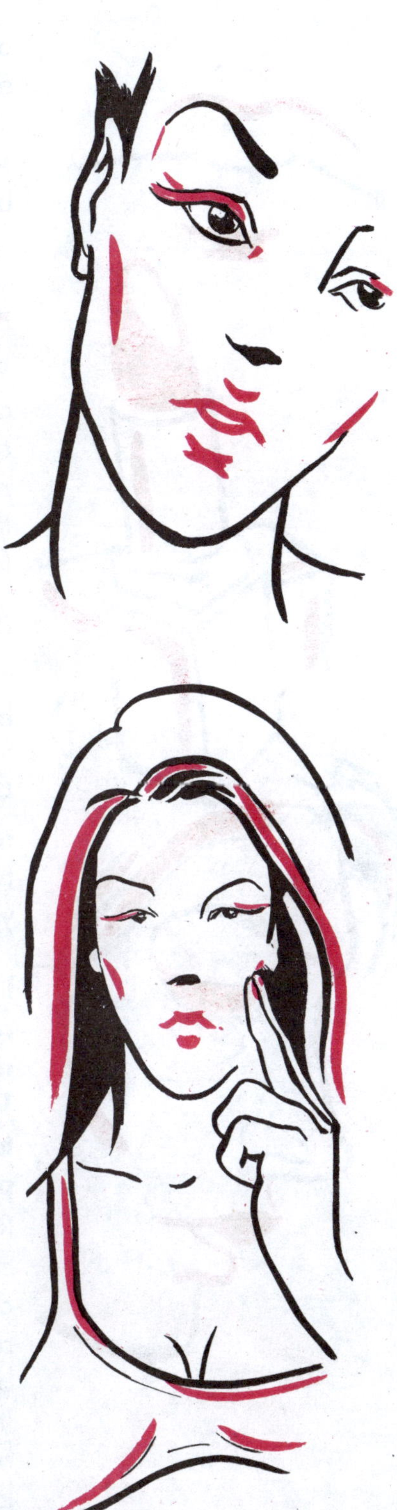

I am a 32-year-old woman. I am troubled about a wart, which has suddenly appeared near my lips. What could I do to get rid of it?

Warts can be hereditary. Sometimes they occur during pregnancy. The problem with warts is that they can be completely removed only with the help of electrocutery but they tend to recur. If they are removed from one spot, they may come up at another spot, at a later date.

I have a habit of biting my lips. As a result, my lips have become quite ugly. The skin that grows is very hard and rough. I cannot apply lipstick as it looks patchy on the rough lips. Will a moisturiser help in making it smooth?

Now that you realise that the habit of biting your lips is causing you grief, it is time to give up the habit. Worries, tensions and shyness sometimes lead to habits like lip-biting or nail-biting. Find out the cause of your bad habit and try to get out of it. Apply a lip salve, at night, to smooth out the roughness. During the daytime, wear a lipstick, which has a built-in moisturiser. There are many foreign brands available which contain a moisturiser. They keep the lips conditioned and give it a gloss.

I am a 27-year-old woman with a dry skin. I have been bleaching my face for the last six years and taking a facial once a month. I read somewhere that a facial is not good when done under the age of 30. Is it true?

Physiologically, the process of ageing begins after the age of 25. This is when the oil and moisture levels start getting

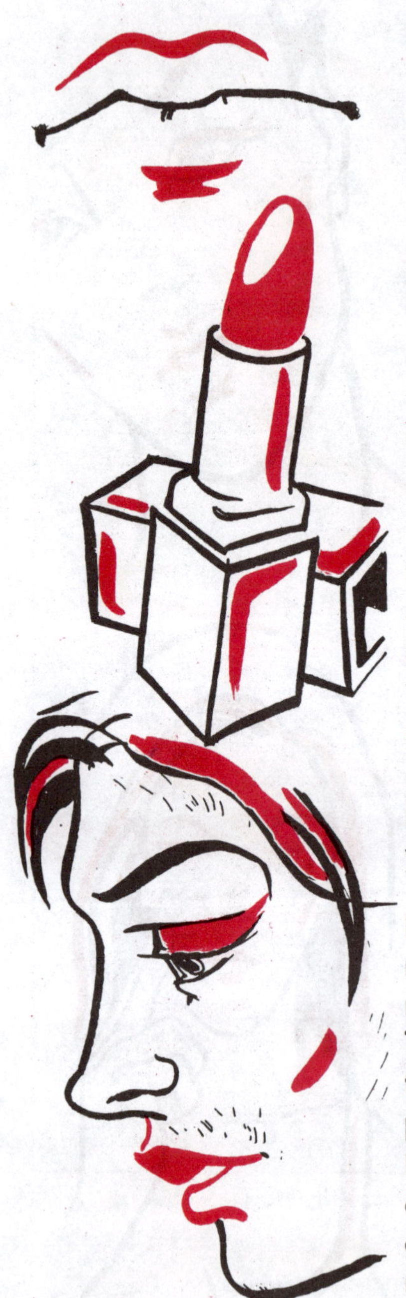

depleted. Ideally, you should get a facial done regularly every month, after the age of 25. A regular facial tones up the muscles, replenishes the oils and moisture levels and scrubs as well as cleanses the skin. However, bleaching can be one of the causes for your dry skin.

SUPERFLUOUS HAIR

With the dresses becoming shorter and the necklines going deeper, no one can afford to be harbouring hairy legs and arms. And the profuse growth of facial hair can rob a person of her self-confidence. It is not difficult to get rid of the superfluous hair. A smooth and hair-less skin is yours for the asking.

I am a 14-year-old girl. I have a lot of facial hair, especially over the lips and forehead. What can I do about it? I have heard of thermolysis, what is it?

You can use an apricot-honey peel off face scrub on your face once a week. You can also try a face scrub of chokker, rosewater and milk. Scrub it off the face and neck region by using circular strokes until the flakes dry and fall off. If yu follow it up regularly, it could discourage facial hair.

I am a young working woman. I have been using a hair removing cream for the last five years. Recently I have noticed that my skin develops rashes after using the cream. These rashes later turn into dark spots. What could I do to remove the dark spots that have developed due to this problem?

Repeated use of hair removing creams can often cause allergies as the chemicals used to dissolve the hard proteins of the hair are very strong. There are other methods of hair removal like using epilators or going in for waxing. It is better for you to switch over from the depilator. However, if you have to continue using the cream, do so sparingly by alternating this method with bleaching. Use a calamine lotion to soothen the irritated areas and take some anti allergy tablets. Moisturise the area with a rich moisturiser.

I am a 15-year-old girl. I need your advice on removing superfluous hair.

You could use methods such as waxing and depilatory creams for removing superfluous hair. Waxing improves the colour of the skin and also removes dust and grime which has settled on the skin. It also softens and removes dead cells. Nowadays, there are good epilators available in the market. These clean up the superfluous hair quickly and efficiently. They are also very easy to use. If you are using an epilator, use a body moisturiser to smoothen the skin

I have thick and rough hair on my face. They make my face look quite ugly. How can I remove them? Is waxing all right for the face? Is there any other method, which will remove the hair permanently?

Firstly, you must examine the cause of such a thick growth on the face. Get some hormonal tests done. Waxing should not be done for facial hair. You could bleach the hair to give it a lighter tone. There are other methods of removing facial hair but they need to be done by experts and may cost quite a bit. Thermolysis is a permanent method of hair removal but it is a gradual process and may need several sitting depending upon the growth of the hair. The method involves the passing of a short wave diathermic current through the tip of a needle inserted in the hair follicle. The current destroys the capillaries that supply nutrients to the hair root.

Is waxing harmful for young girls?

Not at all. Waxing can be done by young girls for removing superfluous hair. Waxing pulls out the hair from the root and has a smooth and lasting effect on the skin. Regular waxing weakens the growth of the hair. It is one of the oldest method of removing superfluous hair and has no side effects.

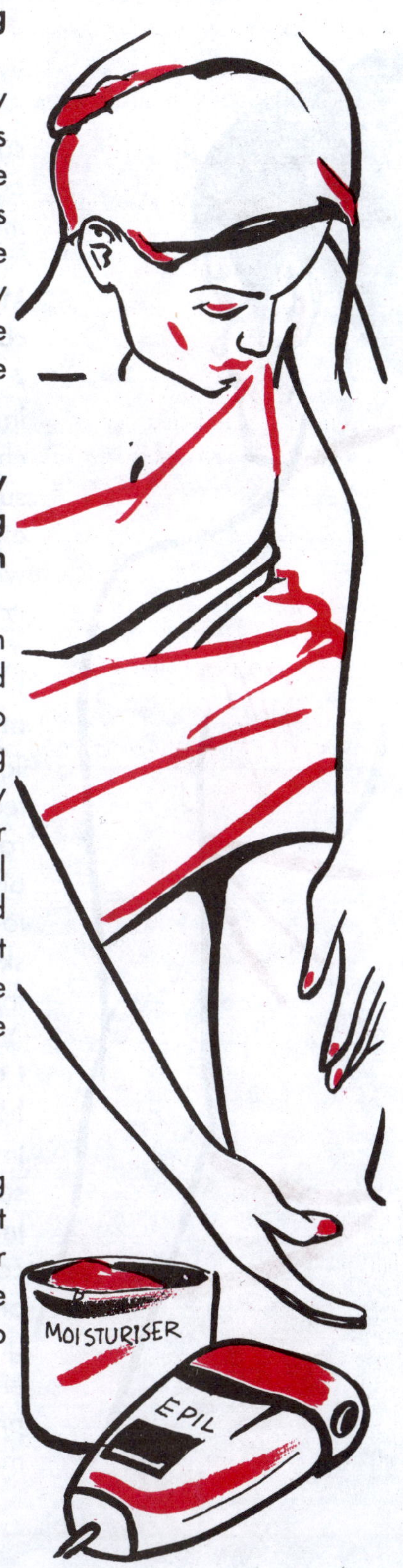

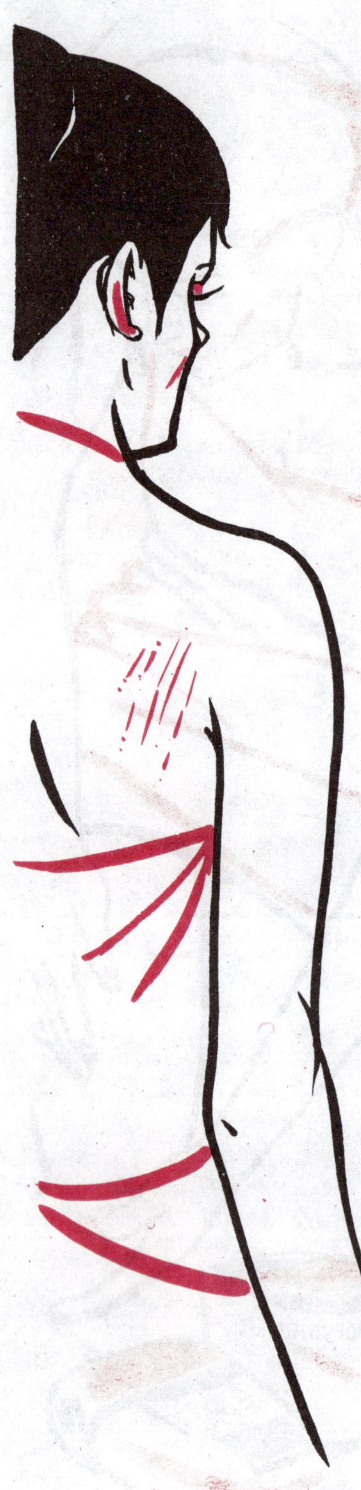

STRETCH MARKS

Whenever a person loses or gains weight, there are chances of developing stretch marks. Pregnancy, teenage fat, sudden spurt in body weight, all can cause these ugly marks to occur. But one can try to prevent the formation of stretch marks and also control them if the correct method is known.

My skin feels very scratchy, especially during winter. What could be the reason for this?

A very common reason for itchy or scratchy skin is the impact of dieting. It could bring about a lot of undesirable changes in the body and the skin. Losing a lot of weight suddenly is not a good sign. Hypo-thyroid patients also experience itchy skin. This condition is aggravated during winter. Iron deficiency or adult diabetes can also cause itchiness.

I have stretch marks on my stomach which came up after my pregnancy. What should I do to get rid of these marks?

To get rid of the stretch marks try this method. Use $^1/_2$-teaspoon of aloes, $^1/_2$-teaspoon papaya pulp, 1-teaspoon rose water, 1-teaspoon sandalwood paste, 10 drops almond oil and 2 drops of lavender oil. Add 2-teaspoon milk cream to these and make a smooth paste. Apply over the affected skin and massage gently before a bath. Do this, at least thrice a week.

I am a 30-year-old woman. Ever since I began dieting, I have noticed that my skin has begun to sag. Please help!

In the 20s and 30s, there is enough elasticity in the skin to sustain weight fluctuation without facing any skin problems. In your case, rapid weight loss could have caused full contraction of the skin. For most women, it takes 3 months of weight maintenance for the flabbiness to disappear. This gives the skin enough time to contract. A balanced diet enables the skin to remain well-hydrated and prevents premature sagging. Calculated weight loss means not losing more than $^1/_2$ or 1 kg per week.

I am a 24-year-old woman and I have prominent stretch marks on my arms, stomach and thighs. Are these a sign of weight gain? Can I get rid of them?

Stretch marks develop when the skin is stretched over a long period of time. This strains the elastic fibres in the deeper layers of the skin to the point where they cannot regain their original resilience and show up when there is a sudden fluctuation in weight or on doing strenuous exercise. There are no lotions or creams that can erase these marks.

I am a 22-year-old woman. The area under my arms and on the inside of my thighs is dark. Can you suggest a remedy for this?

The skin on the inner side of the thighs and the underarms is usually darker in the case of over-weight people. Lose weight sensibly, bleach these areas once a month and use a mixture of creams containing 2% hydroquinone and cortisone.

BODY WEIGHT AND EXERCISES

A beautiful personality requires a beautiful and fit body. With so much emphasis being placed on slender figures, almost everyone has become a fitness freak. Gyms and playgrounds are full of people who are trying to achieve a svelte form. Those who can't reduce by exercises try to do so by resorting to dieting. Dieting can have a positive impact when the body receives all the nutrients, but when one cuts down on the food without balancing the required calories and other elements, it can be dangerous. Lack of nourishment can play havoc with one's hair and skin so one must take expert advice before one begins to diet.

I am 17 years old. I am over-weight and I want to reduce it without exercising. Can you suggest some way to do so?

Exercise is important not only to reduce weight but also to maintain good health. You must do some form of exercise regularly. Choose any form that interests you. It could be

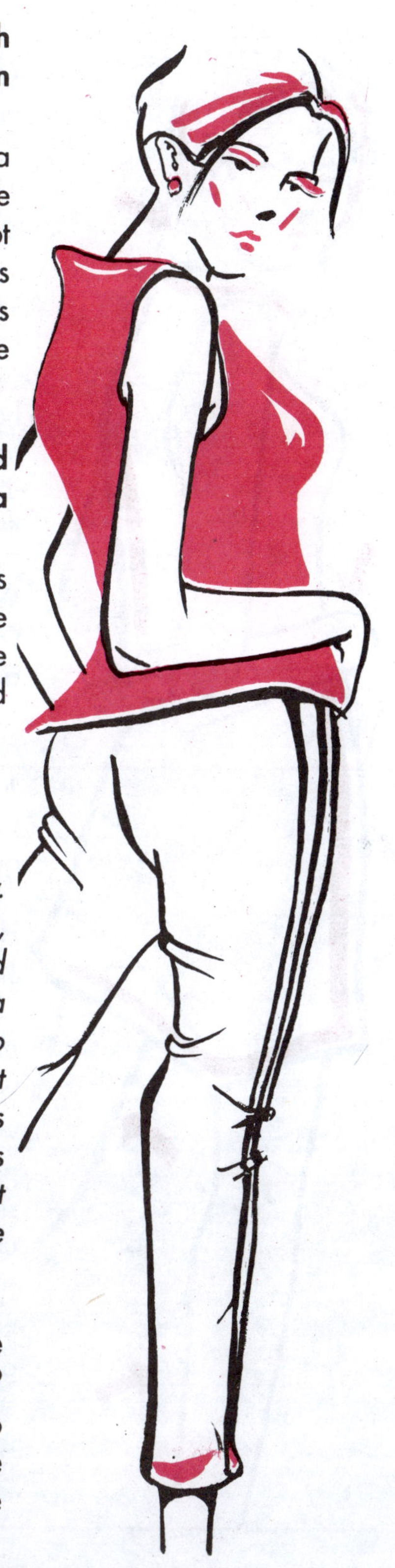

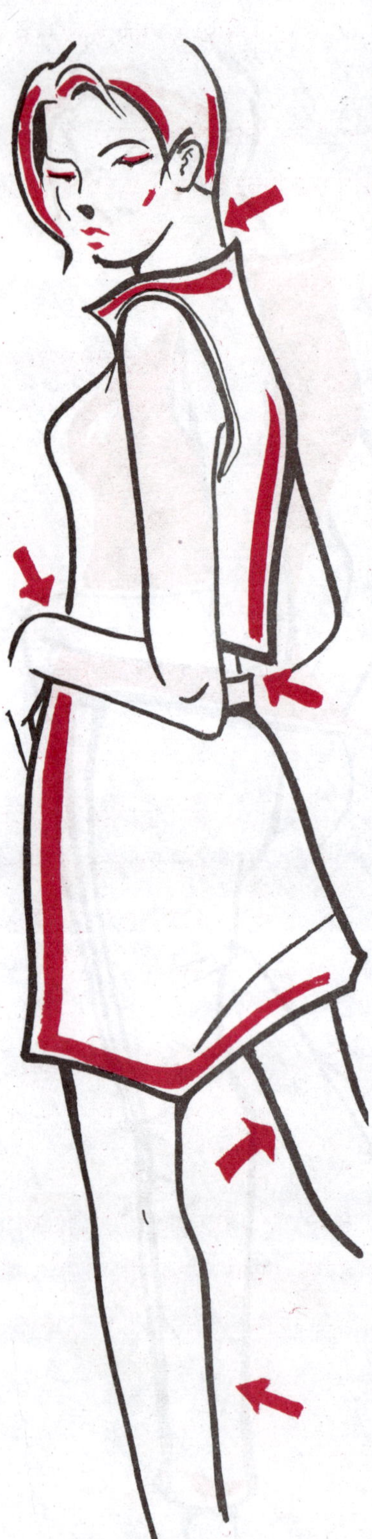

walking, playing some outdoor game, swimming or jogging. As far as diet is concerned, try to eat food that is not fried and is closer to its natural form. Fresh foods like tomatoes, cucumber, salad leaves and fruits are very good for people who want to reduce weight. Avoid all kinds of fast food and sweets.

What is cellulitis?

In beauty parlance, cellulitis denotes that thickening or swelling of the tissue which is characterised by a skin that has the appearance of orange peel and a grating sensation, more or less painful, during massage. Cellulitis is also an inflammation of this same connective tissue due to toxins that the system has failed to eliminate.

Where does it occur?

Cellulitis generally attacks the hips, legs, thighs, abdomen and the nape of the neck.

How do I know if I have cellulitis?

Just pinch and pull the skin between your fingers, if this is painful then you have cellulitis. Cellulitis could be mild, advance or deep-seated.

How do I know what kind of cellulitis I have?

The cellulitis is mild when there is a thickening. The skin adheres to the deeper layers of flesh and will not move freely. Again applying the pinching movement, the tissues will present the characteristic orange peel appearance.

Cellulitis is at an advanced stage when it forms hard patches and is resistant to touch. You can barely raise the skin when you pinch, for it adheres completely to the underlying tissues. Pinching it is very painful and quickly results in bruising.

The cellulitis is deep-seated when you have a sensation of small balls or nodules rolling under your fingers. The surface of the skin has lumps and hollows and it is often impossible to detach the skin from the fibrous tissue, which is the seat of a chronic inflammation.

What are the damages that cellulitis can cause?

Cellulitis can cause a variety of problems.

1. Cellulitis produces deformities: the legs and hips can become greatly enlarged.
2. Bad circulation and even heart problems.
3. Depression, nervousness and fatigue (caused by the toxins in the blood).
4. Pains which can become agonizing, for cellulitis thickens the connective tissues which cause pressure on the nerves.
5. Sciatica, migraine and neuralgia.
6. Insomnia

How can I control the formation of cellulitis?

You can combat cellulitis by:

- by dieting
- by exercise
- by medical treatment
- by massage treatment

How does massage help in combating cellulitis?

One can undertake self-massage to control cellulitis. It helps in the following manner:

- stimulates the return circulation (the venous circulation)
- helps the skin to retract by percussive or 'chopping' movements
- tones up the muscles by rolling movement
- disperses and eliminates the toxins

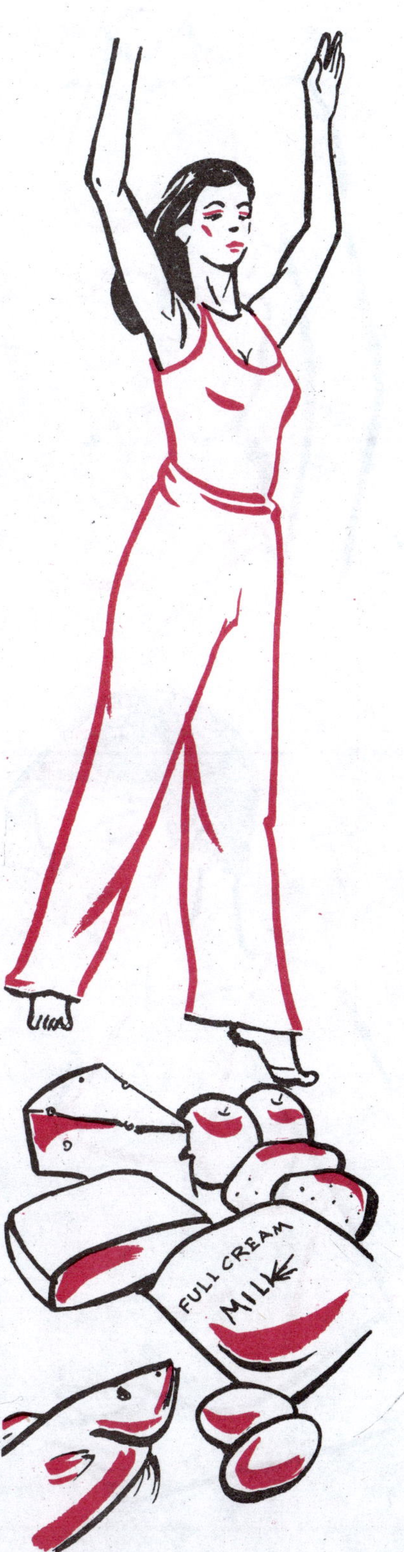

I am a 22-year-old girl. I am under-weight and want to gain some weight. How do I go about it?

First of all, you must check if you have any medical problems or are suffering from some disease. Once that is ruled out, try and follow an exercise regime. Even if you are under-weight, you must exercise regularly. It helps in increasing the appetite. Sometimes inadequate diet is responsible for low weight. Sit with a nutritional expert and work out the daily calorie requirements based on your height and daily

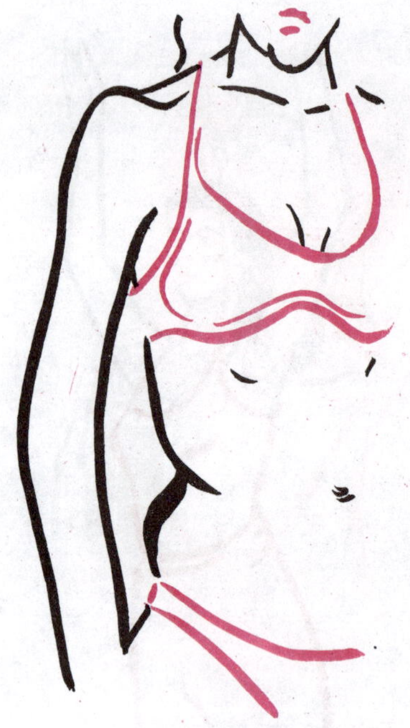

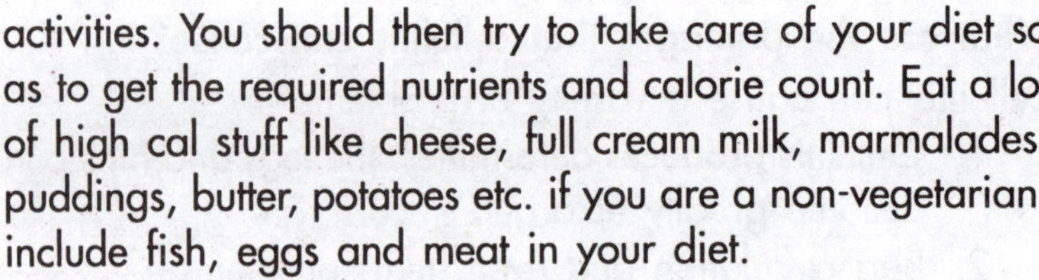

activities. You should then try to take care of your diet so as to get the required nutrients and calorie count. Eat a lot of high cal stuff like cheese, full cream milk, marmalades, puddings, butter, potatoes etc. if you are a non-vegetarian, include fish, eggs and meat in your diet.

I have very fat thighs, could you suggest some exercise by which I can lose weight on my thighs?

Spot reduction is a very difficult matter. One has to lose overall weight in order to make any effect on specific parts of body. However, you must start cycling. Cycling is a very good exercise to reduce the thighs. It strengthens the back, leg and stomach muscles. It also improves cardio-vascular activity. Twelve minutes of cycling will burn about 100 calories. You can also burn an equivalent amount of calories if you run very fast for about 5 minutes. Besides exercise, you must control your diet also. Try and stick to low-fat, low-starch diet and concentrate more on fresh and raw green vegetables and citrus fruits.

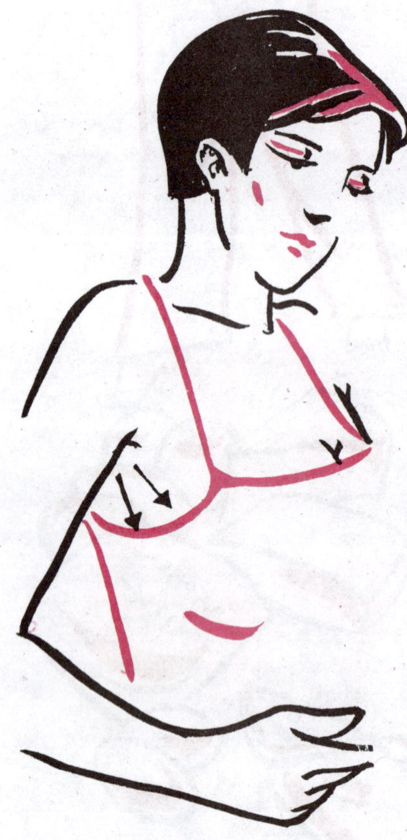

I have a bulge at my midriff. How do I reduce it?

I would like to know your age group and the type of lifestyle that you follow. To reduce excess fat from midriff you have to undertake a strict regiment of exercises because this is the area that is prone to gaining inches and getting them off is the toughest battle possible. There are some simple exercises which need to be done regularly in order to have any effect and results would emerge slowly.

Stand with arms extended at sides and feet wide apart. Keeping the legs straight, bend from the waist and touch each foot with the opposite hand. Repeat for 10 counts.

Stand with your arms raised above your head, feet apart and toes out. Bend from the waist to the left with your left hand touching the left leg below the knee. Return to the starting position and do the same with the right side. Repeat 10 times for each side.

You could also take up yoga, which has several beneficial effects. And don't forget to control your diet.

BODY ODOUR & PERFUMES

The most beautiful person can manage to turn people off if she suffers from body odour (BO). Perspiration and sweat can cause the bacteria to multiply and give out offensive odour. This requires to be controlled by maintaining personal hygiene and using anti-odour products.

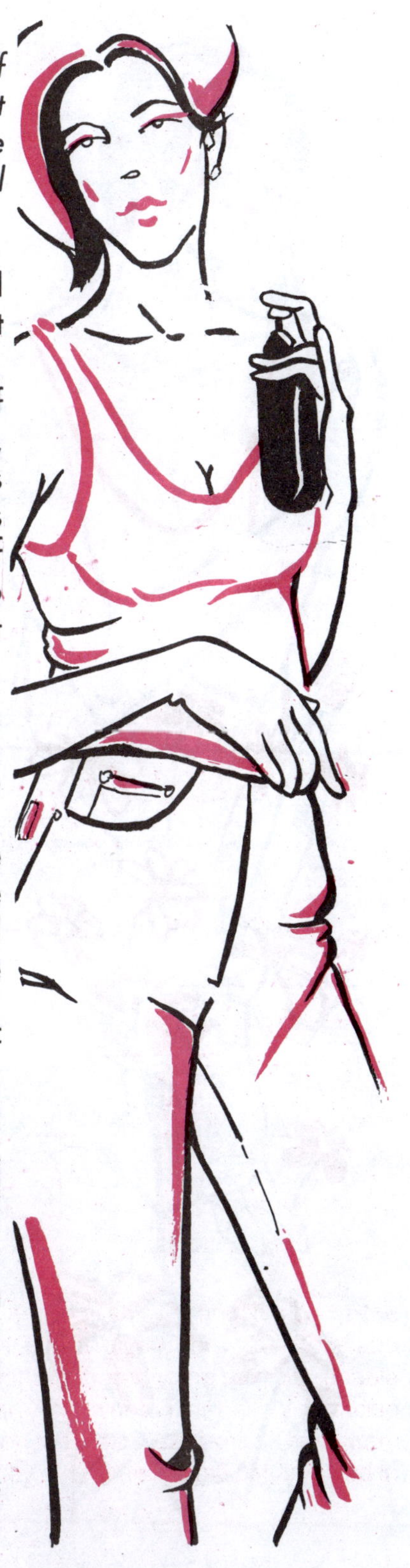

How can underarm odour be prevented? I've tried several brands of roll-ons and spray deodorants but they are not really effective. Please help!

Unpleasant underarm odour is caused due to the action of skin bacteria on the secretions of the aprocrine sweat glands, which are abundant in this area. Sometimes the odour is also caused because of metabolic problems, infections, drugs or spicy foods. Cleanliness is the most important means of controlling this problem. Removing underarm hair helps to reduce the number of bacteria present. It is also important to wear clean clothes. Avoid synthetics and stick to cottons. Deodorants also help but do not replace hygiene.

I am troubled by the excessive perspiration of my body. What should I do to get rid of the sweat problem?

Everyone perspires, some more than the others. There are millions of sweat glands all over our body. Sweating is one of the protective devices of the skin. The skin throws out all the wastes and toxins through sweat and it is also a device for getting the body used to the atmospheric temperature. Soap and water are good for getting rid of the odours of perspiration. A deodorant helps by checking the odour. An anti-perspirant gets to work by sealing the sweat glands in a manner so that the perspiration cannot escape and there are no odours. You can use a good anti-perspirant to avoid excessive sweating.

What is the difference between a bodyspray and a deodorant?

A deodorant is a very functional product. It has anti-bacterial properties, which help to ward off body odour. A bodyspray on the other hand, is a perfume in a spray form. All bodysprays are perfumed and can be sprayed all over the body.

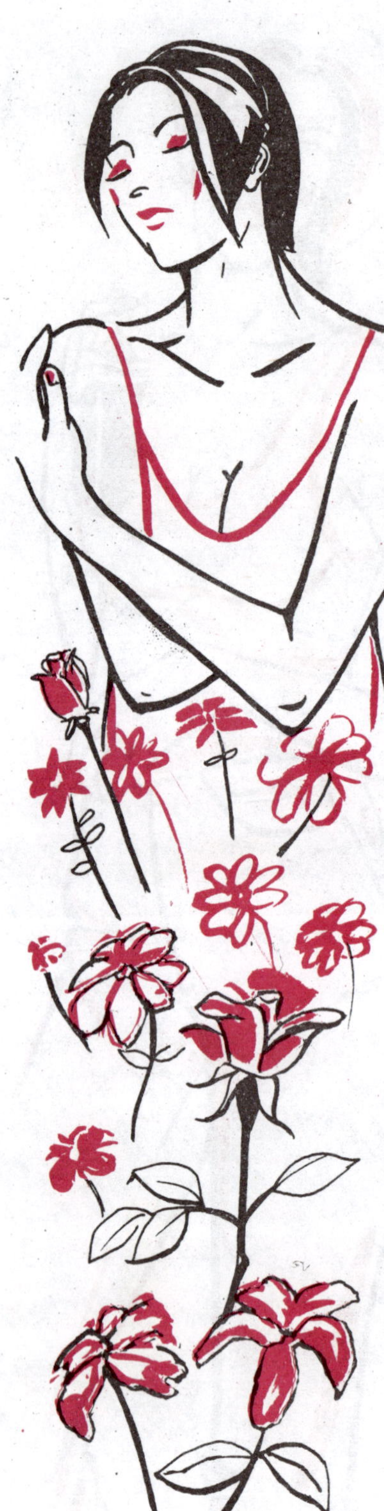

How can I choose the right type of perfume?

To select the right kind of perfume, you must try it out on your pulse spot. The pulse spot at the inner side of the wrist is the best place for trying out the notes of a perfume. Leave it on overnight and you will be able to get the base notes of the perfume as well as its staying power. The perfumes have top notes, which are the scents that appear just after the application. The base notes can be smelt after a few hours of application.

I have heard that a perfume is judged by its notes. What exactly is meant by notes and how can I judge a perfume?

There are three basic notes of a fragrance: the top note, middle note and the base note. The blend of the three notes gives the character to a perfume. The initial whiff that you get from your perfume is the top note. It is more volatile and evaporates quickly, leaving the middle note, which gives body to the fragrance. It is the base note that lasts much longer and gives the retentivity to the perfume. The most popular range of notes are fruity, floral and citrus with base notes of wood, musk or sandalwood.

How should perfume be applied for optimum benefit?

For a lasting effect, the perfume should be applied on the pulse points. The pulse points like the inside of the wrist, behind the ears, nape of the neck and behind the knees as well as the décolletage are the ideal spots. The body heat at these points allows the fragrance to vaporise faster and take effect. Never apply perfume on your clothes.

Does the atmospheric temperature have any effect on perfumes?

During the summer when the temperature is soaring, one must apply the perfume sparingly. The body heat revs up the scent and makes the aroma headier. But you can go lavish with the application during the winter because the only heat will come from your body.

EMOTIONS AND THE SKIN

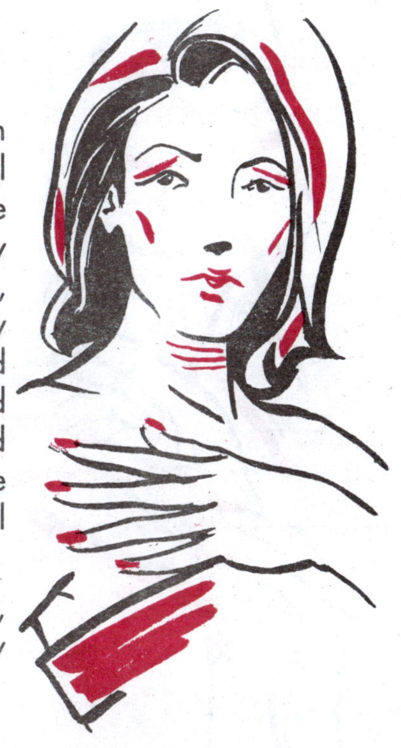

How do emotions affect the skin?

Emotions play a very important role in deciding the condition of the skin. Skin is a barometer of the physical and emotional condition of a person. The state of mind is reflected on the skin. Tensions or unhappiness can cause flaking, patchy dryness and peeling of skin. When we are anxious, depressed, angry or unhappy, the body responds by tightening and constricting the pores, clogging them and preventing the disposal of waste. This destroys the cells and makes the skin surface look dull and flaky. The affected areas are mainly the temples, cheeks, and chin because the sebaceous glands provide more oil and fat under emotional stress.

On the other hand, happiness causes the skin to relax, pores to open and blood circulation increases oxygen supply to the skin, brings a glow to the face.

Does emotional stress have any effect on hormones?

Definitely so. Emotional stress has a very negative effect on the release of hormones in the body. Testosterone, the hormone linked with acne in adolescents increases during periods of stress. This aggravates the acne and other skin problems. Oestrogen, the hormone responsible for fine, firm texture and yourhful skin is also affected by stress. Emotion stress can cause a fall in the level of oestrogen production. And a fall in the oestrogen levels can cause the skin to dry up and become dull and aged.

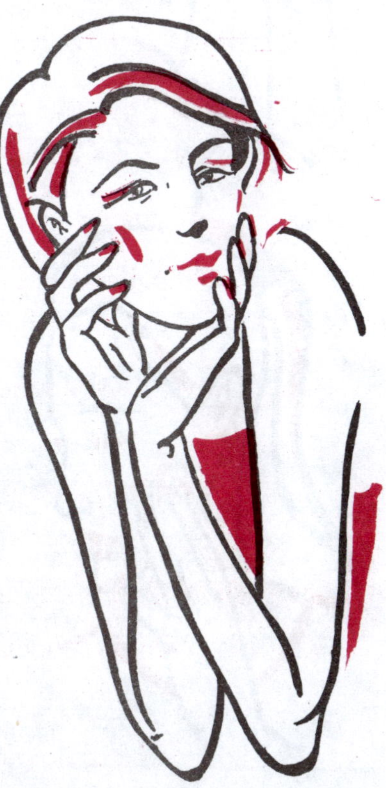

I have deep lines on my neck. How can I get a smooth and slender neck?

Neck is a very important part of a woman. Swan like necks have always attracted attention. But it also happens to be the most neglected part of the body. There are several women who apply creams and oils to the face but ignore the neck.

One must remember to include the neck in all skin care rituals. Once you give it the same attention as you

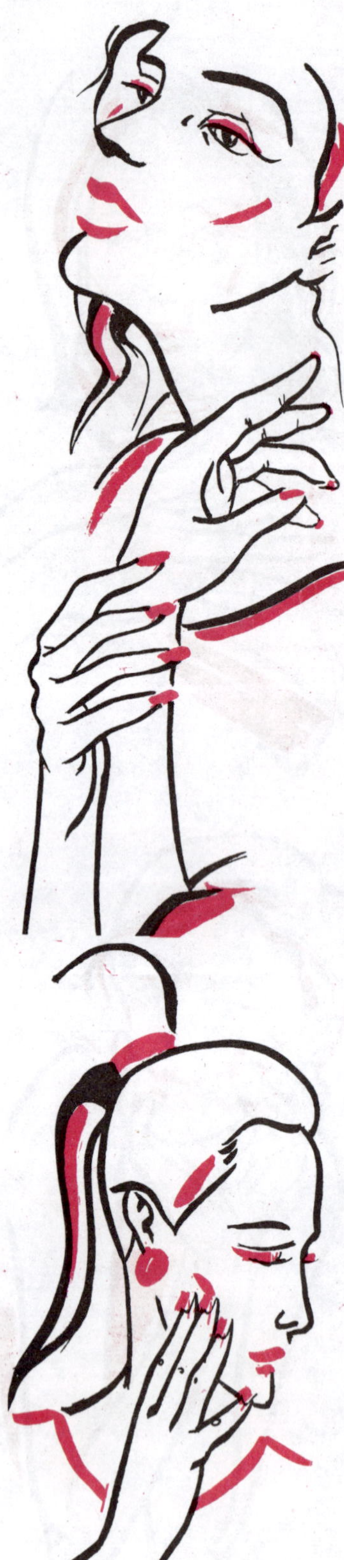

give your face, you will notice the change that occurs. Your neck will be as smooth as your face. Cleanse, tone and nourish the neck just as you do your face.

SENSITIVE SKIN

I have a very sensitive skin. As a result, I can hardly apply any cosmetic products on my face. Please suggest a way by which I can overcome this problem.

The sensitive skin is still a big mystery. Why some skins react to the extremity of temperature, sun, wind, alcohol, fragrance and skincare ingredients is still a grey area. Symptoms, like violent itching, redness or rashes, watering eyes and excessive dryness, occur when the sensitive skin is exposed to any of these elements. Generally it is seen that women who have a fair complexion, blue eyes and naturally light or red hair are more susceptible to sensitivity of the skin. You must take care to choose hypoallergenic range of skin care products and keep the use of chemical based cosmetics to a minimum.

I have heard that sensitive skin ages faster than the other types of skin. Is it true?

Yes, sensitive skin can add years to your life. It ages faster, when it gets irritated, skin becomes weakened and fails to perform its duty of being a protective barrier. It lets moisture escape and the potential irritants enter the skin. Lack of protection from the environmental pollutants leads to the breakdown of collagen and elastin and invites free radical damage, resulting in visible wrinkles and sagging of the skin.

Ever since I began using a cream which contains Alpha Hydroxy Acids, I have become very tanned and my skin itches when I go out in the sun. What could be the reason for this?

Women who are continually using alpha hydroxy acid (AHA) containing cosmetics have noticed that their skin becomes very sensitive to the harsh ultraviolet rays of the sun. AHA evens out the skin texture by exfoliating process, thinning the outer layer of the skin. This makes it more vulnerable to the sunrays and allows the ultraviolet rays to penetrate the skin. The most obvious indications of damage are redness, peeling and irritated patches. If your skin manifests these reactions, stop using the product immediately. Use an extra high ultraviolet sunscreen even on cloudy days to protect the skin from further damage. You must use mild moisturising lotions and cleansers.

My skin is always giving a shiny look. How could I overcome this terrible look?

You must be having an oily skin and must have noticed that the shine is especially visible during hot days. Oiliness increases with the temperature by at least 10% per degree rise in temperature. Hormonal fluctuations can also cause an overproduction of sebum. You must use alkaline soaps because sebaceous glands act against the high pH by giving out more of the oily secretion. Keep away from alcohol-based cosmetic products as alcohol cause extreme dryness, which leads an oily skin to produce more oil. A witch hazel-based toner is very good for an oily skin.

TEETH

A beautiful smile can work wonders for a person's looks. To have a beautiful smile, one must possess a beautiful set of teeth. Today, there have been so many changes in the world of dentistry and cosmetic dentistry that almost all dental problems can be taken care of.

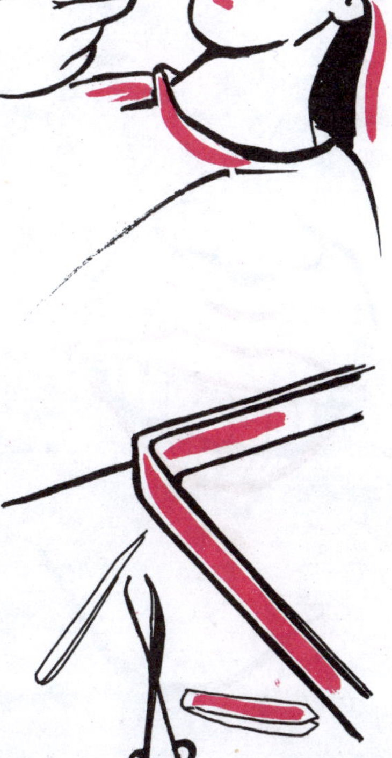

I am to be married in a few months but I am worried about the yellowish look of my teeth. What should I do?

The yellow on your teeth could be 'plaque'. The teeth is susceptible towards picking up stains from the food and drinks you consume every day. It is the deposition of oral bacteria on tooth surface in the form of a fine film. If you fail to remove this by regular brushing of the teeth, the plaque begins to turn yellow. In the long run, if you ignore the plaque, it may cause other problems. Give your teeth a thorough cleaning and they will become sparkling white, once again.

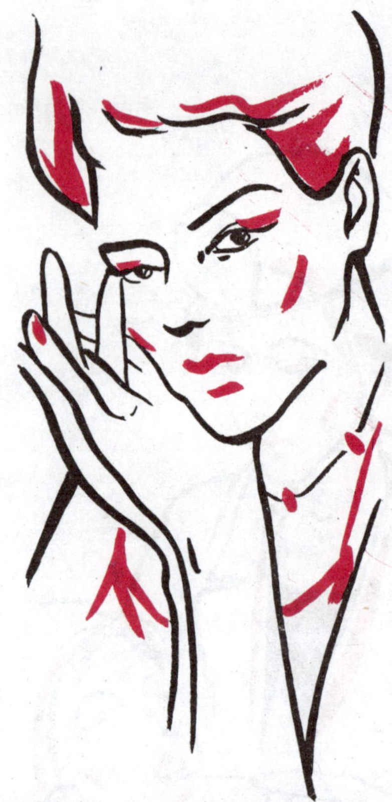

My teeth are slightly discoloured. Initially I thought the discolouration was due to the paan chewing habit that I have. I stopped the habit but the colour of my teeth has not improved. I am very conscious of this fact. Is there any method by which I can whiten the teeth?

It seems that your teeth have been stained due to your habit of taking paan. These stains, once formed, do not get removed easily. You must visit a dentist and seek his expert advice. There are methods by which the teeth can be polished or capped. He is the best person to advise you on the problem.

I have the most awful set of teeth. This makes me very conscious and I can't smile without hiding my mouth. What can I do about my problem?

Do not despair. Science has advanced far enough to take care of such little problems. The orthodentists can change the entire look of a person by resetting the teeth and giving them specialised treatment. Consult a good orthodentist for advice.

I am desperate, please help. My teeth have yellowed in the last two years. What could I do to get the whiteness back in them?

There are many ways by which a cosmetic dentist can work wonders with the teeth. To get rid of the yellowish stains, he would either bleach them or place caps on them. For bleaching, a strong peroxide solution with exposure to heat and light is used. Traditional bleaching will not work if you have stains due to the use of tetracycline. He may also suggest porcelain veneers to cover the teeth. These are thin sheets of porcelain laid over the tooth.

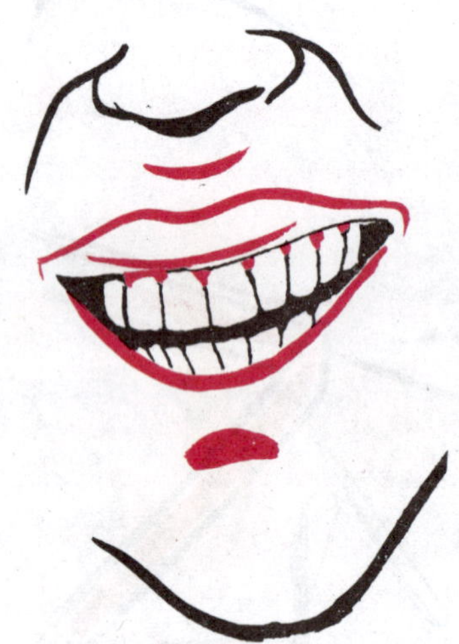

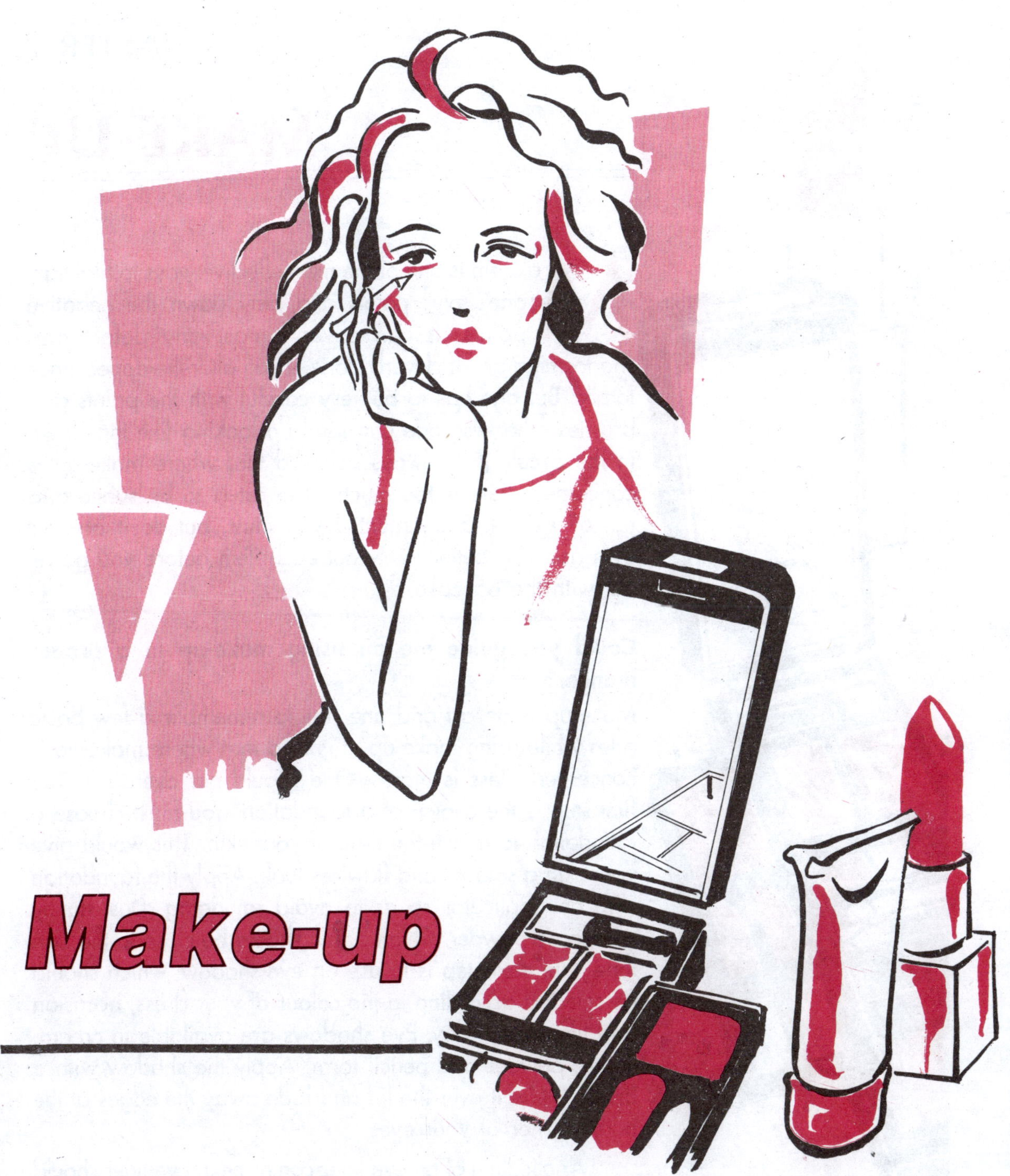

Make-up

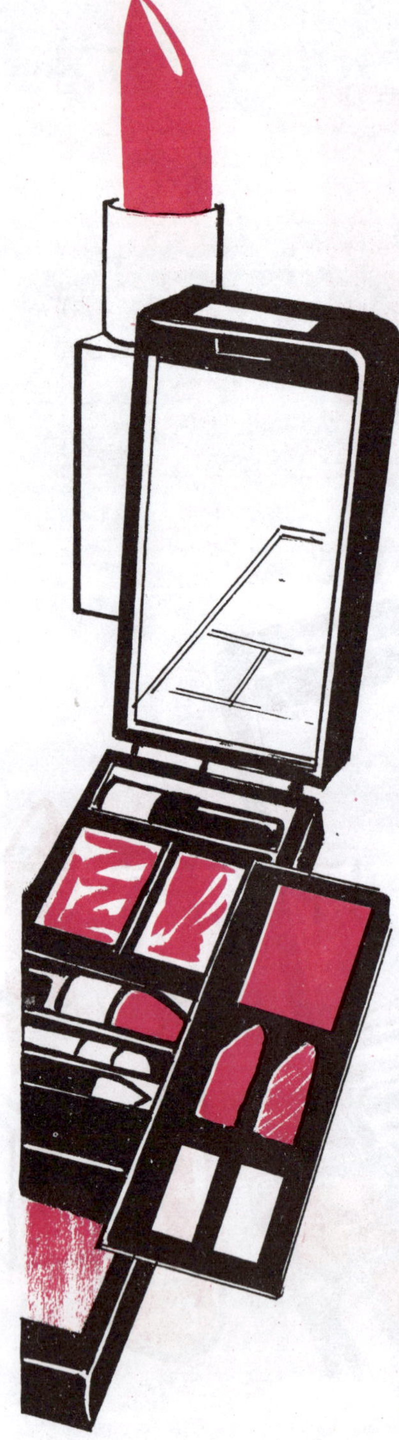

CHAPTER V

MAKE-UP

Make-up is one of the most effective ways to highlight one's plus points and play down the negative points. It can cover almost any defect and shortcoming and if cleverly done, it can alter the appearance totally. But one has to be very careful with the paints and brushes otherwise one can land up looking like the clown in the circus. It is always believed that where make-up is concerned, 'less is too much'. The art is to be subtle and not over-do it. Experiment if you must, but do it at your own risk. It is better to try out each item before you go all out with the pancake.

Could you guide me on using make-up in a proper manner?

Make-up is an art and one has to remember a few basic rules while using make-up. It is said that where make-up is concerned, 'less is more'. One should not overdo it. The first step is the choice of a foundation. You must choose a foundation to match the tone of your skin. This would give your skin a smooth and flawless look. Apply the foundation with an applicator so as to avoid smudging. Dust lightly with loose powder, which again should be close to the skin tone. The next step is to use an eye-shadow, which should be selected according to the colour of your dress, occasion and time of the day. Eye shadows are available in cream, liquid, powder and pencil form. Apply the shadow with a brush. Blend it over the lid and fade away the edges at the outer corner of your eyes.

Application of an eye-liner comes next. Eye-liner should be applied close to the eyelid and not exaggerated too much. Follow the natural lines of the eye contour and emphasise them very subtly. Mascara makes the lashes look thick and long. Apply the mascara with care so that it does not smudge.

For lips, use a lip brush to apply the lipstick. Draw an outline before you fill in the colour. These days there are lip pencils available to match the lipsticks. They give a neat finish to the lips.

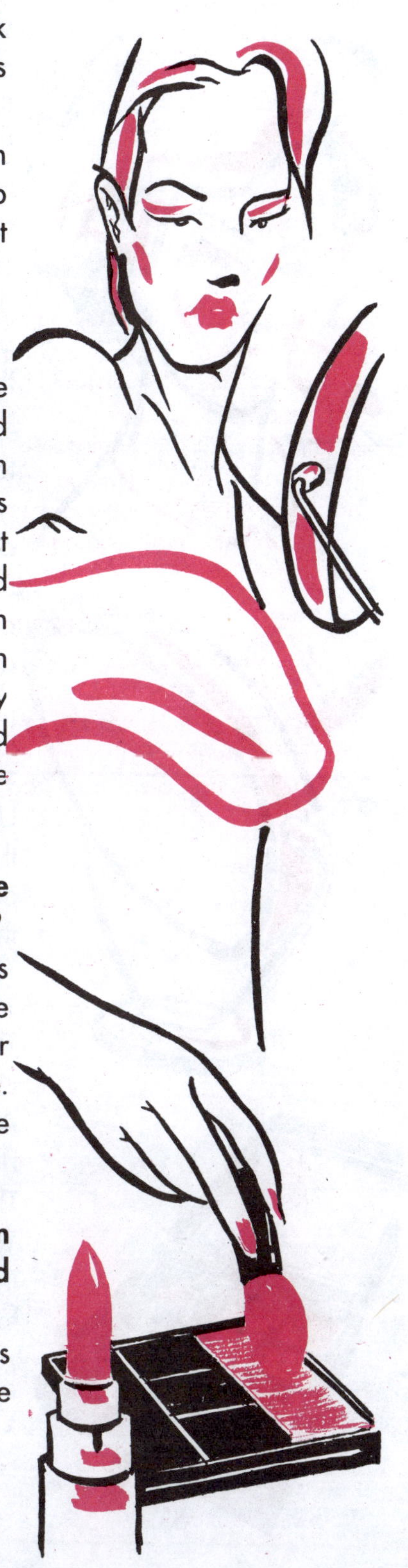

What are the ground rules of selecting a foundation?
Foundation gives a smooth texture to the skin and gives the effect of an evenly toned complexion. A foundation should look natural and not mask-like. The colour of the foundation should be nearest to the skin colour. Sometimes two tints may be blended to lighten or shade an area. Never select your foundation by applying it on the back of the hand because the skin here is always of a different colour than that of your face. The best way to test it is to apply it on the side of your cheek, just above the jawbone. To apply the foundation, dot it over the face and neck and blend with the help of your fingertips. Make use of a damp sponge for blending and ensure that there are no patches.

Can I camouflage facial defects with a foundation? I have a very broad nose. How can I make it look narrower?
You can camouflage the shortcomings on your facial features by using the foundation cleverly. A nose that is too wide can be made to look narrower by using a light colour foundation down the centre of the nose in a straight line. The darker colour foundation is applied on the sides of the nose. Take care to blend it well.

I have heard that clever application of foundation can cover many flaws. I have a heart shaped face. How should I use the foundation to make my face appear perfect?
You should emphasise your chin. If the shape of the face is rather triangular, apply a darker shade to the top of the forehead.

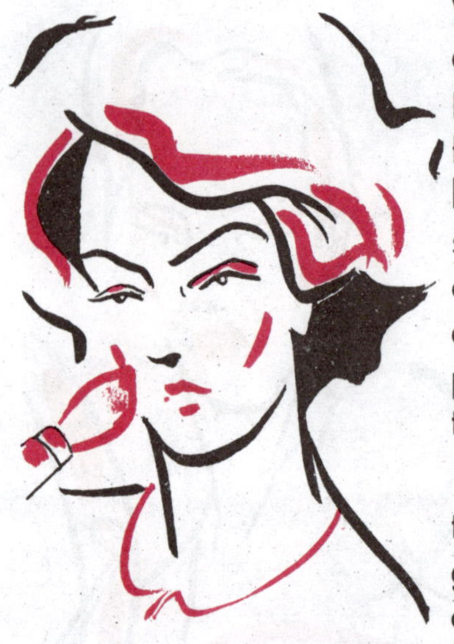

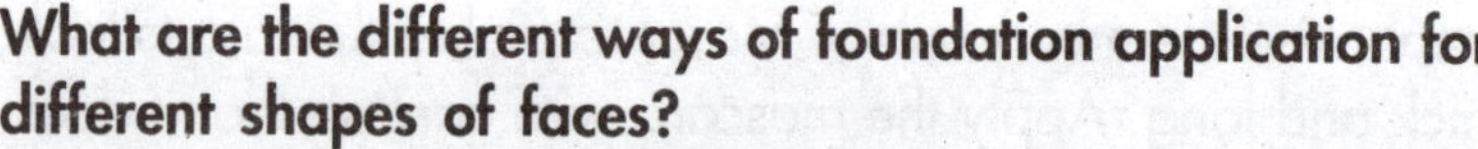

What are the different ways of foundation application for different shapes of faces?

Foundation can be applied in different ways to cover various flaws. If you have an oval face, you do not need any tricks because it is the perfect shape. If the face is round, the stronger shade of foundation should be spread on the cheeks, towards the outer edge, from under the cheekbones down towards the point of the chin. Those who have a pear-shaped face, the darker shade should be spread on the jaw-line and the point of the chin.

An oval, rather elongated face requires the forehead to be darkened. Apply a darker shade on the forehead, graduating the shade towards the eyebrows and the point of the chin. This advice is not to be taken as rigid; try and find out what suits you best and make the necessary correction. Always remember that light shades attract attention while dark shades deflect them.

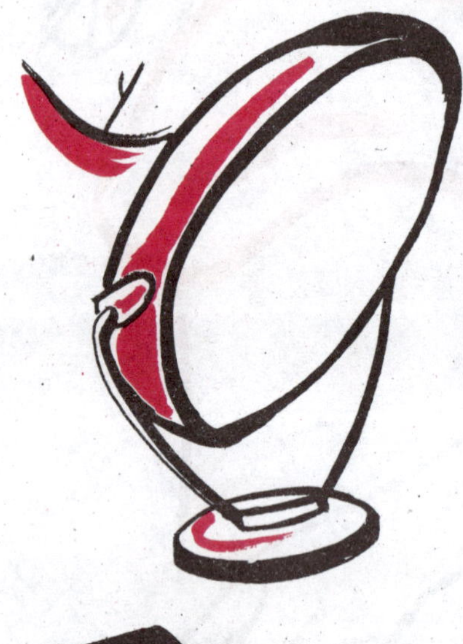

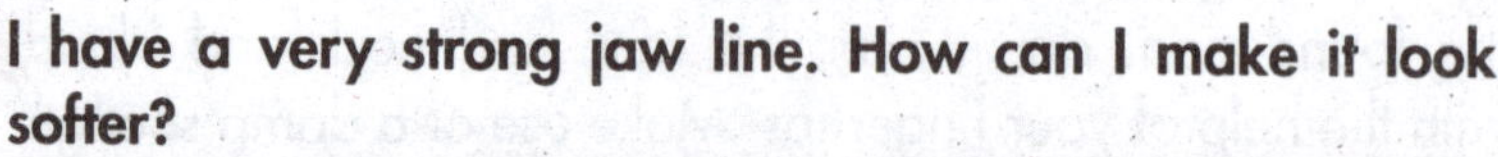

I have a very strong jaw line. How can I make it look softer?

Use a foundation to do the trick. Apply a darker shade of the foundation on your jawbone keeping it just short of the edge. Use a lighter colour on the rest of the face and blend the two tones carefully so that there are no harsh delineation. This will give a softer look to the jawline.

The tips about camouflaging the shape of the face by clever use of the foundation were indeed very interesting. Are there any other tricks one can use to cover up facial flaws?

There are many such tricks that can be used for deception. You can cover up almost all defects if you use the foundation in the right manner. Here are some tips for the right use of foundation.

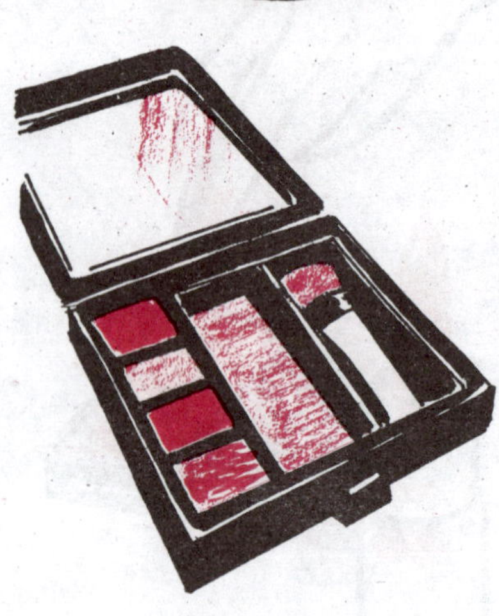

- To make a nose look longer, darken the sides with a vertical line.
- To shorten a nose, use a darker touch on the tips.

- To hide a double chin, darker foundation should be used on the neck, starting from the lobes of the ears and along the jaw-line.
- To conceal bags under the eyes, a light shade should be used on the lower eyelid, or a dab of oil can also be used.
- To widen the distance between the eyebrows, use a light shade between the eyes. This requires great skill of hand and you must be careful that the darker shades blend well with the lighter ones without leaving any line of demarcation. Practise on the face before you step out with the makeover.

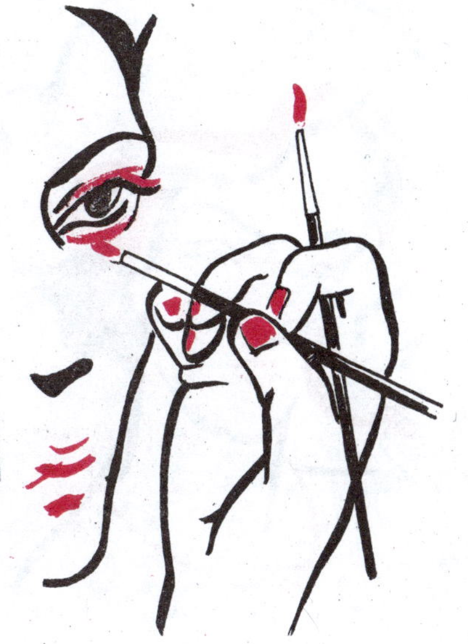

What is the correct method of applying face powder?
You can make your own powder applicators with absorbent cotton and throw them away after use. Ready made powder puffs are not recommended whether smooth or fluffy; with the first one you have to rub the skin hard and the second one is inefficient. Apply the powder generously to the puff and powder the face. Stroke the powder on with light touches, it must cling to the foundation. With another piece of cotton dust off any excess of powder. You may use a soft brush if you prefer. If you have wrinkles, puff out your cheeks when you powder your face.

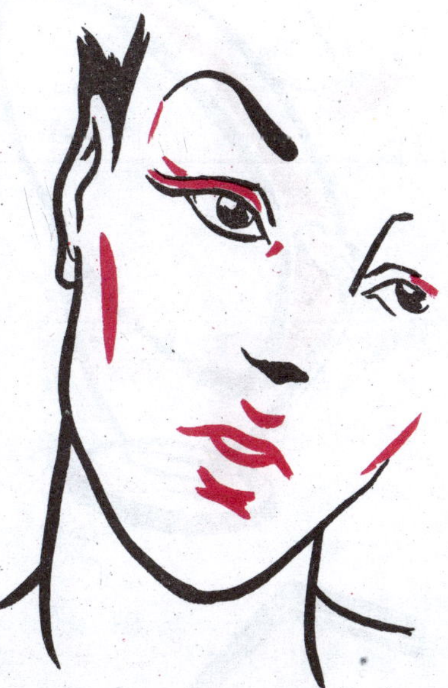

How can face powder be used for a long-lasting effect and also be applied to hold other items of make-up?
Apply a cold damp face cloth to the skin; the make-up will be holed better and give you a velvety natural softness. Take a piece of absorbent cotton, moisten it with toilet water and rub the hairline gently. To hold the mascara better, powder your eyelashes before you apply it. If you powder your lips, the lipstick goes on better.

What is the function of face powder and how should it be applied?
Powder is used to 'set' the foundation. It should be compatible with the shade of your foundation. You can also use a translucent or colourless powder for a matt finish. It

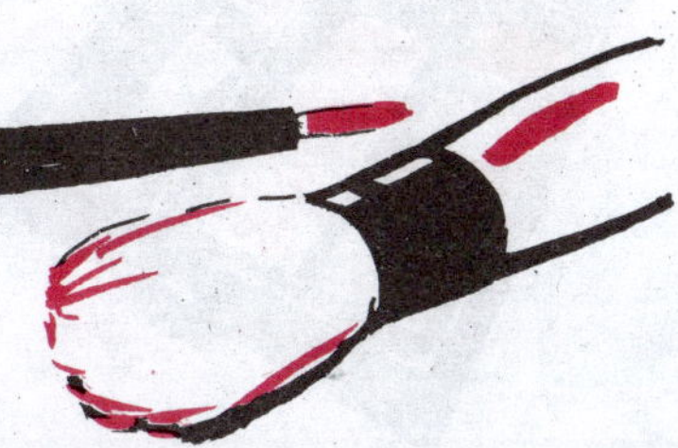

should be applied lightly with a soft puff. Brush off excess with the help of some cotton wool. You could rub a small ice cube over the face to keep the evenness.

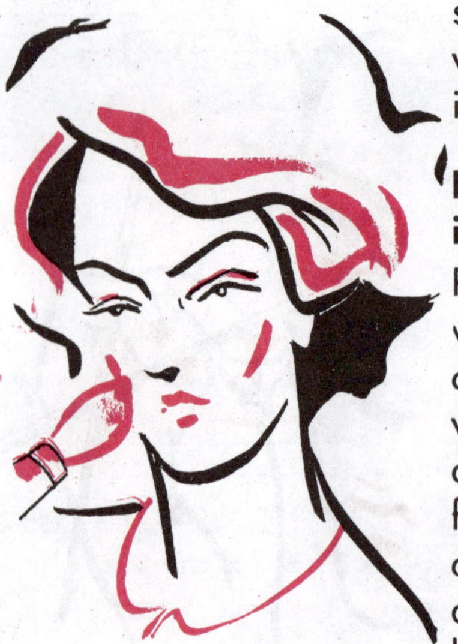

Is the old fashioned rouge still in use? How does one use it for optimum effect?

Rouge has gone out of fashion and now blushers are in vogue. But a little rouge on the cheeks can help to correct certain defects. So, in fashion or not, use it if you think it will improve the outline of your face. First of all, do not apply dry rouge over powder; this is really out of date and far too obvious. Use a good brush for application and with a few light touches, spread the rouge over the foundation and blend in thoroughly. At all costs, avoid rouge with a blue tone.

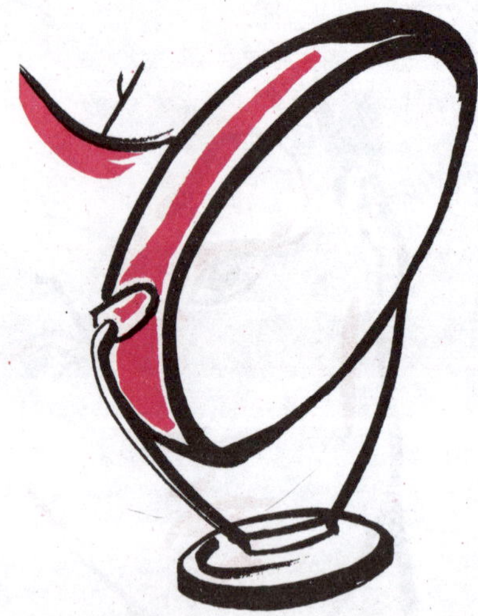

- If your face is oval, you do not need to use rouge to cover the cheeks but if it is an elongated oval, apply a horizontal touch on the cheekbones to break the line.
- If the face is round, a curved line under the eyes, spread vertically down the cheek, would give a very good effect.
- If the face is pear shaped, apply a triangle of rouge between the outer lower edge of the eye and the jaw.
- For a square face, the rouge should be used to make a curved line under the eyes, blended out towards the temples. Whereas for a rectangular face, spread the rouge farther away from the nose, lightly outwards towards the temples.
- For a triangular face you could apply just a touch of blusher over the cheekbones.
- These tricks can be done with a blush-on also.

How should one use blushers?

Blushers give a radiant look to the face. They come in two forms: the cream and powder form. A powder blusher should be applied after the application of the powder and a cream blusher should be applied before the application of the face powder. The blusher must be applied below the cheekbones and never lower than the nose or higher than the eyebrows. It should not be taken inwards further than the iris of the eyes. The cheekbones can be highlighted with a larger colour when they are flat. A blusher can also be applied to perfect the flaws in the shape of the face. For a square face, place the blusher high on the cheekbones and blend it smoothly and softly inwards. To make a round face appear longer, blend the blusher from the cheekbones downwards. Remember to use a blusher sparingly. It should just give the impression of being there and not be strong enough to attract attention to it.

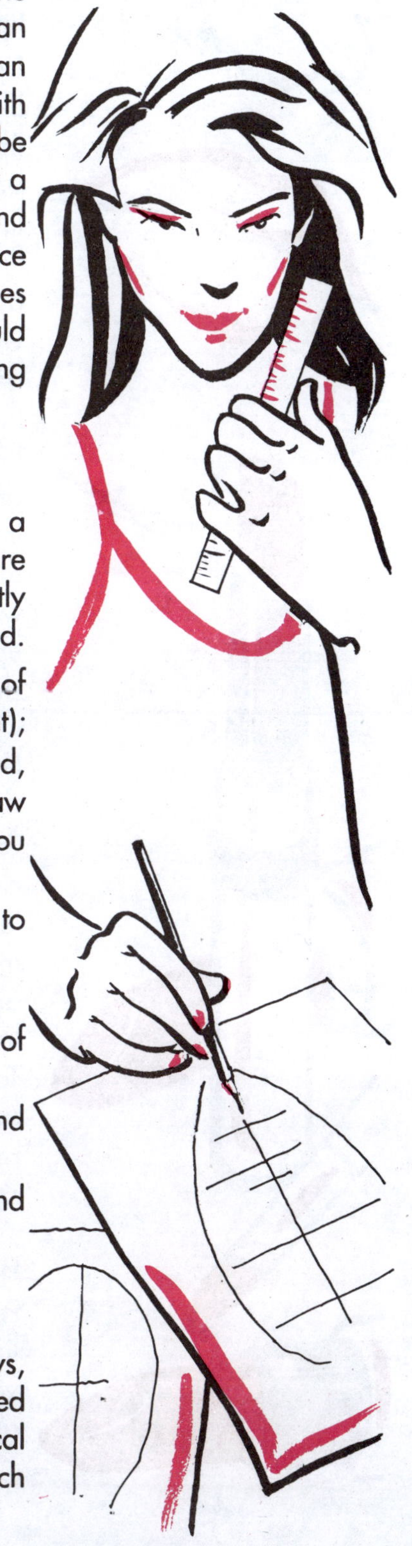

How can I find out the shape of my face?

Take a sheet of paper, the same size as your face and a flat ruler. Brush your hair well back and begin to measure your face, taking great care to keep the ruler perfectly horizontal or vertical, as if your face were traced on a pad.

- Take the total length from the hairline to the point of your chin (draw a line to indicate this measurement);
- Take the total width (at the height of the forehead, the eyes, the cheekbones and the mouth). Now draw the general outline of the face as accurately as you can;
- Take the height of the forehead from the hairline to the eyebrow line (draw a horizontal line there);
- Take the height of the eyes (draw a line there);
- Take the distance from the eyebrows to the base of the nose (a line);
- Take the distance between the base of the nose and the edge of the upper lip;
- Take the distance between the base of the nose and the lower lip;
- Take the width of the mouth;
- Take the length of the chin.
- Draw diagrammatically the curve of the eyebrows, the nose, the mouth, etc. and you have represented your face on the paper. Compare it with the classical oval shaped face and you will see the type to which you belong.

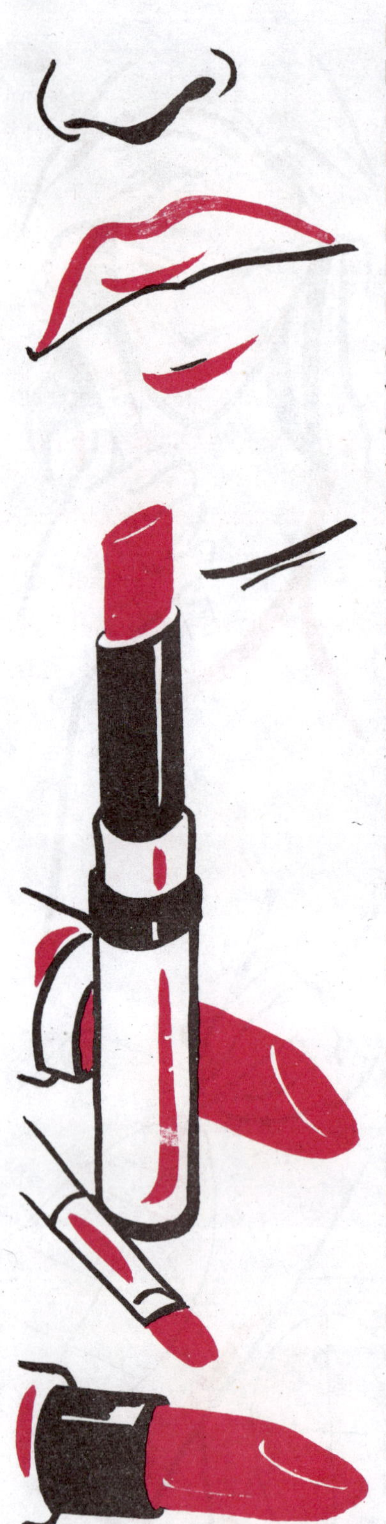

How can one use the lipstick to give an emphasis to the lips and to hide the flaws of the lips?

Lipstick should enhance the beauty of the lips and not appear like a red gash at the opening of the mouth. Always apply lipstick with a lipstick brush. Draw the outer line with the brush or with a lip pencil and then fill in the colour with a lipstick. A darker colour should be used to define the lip-line and a lighter shade should be used to fill in. After application, place a tissue between the lips and press. This will remove the excess colour. If you want a glossy look, use a lip-gloss. But take care not to take the gloss right outside the outer line of the lips. You can use lipstick to camouflage the shortcoming of your mouth. If your lips are small, then draw a line outside the natural line and if your lips are too thick, the line should be drawn inside. A dark colour will make the lips appear smaller while a bright or light colour will do the opposite. If the lower lip is thicker than the upper one, apply a darker colour on the lower one and its shade on the upper lip.

How can I give a neat finish to my lipstick and create the right shape for my lips?

To give a neat finish to your lipstick, clean your lips with cleansing milk. Spread the foundation over your lips and let it dry. With your brush coated with lipstick, open your mouth and without stretching your lips to the maximum, outline the upper lip. Press the lips together; then use the lipstick to outline the lower lip and fill in with the lipstick. Take a tissue and press your lips over it. Powder lightly and start the outlining again; with the darker lipstick on your brush, correct the natural defects of your mouth; the two shades must melt into each other.

How can I correct the outline of my mouth?

Perfect make-up is a studied elegance produced by corrective lines made with a very light hand. Beware of excess just as you should beware of passing fashions. Here are some guidelines for correcting the outline of the mouth:

- For an oval face: follow the natural curve of the upper lip, making the line slightly shorter on the lower lip;
- For a round face: draw both lips generously, right up to the corner.
- For pear-shaped face: the lips should be painted along their whole length, without drawing sweeping or heavy curves.
- For a square shaped face: don't make a heart shaped mouth, but do emphasise the cleft of the upper lip.
- For a rectangular face: design a generous mouth with attractive curves
- For a triangular face: design a full mouth, lengthened at the corners.

How can one design the lips according to the shape of the mouth?

Just as the lips can be designed according to the shape of the face, they can be made-up according to the shape of the mouth. A clever make-up will definitely help in altering the appearance of the mouth and the face.

If you have a drooping mouth: powder the corners and emphasise the dip at the centre. Put a touch of a darker lipstick at the corners of the upper lip. Finish off with the slightest trace of vaseline or gloss at the centre of the mouth.

If you have pouting lips: paint out the dip. Accentuate the depth of the upper lip. A slightly darker shade for the lower lip, drawn a little within the natural contour of the lip.

If your mouth is too small: use a darker shade on the upper lip, draw in the cleft but don't accentuate it. The lower lip should be given a squarer shape, with a touch of gloss or vaseline near the corners.

If your lips are too thin: outline the mouth well and fully, going a fraction beyond the limits of the lips. Use the darker shade on the lower lip. Draw the corners upwards, outline the cleft distinctly and smile all day!

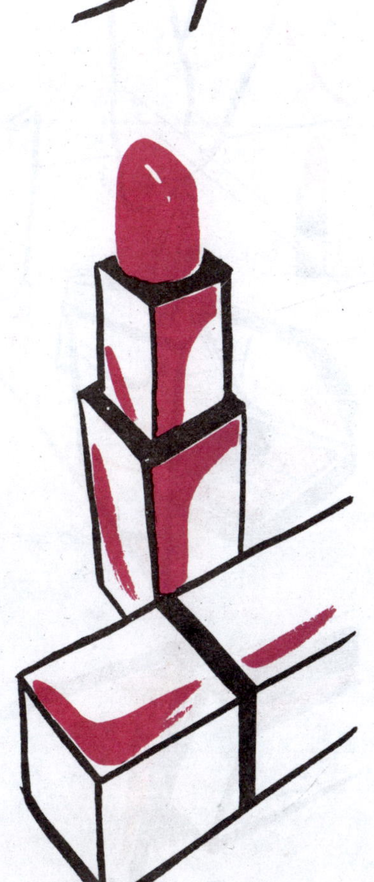

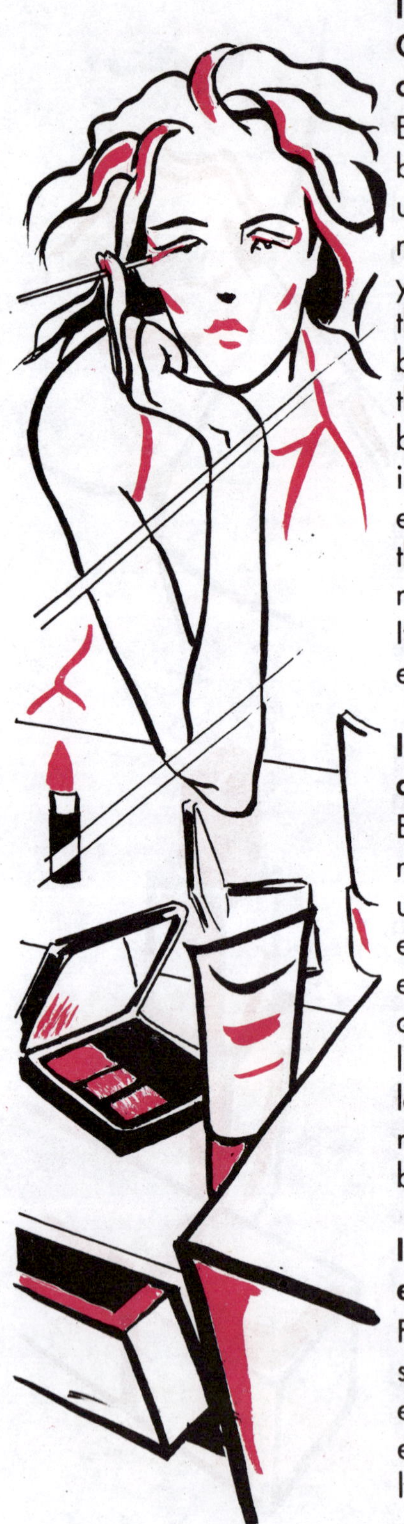

I love applying eyeliner but I am not very good at it. Could you give some tips on how to apply eyeliner correctly?

Eyes are the most prominent features of the face and beautiful eyes can attract everyone's attention. Eye make-up needs a lot of care and expertise. Badly applied eye make-up can ruin the entire look. One ground rule is that you should never over-do any sort of make-up and so with the eyes. For correct application of the eyeliner, dip the brush into the bottle and drain off the excess. Sit down at the dressing table, lean on your right elbow, holding the brush lightly between your fingers. Have a magnifying mirror in front of you to give you a better view. Half close your eye and start from the middle of the eye to outer corner of the eye. Then, start from the inner corner of the eye to the middle. Spread it evenly so that there are no rough strokes. If you like, you can thicken the line at the outer edge of the eyes. Do this if you have small eyes.

I would love to apply proper eye make-up but I am not able to do a neat job. How should I apply eye-makeup?

Eyes are the most expressive features of our face and one must attempt to enhance their beauty by proper eye make-up. To get an effective result, begin by an application of eye shadow. Apply the lighter colour to highlight the entire eyelid and the area below the eyebrow. Then use the darker colour to put an accent. This can be done by drawing a line starting from the middle of the eyelid, just above the lashes, moving outwards till the corner of the eye, and then reverse it in a V-shape defining the eye contour. This should be followed by the application of an eyeliner and mascara.

I have bushy eyebrows. What is the perfect shape of eyebrows and how can I achieve it?

For a perfect eyebrow, use a pencil. Your eyebrow should start where the pencil makes an alignment with the outer edge of your lip and the inner corner of your eye. It should end at the alignment formed along the outer edge of your lip and the outer corner of your eye. Always pluck stray hair from underneath the brow, never from the above because doing so will ruin the shape of the brows.

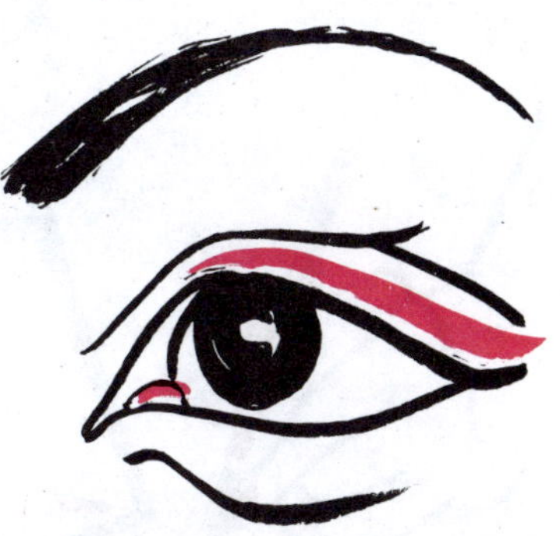

How can I get the best shape of eyebrows? What are the basic rules one must follow while shaping the eyebrows?

Eyebrows can give expression to the face and highlight the eyes, too. A downward line suggests sorrow and makes you look old. The following rules will help you create a neat eyebrow line:

- The eyebrow should never weigh heavily on the eye, but should arch over it in a gentle curve.
- Don't pluck your eyebrows completely or pluck them too often, for you may destroy the roots.
- The most natural line is the one parallel to the line of your upper eyelid.

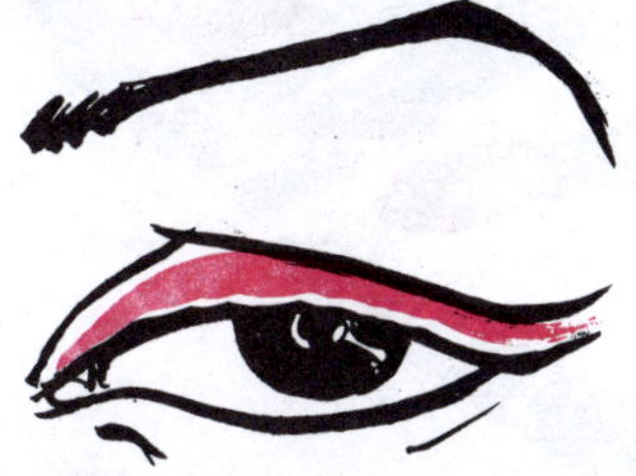

- The end of the line should taper off towards the temple, so look carefully at your profile.
- Each eyebrow should begin exactly over the tear duct.
- To touch up, sharpen your pencil carefully and try to draw tiny hairs rather than one continuous line; it will look more natural.
- If your nose is too long, do not draw your eyebrows too high.

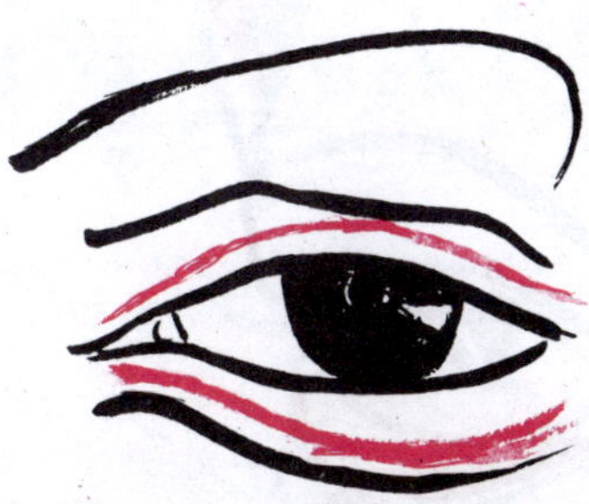

- High and finely drawn eyebrows make the eyes look smaller.
- With a small brush and a drop of oil, brush your eyebrows upwards everyday.

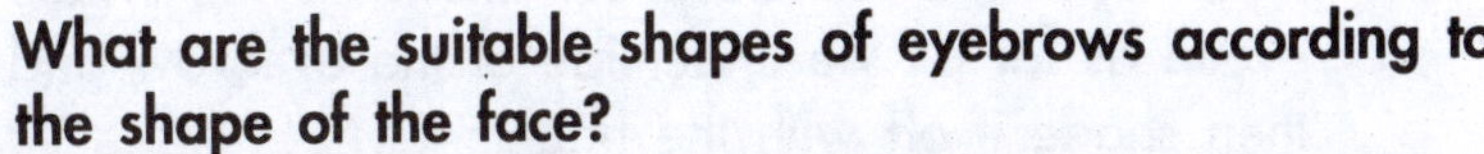

What are the suitable shapes of eyebrows according to the shape of the face?

For a round face – long and slightly arched eyebrows;

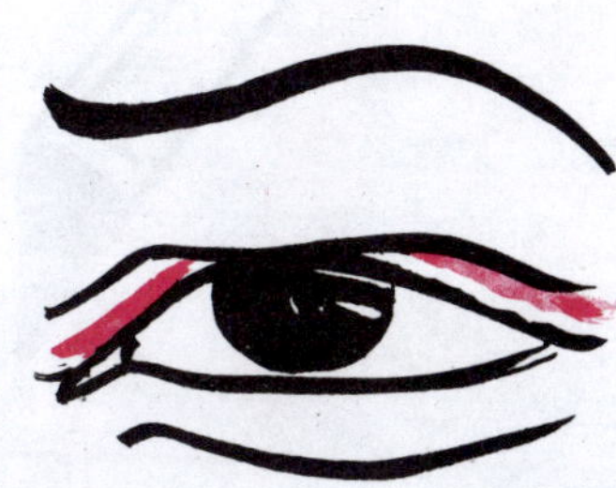

- For a square face – not a straight line but a gently arched curve;
- For a rectangular face – the same as the square face, except that it should start as a straight line and the curve should begin at the centre of the eye;

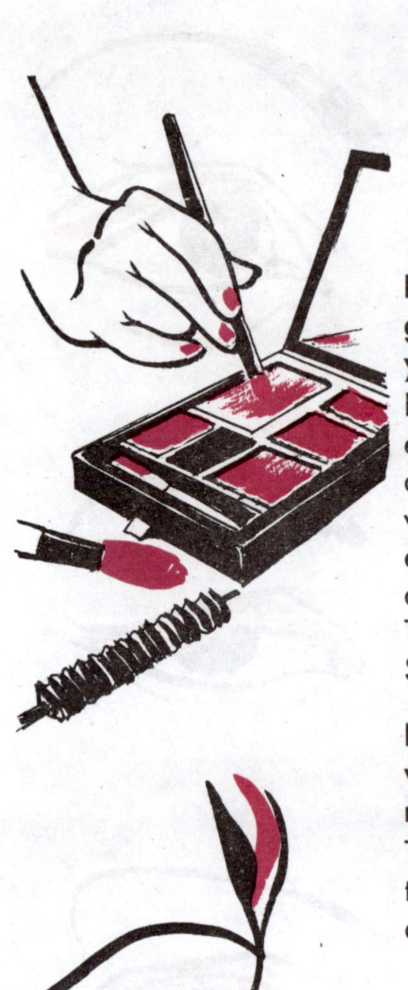

- For an oval face – a line following the shape of the upper lid; draw it out a little towards the temple;
- For a pear-shaped face – widen the forehead with rather straight eyebrows, not too long;
- For triangular face- straight eyebrows, curve the ends slightly downwards.

I am very fond of using eye shadows but I need some guidelines towards the proper use of eye shadow. Could you please explain some basics?

Eye shadows are used to enhance the mystical effect of eyes. If used properly, they can give a very attractive effect and depth to the eyes. Some of the basics to remember while using eye-shadows are – they should enhance your eyes and not dominate them. The colour of your eyes should always be more prominent that the colour of the shadow. To choose the right colour, observe the colour of your iris. Select a colour, which will complement your complexion.

Like the eyebrows, should the use of eye shadow also vary with the facial features? If so, what are the ground rules?

The application of eye shadow does make a difference to the appearance of a person. It can enhance the eyes and also correct some flaws, if used cleverly.

- If your eyes are too close together: apply the shadow from the middle of the eyelid towards the outside;
- If they are too far apart: apply the shadow all over the eyelid, but very lightly; darken the shade a little towards the bridge of the nose;
- If the eyes are too deep set: make-up the whole eyelid as far as the underside of the eyebrow and then shade it off with the finger;
- If you have dark-circles under your eyes: avoid eye-shadow, but spread a light foundation or a special preparation for dark-ringed eyes under the lower eyelid;
- If your eyes are surrounded with fine wrinkles: shade off the shadow towards the outside of the eyelid; it is advisable not to use eyeliner.

How can I apply the mascara for a dramatic effect?

To apply mascara effectively, coat the upper and lower surfaces of the lashes. Tilt your head down and look down into the mirror. Draw the wand across the top surface of your upper lashes. Then tilt your head up, look up into the mirror and coat your lashes from the root to the tip. Then, looking straight into the mirror apply the mascara lightly to the bottom lashes, first with one horizontal stroke from the inner to the outer corner of the eye and then with short vertical strokes from root to tip. Switch off the fans while applying mascara, as the air will dry it up. Wait for each coat to dry before applying the next.

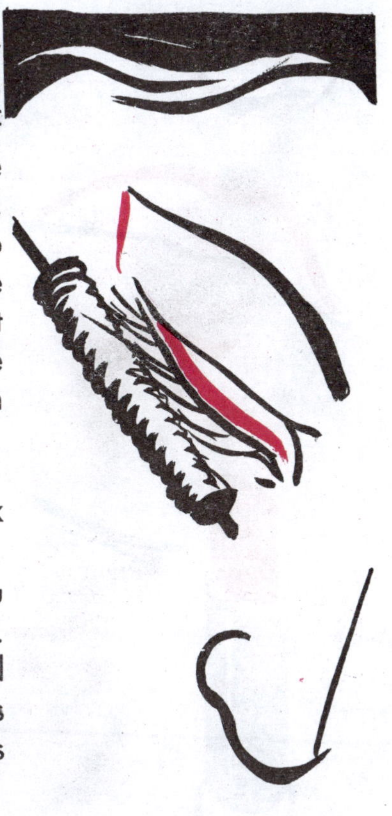

How should mascara be removed without getting black smudges around the eyes?

Remove mascara properly with an oil based remover. You could also use petroleum jelly for removing the mascara. Wipe gently on to the lashes; leave for a few seconds and then gripping the lashes gently between your fingers wrapped in tissue remove the mascara from root to tip. This will not pull out your lashes if done carefully.

I am a middle-aged woman. I like using a make-up but it gives me a very old look. What is the right type of make-up for my age?

For mature age women, it is necessary not to over-do the make-up. Overdoing will make them look older. Remember to choose a foundation that is lighter in texture because the heavy formulas accentuate wrinkles. Matt eyeshadows are more flattering than the frosted or pearly shades. Browns, greys and mauves look nice on aged women. When wearing a strong lip colour, apply the lipstick before the eyeshadow to get the balance right. Avoid using very bright shades of lipstick because that can give a very ageing effect.

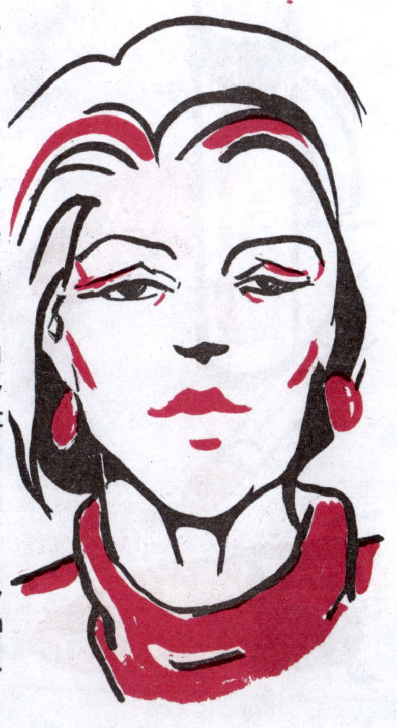

What is meant by base make-up?

Base make-up comprises of a set of products like foundation, compact and concealer. These are used to give a smooth and even tone to the skin and cover the minor imperfections.

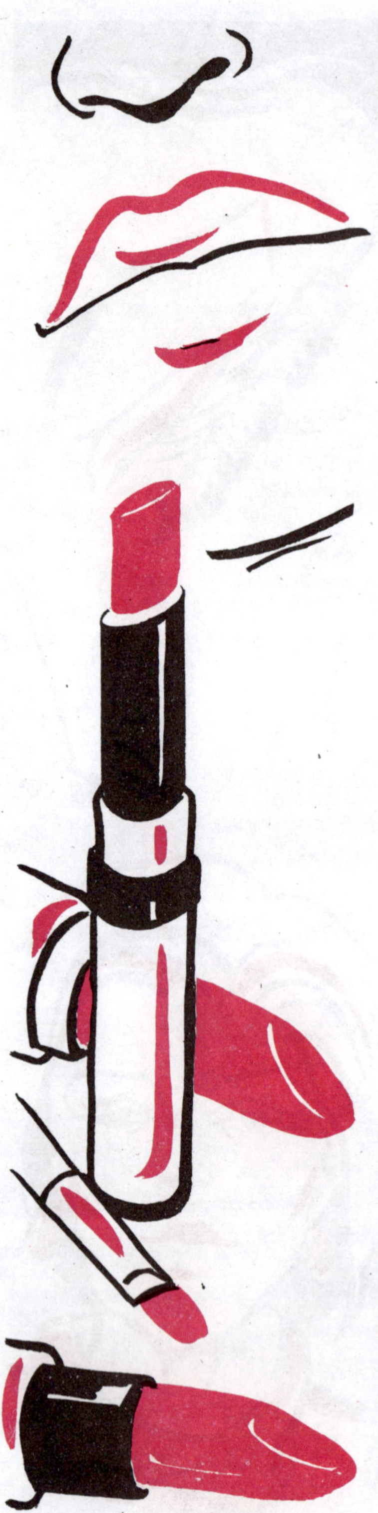

Can you give a step by step guidance for getting made up in a hurry?

Here is a step by step guide for coping with the lack of time.

- Put a tonic lotion or cold water on your face, wet a face cloth and pat your face briskly with it. Then dry it without rubbing.
- Then spray your face with rose water and let it dry naturally.
- Apply your base cream (slightly warmed in the hollow of your hand), or use a moisturising lotion if the skin is sensitive.
- Spread over your face a liquid foundation, which does not contain powder, or if your complexion is good, do not use foundation in the morning, just powder your face.
- Powder the eyelashes and lips
- Apply mascara to the outer edges of your eyelashes and with a very fine line, draw the eye-liner along the roots of the lashes
- Brush your eyebrows with castor-oil
- Draw the outline of your mouth with a lip brush, press your lips on absorbent paper and fill in with lipstick.
- With a damp face cloth, dab cold water on your powdered face, this will give a natural brightness to your complexion.
- Comb your hair neatly, and you are ready for the show.

I am a working woman and I don't have much time to do a proper make-up. After the entire day's work I generally look tired and dull. Sometimes I have to go out for a function and I do not know how to look beautiful. How can I achieve a perfectly made up look within a limited time?

Here is a way by which you can look ravishing within an hour's time.

To begin with, go in for a relaxing shower. To look beautiful, it is necessary to get rid of the tiredness and tension of the entire day. Let the water run down your spine. Spray cold water on one foot and then the other. Then up the legs to the stomach, arms and chest. You are now as fresh as a rose.

Rub your body with a hard bath glove moistened with water.

Remove all make-up and apply a skin toner.

Dab some cold water on your face and quickly brush your nails.

Start with the mask: You can buy ready-made masks specially designed to revive a tired face. Apply the mask and lie down for some 15 minutes with your feet at an elevated height. Place two pieces of cotton moistened with rose water on your eyes. Let your arms fall to your sides. Relax completely.

Remove the face mask after 15 minutes with warm water, splash your face with cold water and begin your make up as given above.

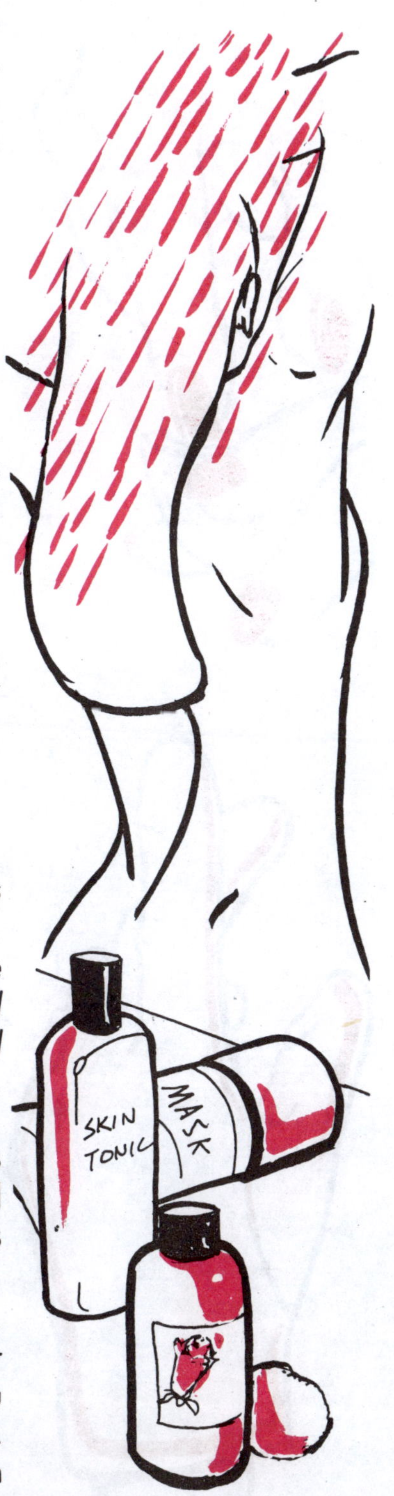

MANICURE AND PEDICURE

A beautiful face without good-looking hands or feet, reminds one of the peacock which is so beautiful but has ugly feet. Without the soft hands to flash your diamond rings and the smooth feet to display the expensive sandals, you would feel rather self-conscious. It is quite easy to achieve soft and smooth hands and feet, if one were to make a little effort.

My hands and feet perspire a lot during the summer. As a result, I feel uncomfortable when I have to hold something in my hand. What could I do to get rid of this problem?

You could rub an ice cube on your palms three times a day. Place some cologne soaked tissue paper on the palms for a few minutes and then dust with a talcum powder. You could use cologne sticks, which are available in the market. Cologne has a very instant refreshing effect. Wear cotton

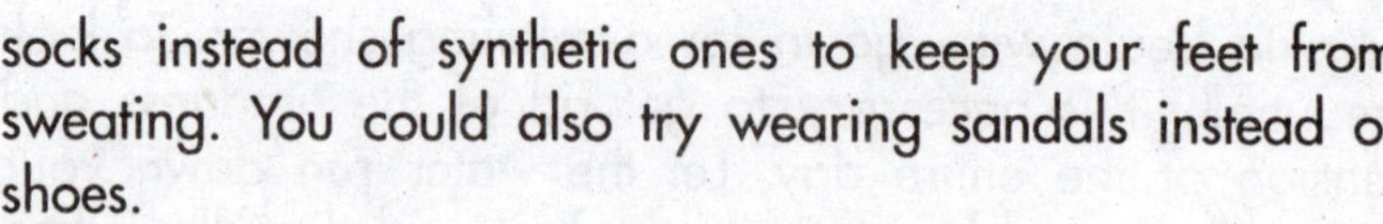

socks instead of synthetic ones to keep your feet from sweating. You could also try wearing sandals instead of shoes.

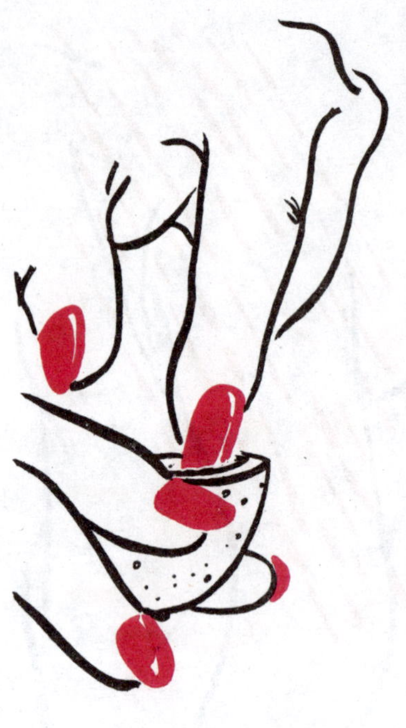

I want to have soft and silky hands. My hands are rough and callused. How can I have the desired softness in my hands?

For silky soft hands, rub in moisturising cream and wear cotton gloves overnight. The heat will ensure maximum absorption. You must also wear gloves while gardening and washing so that your hands are protected from the harmful effects.

My nails are very brittle. I want to grow them but they keep breaking. What can I do about this problem?

Your nails could become stronger if you take 1-tablespoon of unflavoured gelatine every day. You could also try taking 2-3 kelp tablets every day. Blue iris flowers steeped in water overnight and brushed regularly on the nails will help in strengthening them. Alternatively, make an infusion of elm leaves; soak the nails in this preparation everyday to prevent brittleness.

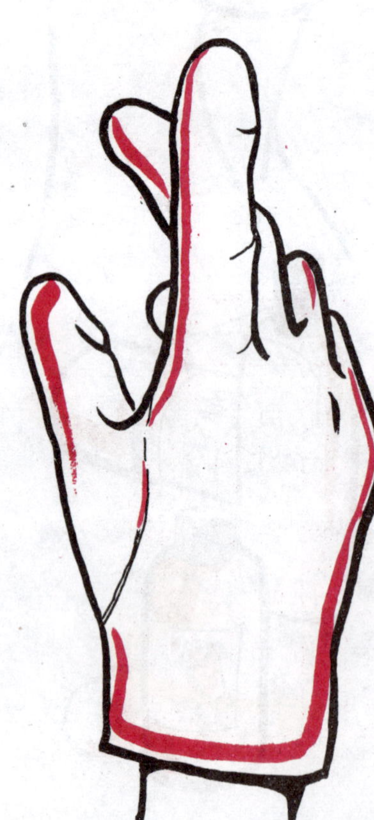

My nails are in a very bad condition. Can you give some tips on nail care?

For a complete nail care treatment; you should follow the regimen given below–

Take a lemon rind and rub the insides on your nails. This will discourage the dislodging of the skin around your nails. Then you would not be tempted to bite your nails to the quick.

Use nourishing or moisturising cream as often as possible on your hands. The detergents used in washing up dissolves all the natural fat secreted by the skin, as well as the keratin of the nails.

Massage your finger joints and make them flexible with frequent exercises.

When you do your washing, wear rubber gloves to protect your hands from the ill effects of successive cold and hot water.

When you prepare mashed potatoes, apply some on your hands when still warm. It is an excellent 'mask' for the skin.

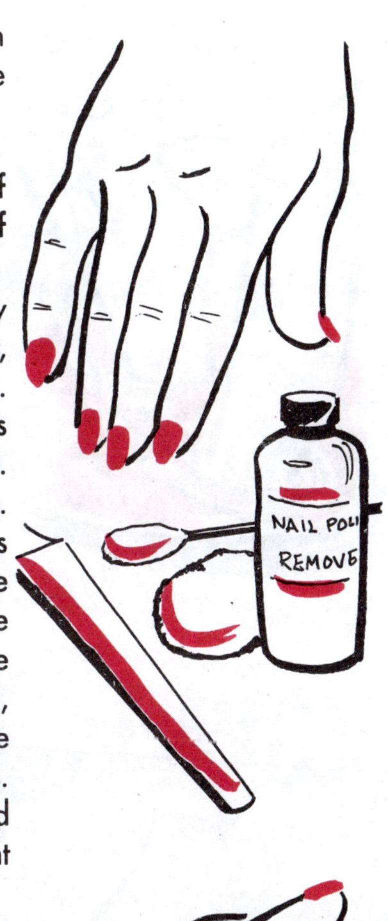

My hands look quite awful and I am very conscious of them. I never like to shake hands with anyone because of this reason. How can I make my hands look good?

The illusion of a well-groomed and beautiful woman may be shattered if her hands are uncared for. Rough, chapped, wrinkled and callused hands are a sign of bad health. Detergents, soap and water constantly dry the skin, so always wear rubber gloves while doing housework in the kitchen. Protect your hands from extreme change in the temperatures. If you work with hot water and then with cold water, it is bound to have an effect on your hands. When you have had your hands in water, dry them and smooth on some hand cream or lotion on them. Lemon juice is one of the best ingredients towards care of the hands. They soften, clean and bleach the skin. Hand massage and exercise both help the circulation and relieve tension and stiffness. Always massage towards the wrist using the thumb and index finger. Make small rotary movements on each joint with the little finger.

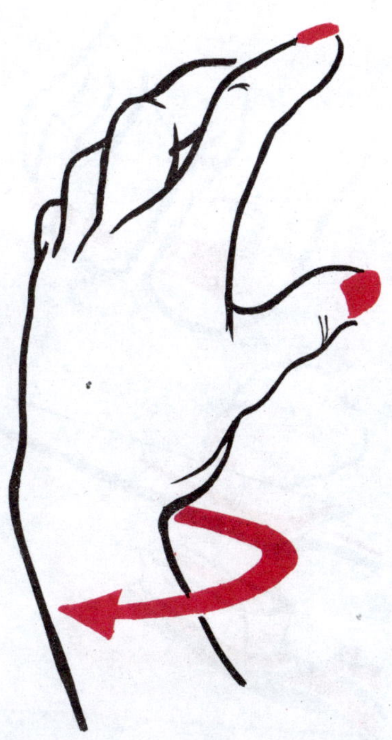

Is it essential to go to a beauty parlour for a manicure? Can I do it at home?

It is not at all necessary to go to a beauty parlour for a manicure. You could easily do a manicure at home. With a piece of cotton wool soaked in nail polish remover, wipe out the traces of your nailpolish. Shape the nails by filing them with a filer from sides to the centre. If the nails are brittle, file them short. Brush the nails clean and apply a little cuticle cream. Soak the fingertips in warm soapy water for a couple of minutes.

Dab the hands with a clean towel and using a good nourishing cream or olive oil, massage the hands with your thumb and index finger.

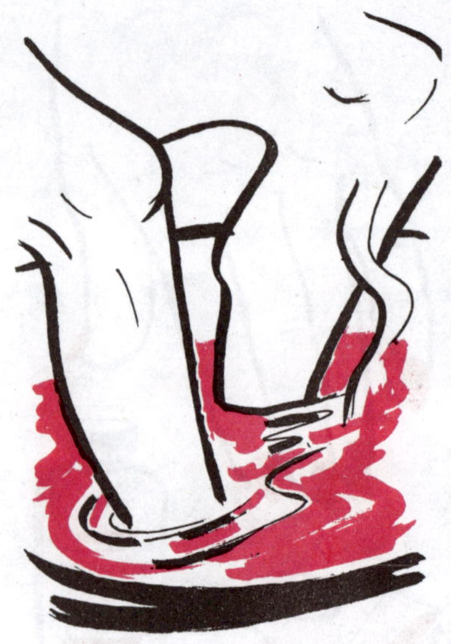

Twist a little cotton wool around the tip of a stick and with this, work a little cuticle remover around the nail, gently pushing the cuticle back, lifting it slightly but being careful not to damage the new nail which is under it.

Before varnishing and polishing the nails they must be cleaned of any remaining grease. To help the varnish to last, a coat of polish base must be applied. Let the base dry thoroughly before applying the next coat of your nail polish. Paint on the final coat using strokes in the upward direction.

What are the benefits of a hand exercises and how can I do them?

Exercise meant for the hand help in promoting better circulation. They also help in relieving tension and stiffness from the hands and fingers. You can try these exercises for a good effect. The hand exercises can be done at any time and at any place. In fact, whenever you feel tired, especially if you have to write for long hours, type or work on the computer, these exercises are extremely beneficial for you.

Stretch your fingers out as tautly as possible, relax and throw them out again. Repeat this several times.

Circle your hands from the wrist, making the circle as wide as possible. Repeat this exercise several times a day.

How can I take care of my feet? They look so bad that I am ashamed to take them out of my shoes when I have to go to a shoe shop to buy a new pair. What can I do to make them presentable?

Feet are a very important part of our body. They bear our weight and keep us upright. Neglecting the feet can not only give a bad personality but also cause a lot of strain and tiredness. Tired and aching feet can mar your efficiency. A good pedicure should help you improving the appearance of your feet. Also remember not to wear high heels, tight shoes and shoes with pointed toes as these cause a lot of harm and tiredness to the feet.

What is pedicure and how can I do a pedicure by myself?

A pedicure is a treatment meant to relax, beautify and improve the condition of the feet. It is a very simple treatment involving the cleansing, massage, nail care and heel care of the feet. Pedicure can be done easily at home. To do so, soak your feet in warm water to which a few drops of a disinfectant has been added. You can dissolve a tablespoon of shampoo in the water too. Scrub the toe nails with an old toothbrush. Treat the hard skin of the heel with a pumice stone to dislodge all dead skin. Wipe the feet dry, especially between the toes.

Next, massage the feet with a good cream or olive oil and apply cuticle cream around the nails. Wrap stick with a cotton wool and dip it in cuticle remover. Gently press the cuticles back. The cuticle should never be cut unless the edges are ragged.

Cut the toe nails straight across and smoothen the edges with a filer. Don't try to cut the nails too close on the sides. Next wipe the nails clean and dry them with a clean piece of cotton wool.

Your feet are now ready for the nail varnish. Put some cotton wool pads between the toes to avoid smudging the nail polish and then apply the desired shade carefully on your toe nails.

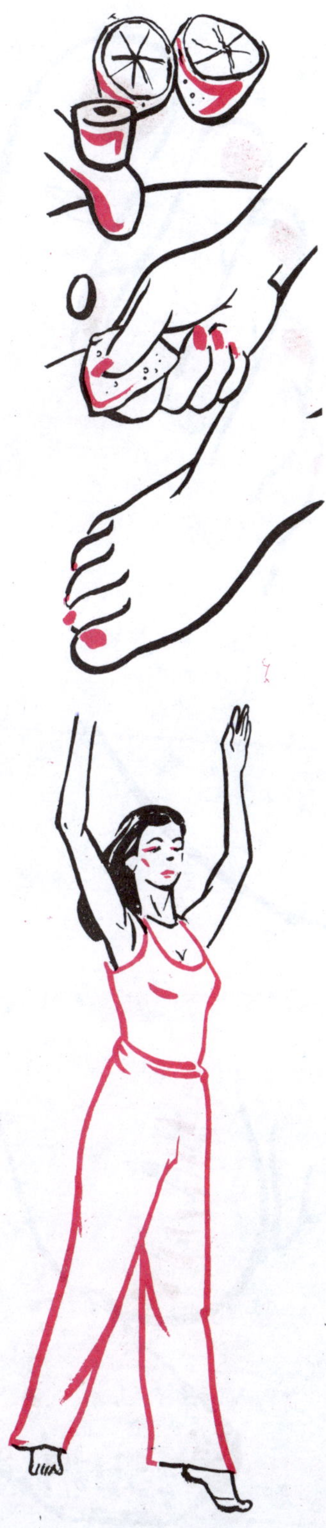

Are there any exercises for the feet to take away the tiredness and give them flexibility?

There are several types of exercises to give flexibility to the feet.

Spread some marbles on the floor and try to lift them up with your toes. This exercise will help in strengthening the muscles of your feet.

Sit with your legs crossed and rotate the feet six times towards each other and another six times, away from each other.

Put a pencil on the floor and try to pick it up with your toes.

Sit comfortably on a chair and spread out the toes as far as possible. This exercise tones up the muscles of the feet.

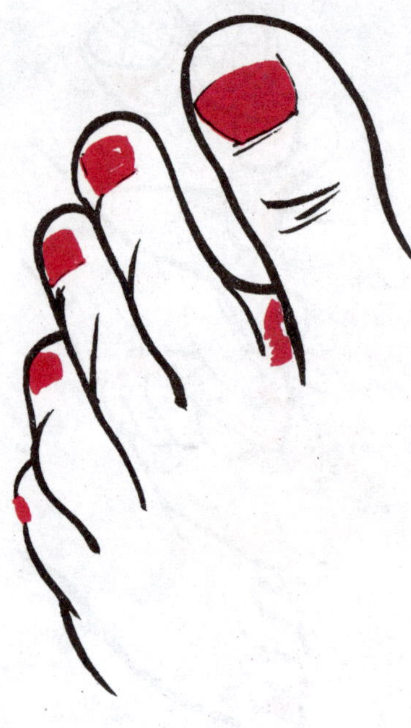

What are the common foot problems and how can one avoid/treat them?

The most common foot problems are corns, fungal attack and blisters. Applying a little white iodine can treat corns at home. Avoid wearing tight and uncomfortable shoes. Wearing the wrong kind of shoes or new shoes also causes blisters. You can apply a little vaseline to the inner part of the shoes before wearing them. If the problem of corns persist, it is better to take the advice of a chiropodist. Fungal problems generally occur because of the build up of fungus, between the toes. This problem is quite common during the monsoon and in humid conditions. Always dry the area between the toes and dust it with some talcum powder. This will prevent the fungus from building up.

I suffer from cracked heels. How can I take care of my feet and get rid of the cracks?

Cracked heels is a common occurrence because the foot is not completely covered. Cracked heels are caused due to excessive dryness of the skin. The heels are especially susceptible to cracks as they are subjected to constant friction and pressure. You can soak your feet in hot water with a few drops of oil or a moisturising lotion added to it. Pat dry and remove any dry flaky residue with a pumice stone. Rub in a moisturising cream or petroleum jelly, at night, and wear a pair of old socks while going to bed.

I have deep cracks on the soles of my feet. They are so painful, especially in winter that I cannot even walk. What can I do about this problem?

Cracks on the soles are due to prolonged neglect of the area. You need a regular pedicure to combat the problem. Pedicure can be done at home or by a chiropodist. Since yours is quite a grave problem, I suggest that you get the first treatment done by a qualified chiropodist. Once the feet are a little better, you could follow up with a regular pedicure done at home. For the pedicure: soak your feet in warm soapy water for 15 minutes. Lightly scrub the heels with a pumice stone and wash with plain water. Dry the feet on a towel and massage them well with a nourishing cream. Repeat the treatment twice a day. Lastly, apply anti-crack cream at night and wear a pair of cotton socks. Regular pedicure will control your problem.

I am a 40-year-old woman. My legs and hands are very rough. What should I do to make them soft and smooth?

As one grows older, the skin becomes rough and dry. The internal moisture and the oil of the skin starts depleting and you have to replace it externally. Rub your legs and hands with baby oil or olive oil after bath. Apply a nourishing cream containing vitamin E, thrice a day, especially at bedtime. A massage done daily with any vegetable oil will also improve the condition by stimulating the blood circulation.

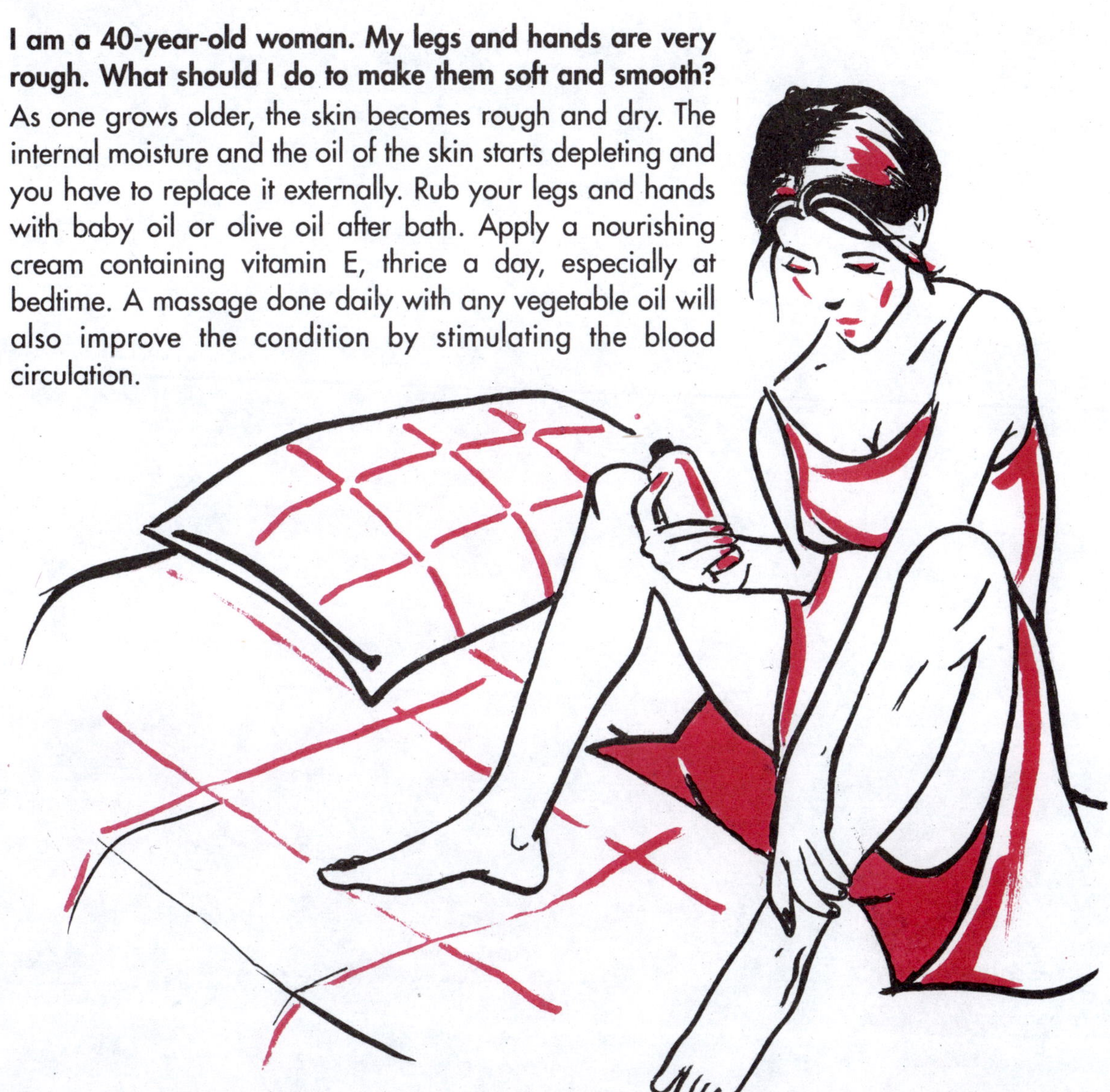

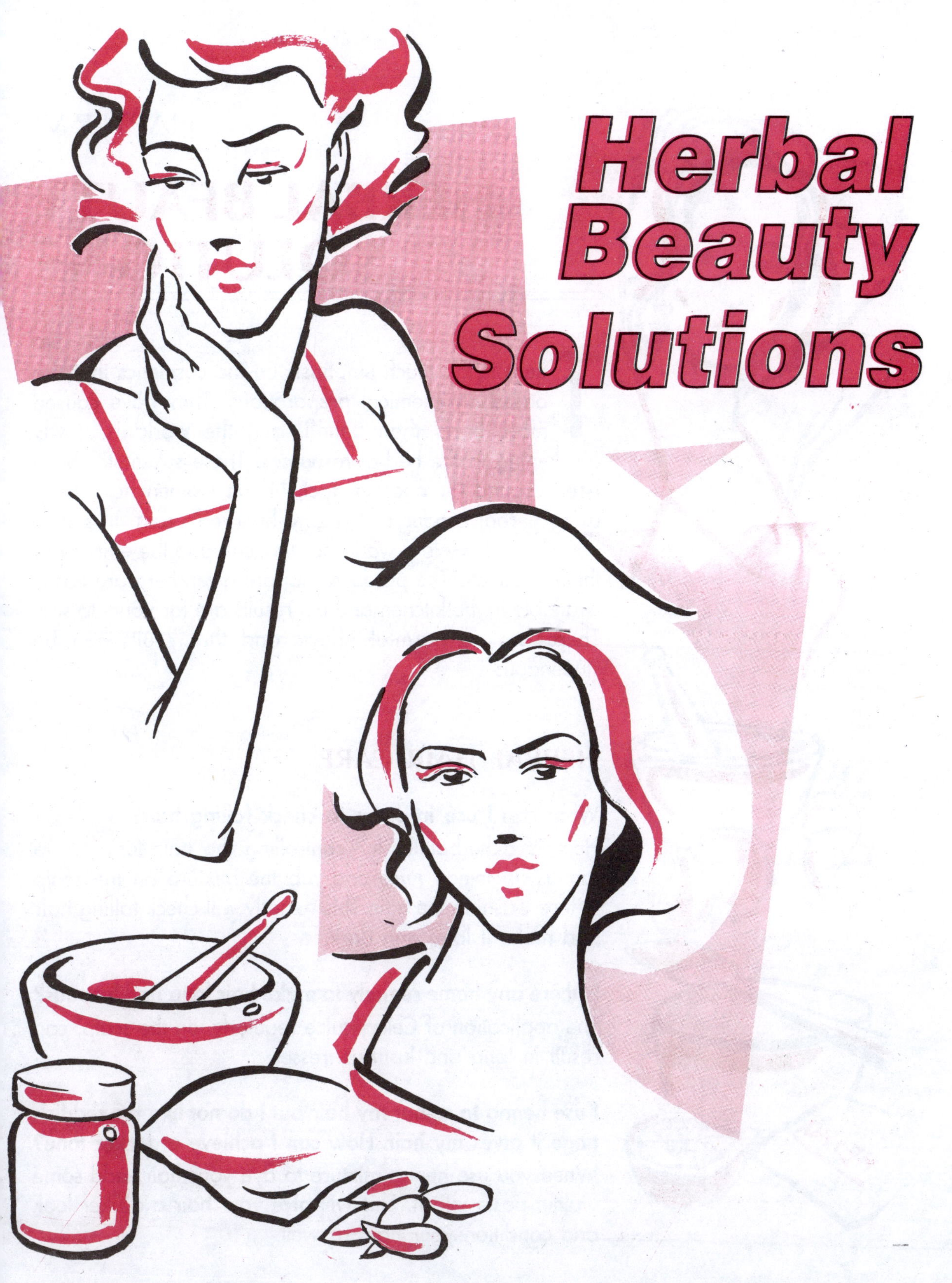

Herbal Beauty Solutions

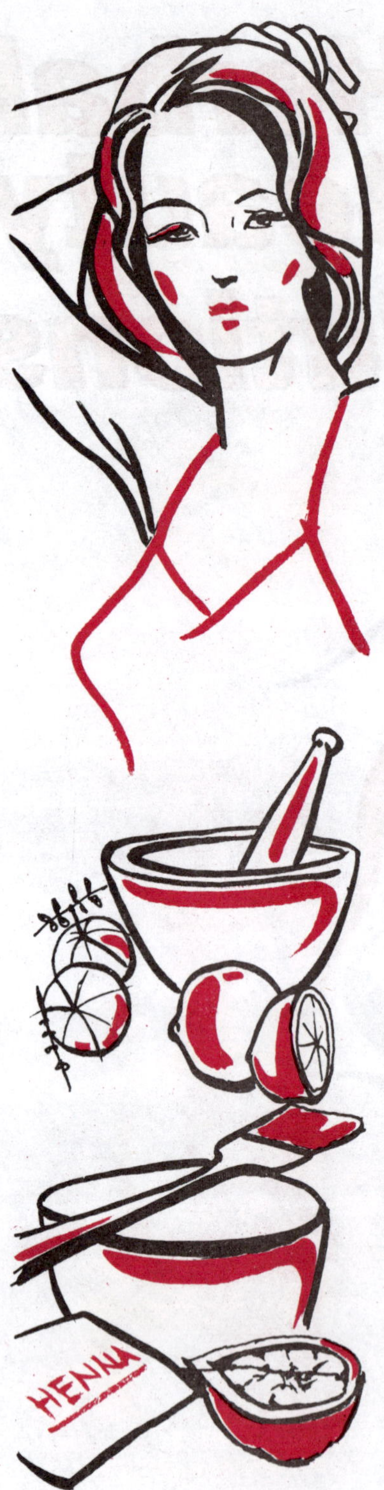

CHAPTER VI

HERBAL BEAUTY SOLUTIONS

There is too much emphasis on the cosmetics that are based on chemical preparations. They have caused more harm than benefit and the world is slowly awakening to the herbal resources. These substitutes have been around for ages; in fact, Indian women have been using herbal products for many hundred years. It is only now that the western world has woken up to the efficacy of these products. The products that are given here are easily available in the kitchen and the results are for yours to see. There are no harmful effects and the results can be stupendous.

HERBAL HAIR CARE

What can I use in order to check falling hair?
Here is a herbal tip for controlling the hair loss. Grind 'amlas' in lemon juice and rub the mixture on the scalp before washing the hair. This remedy will check falling hair and make it long and dark.

Is there any home remedy to make hair long and lustrous?
The application of Celery juice regularly, on the scalp, can result in long and lustrous tresses.

I use henna to colour my hair but I do not like the reddish tinge it gives my hair. How can I achieve a darker tone?
When you use henna mixture to dye your hair; add some walnut paste into it. This will give your hair a darker look and condition your hair, as well.

When I use henna on my hair it gives a red colour but I have seen many women who achieve a coppery tinge with henna. What is their secret recipe?

There is nothing very secret about the coppery colour. To get a rich coppery colour in your hair all you have to do is to add a few drops of eucalyptus oil to the henna mixture before applying to the hair. This will also help you to get rid of dandruff and leave it shining.

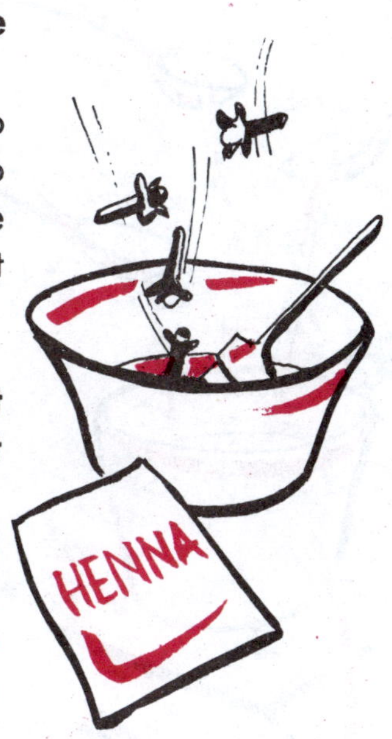

I would love to give my hair an auburn tinge but do not know how to bring that effect. Could you please suggest a way to do so?

To give your hair an auburn tinge, boil grated beetroot with 1/2 teaspoon 'kattha', 1-teaspoon methi powder and water. Strain and add it to the henna powder mixed with a teaspoon of coffee powder. Let it stand overnight in an iron vessel. In the morning add 1/2 cup curd to the concoction, mix well and apply to the scalp. Wash off after 3 hours.

Each time I henna my hair, I end up with a cold. How can I prevent it?

If you end up with cold every time you apply henna on your hair, add a few cloves to the henna mixture.

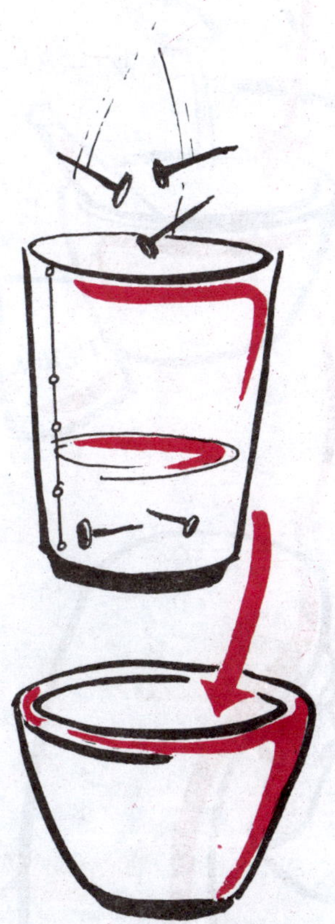

Is there any other method of dyeing the hair apart from using henna?

You can use this method. For natural hairy dye, soak rusted iron nails in water in an iron container. Strain the water, make a paste with 'trifla' (all spice) powder and apply on the scalp for 2 hours. Wash off with water and you will have shiny, black hair.

Could you give a good recipe for henna mixture to colour the hair?

For a lovely black sheen to the hair, boil 8-10 pieces of amla, 2-3 pieces of shikakai, 25 gm harar, 25 gm bahera and soak overnight in an iron vessel. Sieve the water and mix henna powder. Apply for 2 hours and then wash it off.

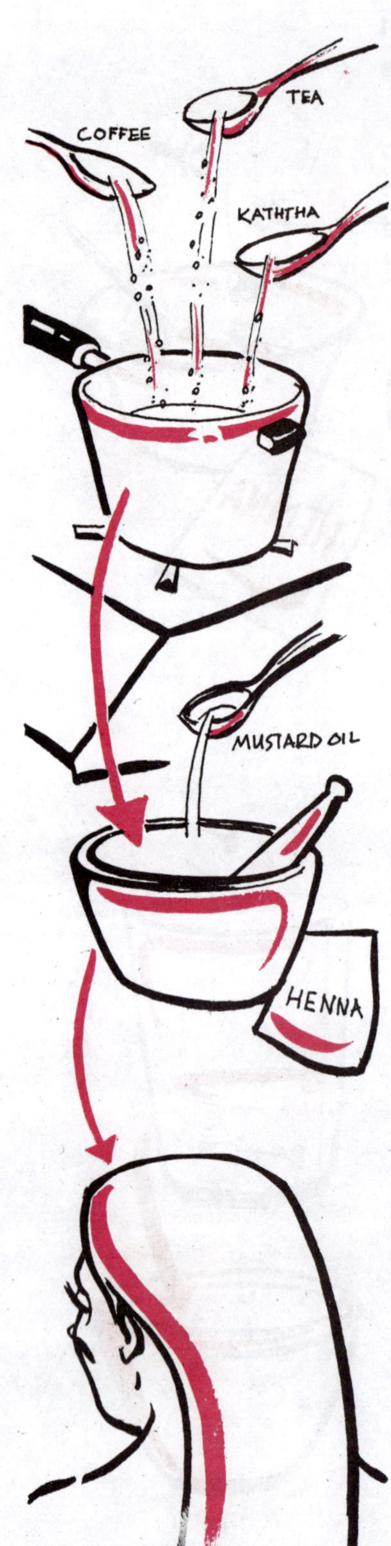

What does one do when there is no time to apply henna to the hair? I am required to go for parties and sometimes I just don't have the time to apply henna and wait for two to three hours before the colour takes effect.

For an emergency henna of hair, sprinkle a little brown powder blush-on and apply on the hair. The hennaed effect will last till the next shampoo.

How can I colour my hair into a rich burgundy colour, without using any chemical hair colour?

For a rich burgundy sheen to your hair, boil 2-3-teaspoons of tea, 1-teaspoon coffee, $^1/_2$-teaspoon of 'khattha' powder and red sandalwood in water. Mix this red water with henna powder; add 2-teaspoon of mustard oil and 1-teaspoon of eucalyptus oil (optional). Apply this to the hair for at least 2 hours and then wash.

What is the easiest method of making a henna mix for colouring grey hair?

Mix one cup of henna with one cup of tea. To this paste add an egg and a tablespoon of castor oil. This helps the paste to stick nicely to the hair. You may also add a spoon of coffee powder and a spoon of amla powder for better effect. Keep the paste in an iron vessel overnight. Apply to the hair, in the morning. Keep it on the hair for about 2-3 hours for a nice tint. Wash off with cold water.

I am tired of my dull and lifeless hair. Is there any home remedy that I can use to bring a shine to my hair?

For glowing hair, grind a few whole green grams, lemon peels, a handful of curry leaves and a few 'reethas' to a paste and apply to the hair before washing off.

My daughter brings back lice from the school. I have tried to eradicate them but they keep coming back. I hate using any chemical product on her hair. Is there any other method of getting the nits out of her hair?

There definitely is a method, which works very well. To get rid of nits in the hair, mix equal quantities of vinegar and water and apply on the hair and scalp. Leave for an hour before washing. Brush your hair backward with a fine toothed comb. Doing this for a few days will get rid of the nits.

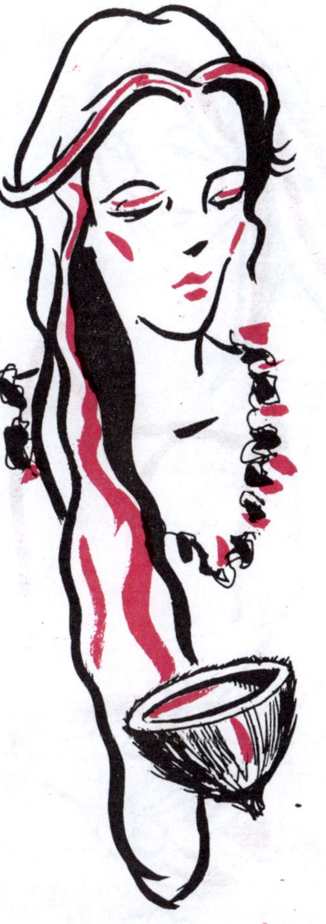

How can I bring lustre to my lifeless hair?
Rinse lifeless hair with a solution of 100-ml light tea mixed with $^{3}/_{4}$-teaspoon vinegar. This helps in adding bounce and lustre to the hair.

How can one keep the hair free from lice and keep the scalp cool, too?
A few crushed camphor tablets added to hair oil will keep the hair free from lice and infection apart from keeping the scalp cool.

Lice can also be removed from the hair by wrapping the hair in a towel full of basil leaves and leaving it overnight. Do it for a week.

I am wonderstruck when I see the long and dark hair of my friend who is a Keralite. She tells me that coconut is the best thing to use. How does one use it?
Coconut in its natural form is a very good element for the hair. For long and healthy hair you could wash it with tender coconut water.

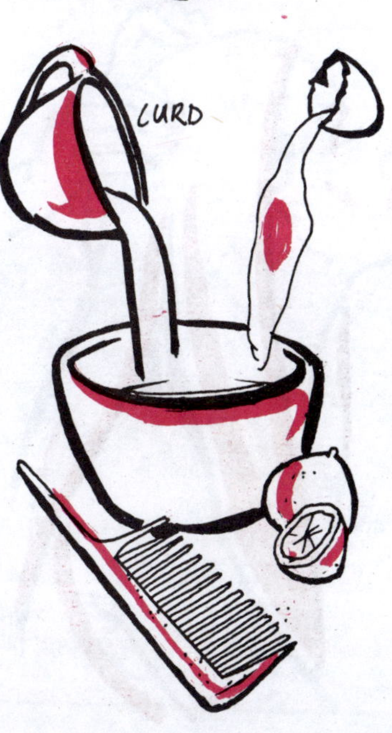

I am fed up of my falling hair, please help.
Don't despair, try this remedy. To prevent hair fall, rub amla, neem and fresh coconut milk to the scalp.

The other method is to boil a handful of curry leaves in 100-ml. coconut oil and massage this oil into the scalp, twice a week. This prevents loss of hair.

How can one arrest the hair loss by using kitchen products?
Grind together the peels of lemon, orange and pomegranate. Dry these in the sun. Mix it with coconut oil and apply on the scalp. Using it regularly will help in arresting falling hair.

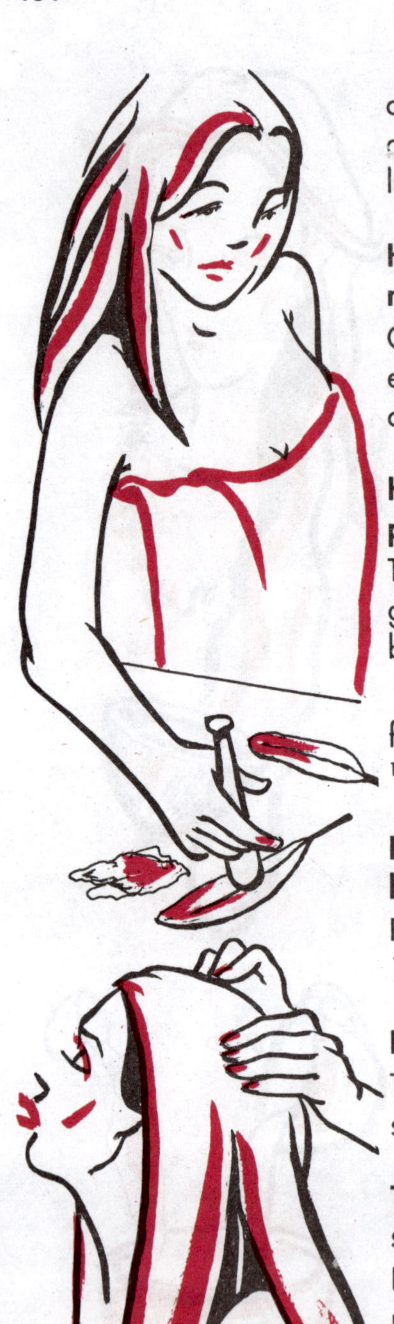

Another method is to mix coconut, castor and mustard oil in equal quantities. Heat this and apply with the help of a cotton swab to the roots of the hair. The hair will become lustrous and stop falling.

How can I get rid of dandruff from my hair? Is there any method by which one can prevent greying?
Get rid of dandruff with beetroot juice or a mixture of curd, egg and lime. To prevent greying of hair, rub a mixture of curry leaves, amla and fresh coconut milk to the scalp.

How can hair follicles be stimulated and dandruff be prevented by using material from the kitchen?
To stimulate hair follicles, take 2-teaspoon fenugreek seeds, grind and add to the henna mix. The methi seeds, can also be mixed with curd and applied, to prevent dandruff.

You could also massage the paste of 1-tablespoon fenugreek seeds, 1-teaspoon black pepper powder and $^1/_2$ cup milk, gently into the scalp, to get rid of dandruff.

I have always envied women who have soft and silky hair. How can one achieve it?
For soft and silky hair, rinse it with tea decoction to which 1-tablespoon of lime juice has been added.

How can one use a home remedy to condition the hair?
That's very easy. All you have to do is to use crushed spinach leaves. They make an excellent hair conditioner.

This is an SOS. I am losing hair by the dozens. Please suggest a remedy before I become bald.
I am sure it will not come to that if you use the following method. To prevent hair loss, dry, powder and mix together bay and neem leaves and 25 gms of tulsi leaves. Add 5-teaspoons of this mixture to 50-ml water and apply to the scalp once a week.

Here is another one, just in case you can't be satisfied with one method. Dry, powder and mix together lemon peels, rose and hibiscus petals, curry leaves and shikakai powder. Mix a tablespoon of this mixture with egg white and use as a conditioner to arrest falling of hair.

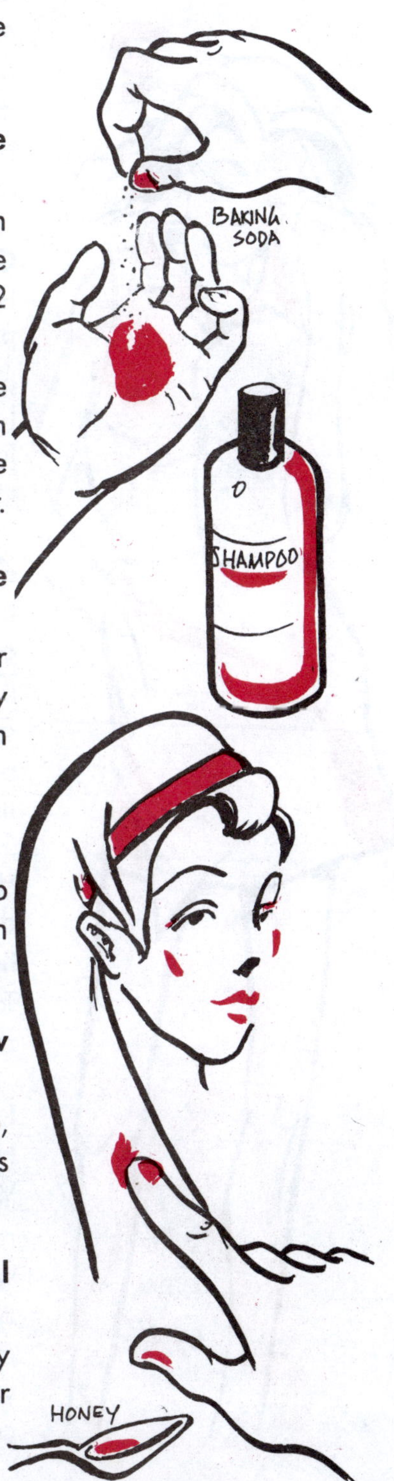

I have been suffering from split ends. My hair is coarse and rough. How can I control these problems?

To control split ends and treat rough and coarse hair, warm a combination of castor, mustard and olive oil and massage into the scalp for 20 minutes. Steam with hot towel after 2 hours.

There is another method to get rid of split ends in the hair. Mix together 1-tablespoon of almond oil, 1-teaspoon of honey, 1 egg yolk and smear all over the scalp. Leave it on for about 30 minutes. Wash off with lukewarm water.

Are there any home products which can be used to style the hair?

There definitely are. Try this method. Boil $^1/_2$ cup water with 12 lemon slices in it. When the volume is reduced by half, mix in a teaspoon of Vodka and cool. Use this solution to style hair.

How can I revitalise my stressed hair?

Massage the contents of a vitamin E capsule into the scalp to revitalise and condition stressed hair. Leave for half an hour and rinse thoroughly.

I would love to feel that my hair is squeaky clean. How can I achieve that effect?

Once a week, mix a little baking soda with your shampoo, work up a good lather and leave for a minute. This leaves the hair shiny and squeaky-clean.

Every summer, my daughter gets rashes on her scalp. I guess it is due to the heat. How can it be cured?

To prevent summer rashes on the scalp, mix castor, gingelly and coconut oil in equal proportions, leave on the scalp for some time. Wash away with cold water.

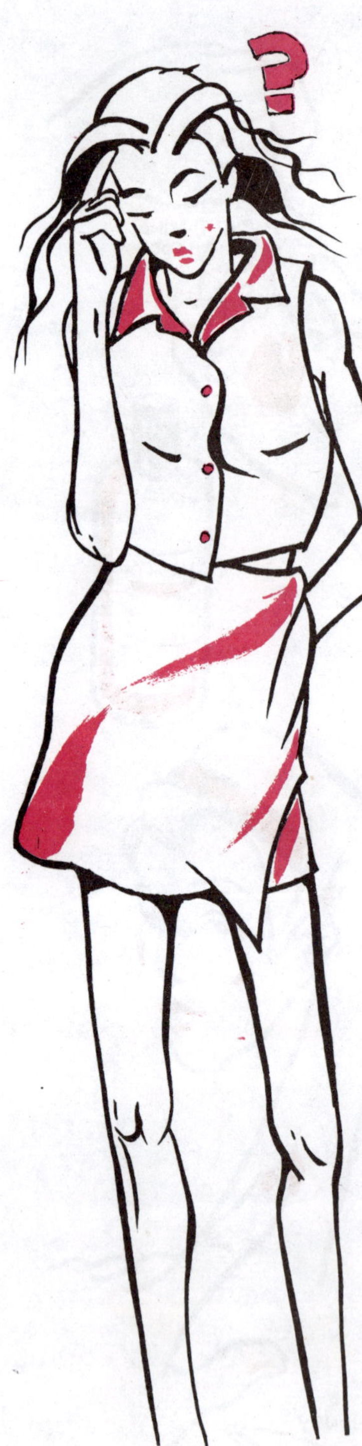

Could you suggest a way to make my dry hair manageable and soft?

Mayonnaise is a good way to add oils to dry hair. Massage it into the hair and wash off after $^1/_2$ an hour. Do this about twice a month. This will make your hair soft and manageable.

Can the goodness of Aloe Vera be used for the hair, too? How does one use this plant to add moisture to dry hair?

Pluck off a leaf from aloe plant, take the hard green covering off with a knife. The jelly like substance that you get should be mixed with 2-tablespoon Vaseline and applied to the hair for moisturing effect.

I have a very hectic social life and have to go for parties quite often. Sometimes I do not have time to shampoo my hair. Could you suggest an emergency method to take care of my problem?

If you don't have the time to wash and dry your hair, sprinkle talcum powder on it and brush vigorously. The powder soaks the excess oil and leaves the hair dry and fluffy.

How can I remove chewing gum from the hair? My daughter often comes home with chewing gum in her hair.

To remove chewing gum from your daughter's hair just rub a little honey over it.

I have heard that eggs can be used to shampoo the hair. How does one do it?

You have heard right. Eggs are full of proteins and they revitalise the hair while cleaning it. Simply wash your hair with egg. To do so, beat up one or two eggs with a cup of water and massage this into your wet hair for about ten minutes. Rinse off thoroughly. Don't use hot water or you will have a poached egg on your hair. As a last rinse, you can use the juice of one lemon in a cup of lukewarm water.

What is hot oil therapy?

Hot oil therapy is a method to check dandruff. Massage hot oil into the scalp at bedtime. Next morning an hour before bath, rub lemon juice mixed with pure vinegar (1:2 ratio) on the scalp. Then follow it up with a shampoo. If you cannot keep the oil, overnight, in the hair, wrap a steamed towel around the head and keep it for about 5 minutes.

Can you suggest some recipe for a home-made shampoo?

You can make several types of shampoos at home. One of them is the Rum shampoo. For this, combine two egg yolk with 2-dessertspoonful of odourless linseed oil and 2-dessertspoon of rum. Soak the hair and the scalp. Keep this concoction on the hair for about an hour. Rinse off with warm water. This is especially good for dandruff and dry hair.

To make an egg shampoo at home, beat 2 egg yolks in a glass of hot water. Strain, and apply to the hair and scalp. Keep it on for an hour and rinse off. This is one of the oldest recipes of making a home made shampoo.

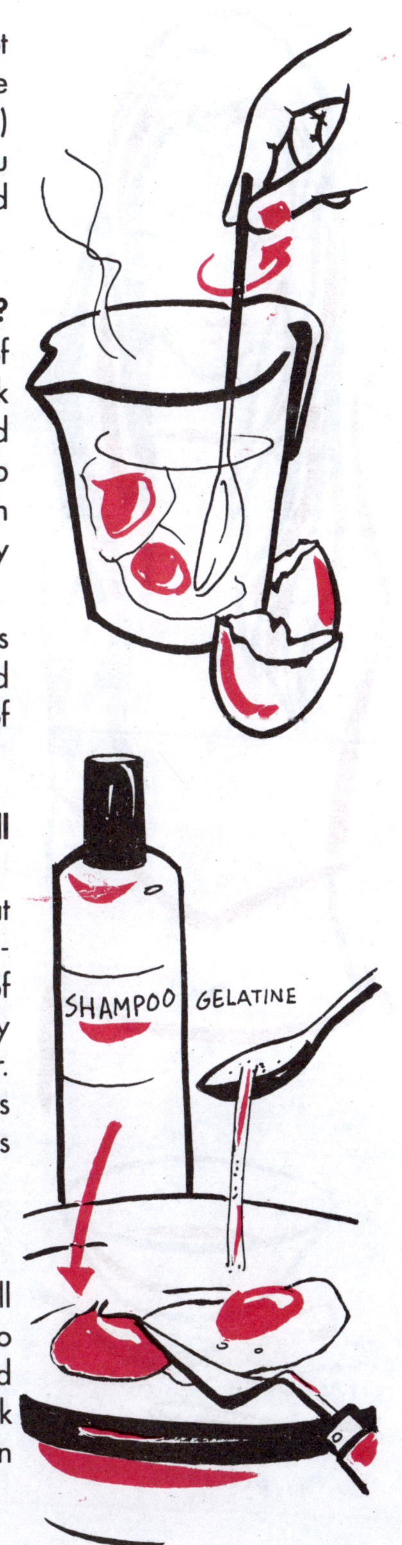

Is it possible to make a shampoo at home, which will condition the hair?

It is definitely possible to make a conditioning shampoo at home and its quite easy to make. Blend together 1-2-tablespoons of any shampoo, 1 egg and 1-tablespoon of unflavoured gelatine powder. Take care to avoid any formation of lumps in the mixture. Use it to wash the hair. Since egg and gelatine both are a source of protein, this mixture will make the hair thick and lustrous. Besides cleaning the hair, this shampoo will condition it also.

Can I make a herbal shampoo at home?

Using any herbal product for the making of a shampoo will give you a herbal shampoo. One of the easiest ones to make is the one with shikakai. Wash 200 gms of dried olives and 200 gms of shikakai in cold water and soak them in an iron vessel. The next morning, boil the decoction

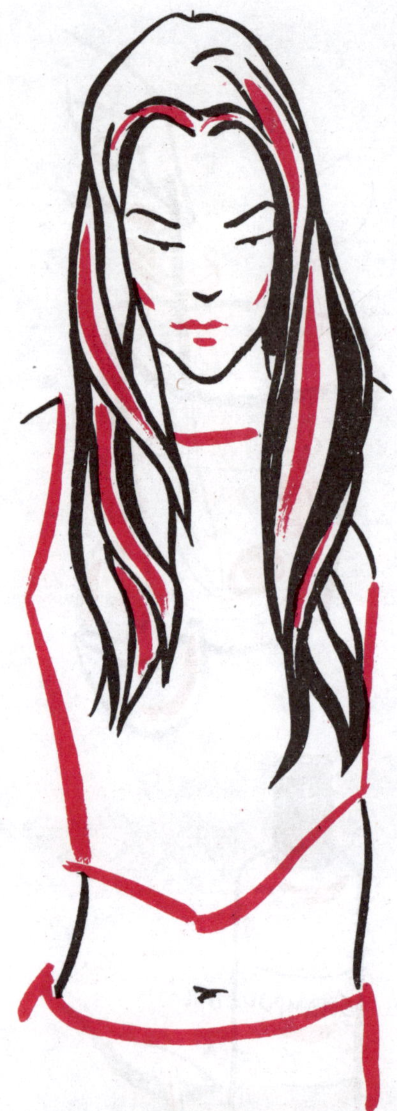

for about 10-15 minutes. Mash the thick residue into the water and strain. Use this to wash the hair. This shampoo leaves the hair soft and silky.

You can also make a home-made herbal shampoo by using reetha and shikakai. Soak 125 gms each of reetha, shikakai and amla in 1 litre of water. Keep it aside for about 24 hours. Boil and allow the mixture to cool. Strain and use it to shampoo the hair. It is a very good way to wash the hair without harming it.

How can I make a conditioner at home?

To make a hair conditioner, you will need 2-tablespoons of lanolin, 3-tablespoons of castor oil, $^1/_2$-tablespoon of coconut oil, 1-tablespoon of vegetable lard, $^1/_2$ cup water, 1-teaspoon vinegar, 1-teaspoon glycerine and 1-teaspoon shampoo. Melt the oils and lanolin in a pan and heat water in another pan over a water bath. Add water quickly to the oils, beating continuously until they are thoroughly blended. These ingredients are sufficient for making a large pot of a very nutritious hair conditioning cream. To use this cream, apply 2-tablespoon of it to your hair and steam it. If you add an egg to this cream, it will restore the driest of the hair to a peak condition.

I want to make a hair conditioner at home but I want the recipe to be a simple one which will not take too much of my time. Can you suggest one?

Here is a conditioner you can make in very little time. Mix together 1 egg, 2-tablespoon castor oil, 1-teaspoon vinegar and 1-teaspoon glycerine. Beat constantly till they blend well. Apply in on your scalp and massage lightly. Wrap your head in a hot towel and steam the hair. Wash off with cold water. This conditioner makes the hair soft, shiny and manageable.

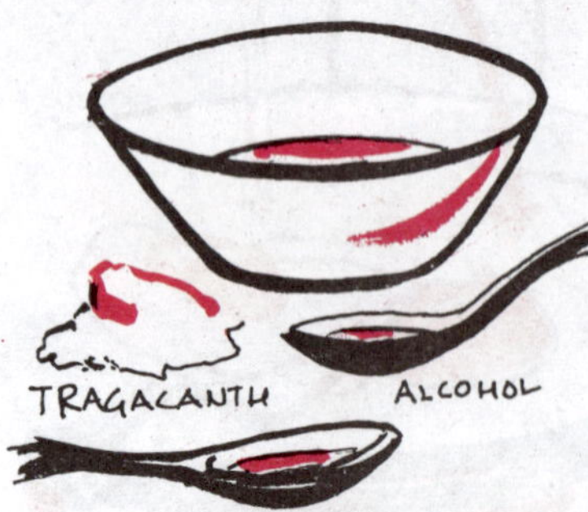

Is there any method by which I can make a hair-setting lotion at home?

You can make a hair setting lotion at home by using the following ingredients: 1-teaspoon of gum tragacanth, 8-

tablespoons water, 1-tablespoon alcohol and $^1/_2$-teaspoon glycerine. Crush the gum tragacanth with a pestle and mortar. Add water to it and stir until the gum dissolves and you have a smooth solution. Now add alcohol and glycerine to it. The lotion will thicken after a couple of hours and be ready for use.

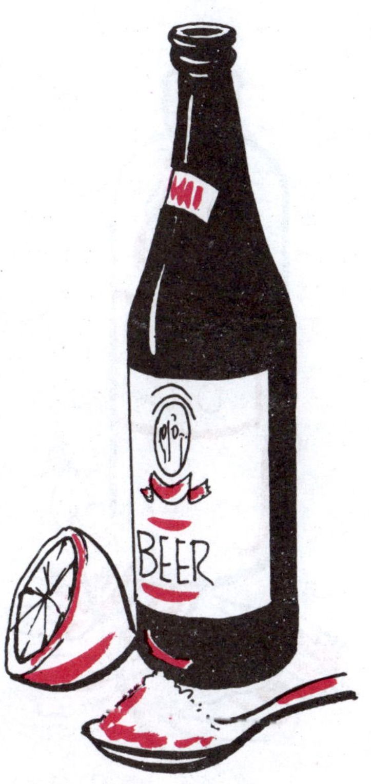

What other materials can be used for setting the hair?

Beer is a very material for setting the hair. Simply wet the hair before setting it. It gives a strong holding and helps in setting the hair neatly. The other items that can be used as setting lotions are gelatine and lemon. Lemon juice makes a good setting lotion, especially for greasy hair. Squeeze a lemon and use the diluted juice to obtain a firm set. It also makes the hair soft and shiny. Since lemon juice dries very fast, it can be used as an effective hair lacquer. To make lemon hair lacquer, cut a lemon in pieces and boil it with a cup of water until it reduces by half the quantity. Strain and use this as hair lacquer. If you add a few drops of alcohol or Vodka, this lacquer can be kept for some time.

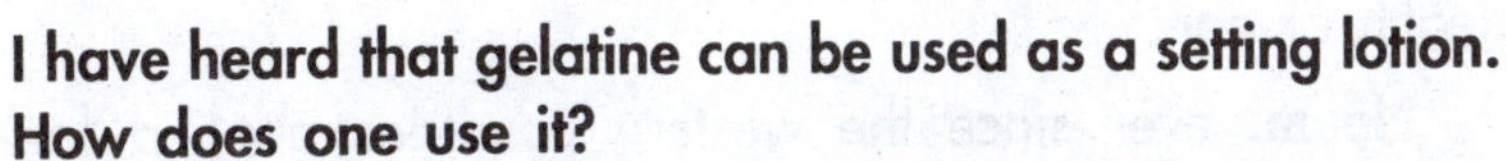

I have heard that gelatine can be used as a setting lotion. How does one use it?

Gelatine is an excellent material for making a setting lotion. It gives body to limp hair and being a source of protein, it nourishes the hair. Dissolve 2-tablespoons of gelatine in 2 cups of boiling water. Use this for the final rinse of the hair.

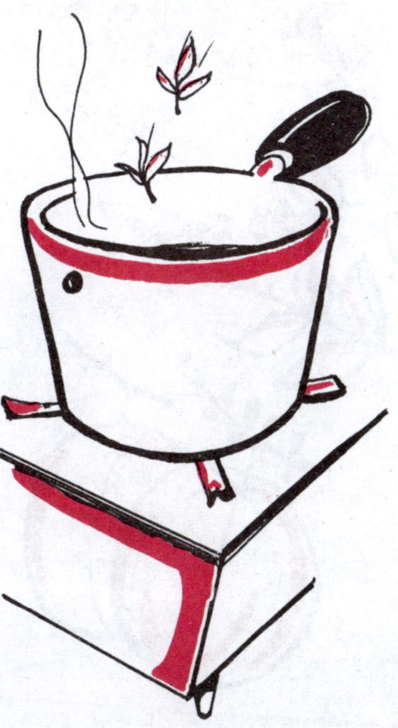

I have heard that used tea leaves are good conditioners. How does one use them?

You have heard right. Tea and lemon rinses are good for the hair. Boil used tea leaves again, in enough water, cool the liquid and strain. Use it as a rinse after your shampoo.

HERBAL HAIR OILS

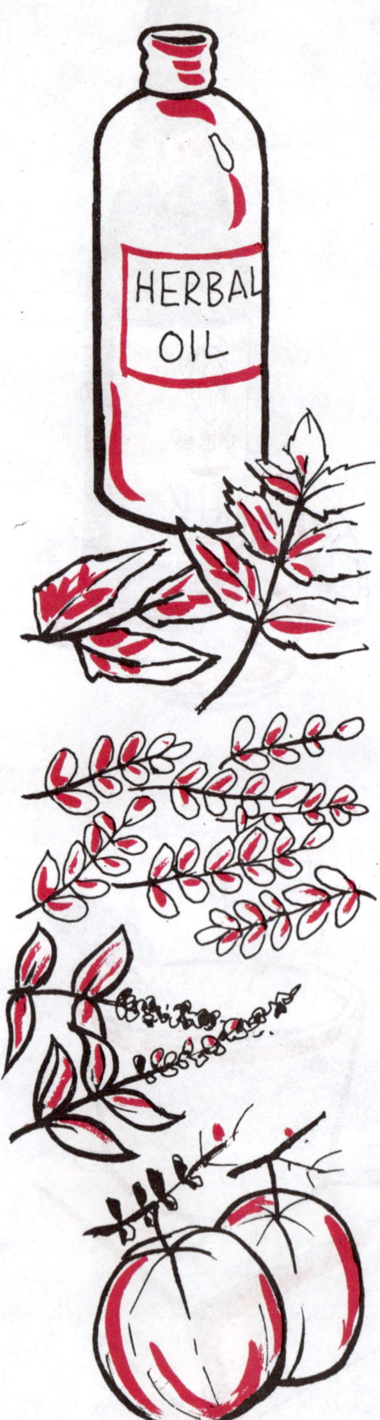

Can I make herbal oils at home? What are the different types of herbal oil that can be made at home and how can I make them?

Any of the following can be used to make herbal oils with base oils such as coconut, mustard oil, castor oil, olive oil, etc. Sometimes two of them can be mixed to make the herbal oil. Hair massage can be done with these hair oils with a touch of water or a drop of lemon juice.

Bhringraj: also called 'maka', the fragrant leaves of this plant are very useful as they can be used to make a very beneficial herbal oil which has a strong cooling property. This oil helps the hair to grow as well as refreshes the eyes. Since it cools the scalp, this oil can be used for curing headaches.

Jabakusum: the common hibiscus is a great source of hair oil with excellent properties. The leaves as well as the flowers of this plant are used to darken greying hair and the oil made out of it helps in hair growth as well as the health of hair.

Neem: ever since the western countries applied for patents of neem products, we have woken up to the benefits of this plant. Oils made out of the leaves and the berries cure headaches, baldness, increase hair growth and strength.

Brahmi: it is a herb, which grows wild everywhere in India. It is the commonest ingredient in hair oils. It cools the head, removes stress and helps hair growth.

Parijat: also called 'harsingar', this tree has orange, white, fragrant flowers. The juice of these flowers cures dandruff and strengthens hair roots.

Tulsi: the leaves of this plant when used in oil add lustre to hair.

Castor seeds: hair oil made of these seeds brings about sound sleep and healthy hair.

Henna: henna leaves are used to darken the gray hair. They nourish and condition the hair.

Curry leaves: also called 'meethi neem'; the leaves when eaten regularly prevent greying. They nourish the roots and restore normal pigmentation of the hair. The leaves can be eaten raw in chutney or their juice may be added to buttermilk or yogurt.

Amla: enriches hair growth and pigmentation. Amla water makes a good rinse for the hair.

HERBAL SKIN SOLUTIONS

Can I make some face packs at home? If so, please give me the ingredients to make one?

You can make a very good face pack by mixing bitter almonds with sandalwood powder and 'multani mitti'.

Face masks made with 'dal' are great softeners for the skin. Grind any dal with a pinch of turmeric. Add a few drops of lemon juice and a tablespoon of milk. Apply this paste on the face. Leave it on till dry and then wash off with lukewarm water.

I have very rough palms, is there a home remedy to make them soft?

For soft palms, apply a mixture of sugar and olive oil and rub for a while before washing it off.

My skin has got badly tanned due to the outdoor activities. How can I get rid of the tan by using a home product?

If your skin has got badly tanned, apply raw potato juice to get rid of the tan.

For a very tanned skin, mix the juice of a lemon with sugar, add a little glycerine and scrub gently in circular movements. This will not only get rid of the tan but also soften the skin.

To prevent the effects of sunburn, mix 1-teaspoon potato juice with 1-teaspoon lemon juice and leave it on for 15 minutes. Wash after some time. Repeat for a few days to get rid of the tan.

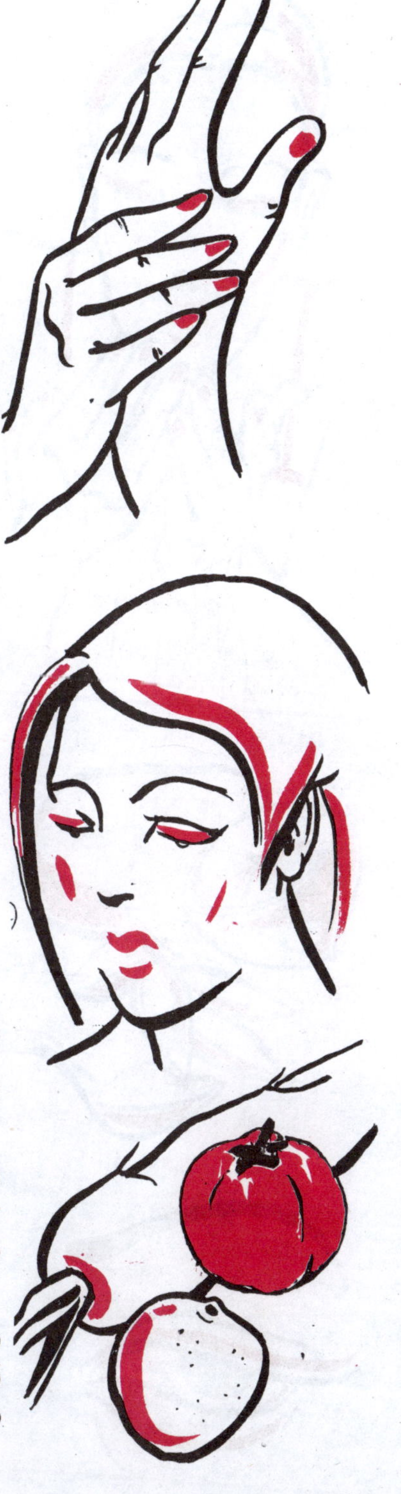

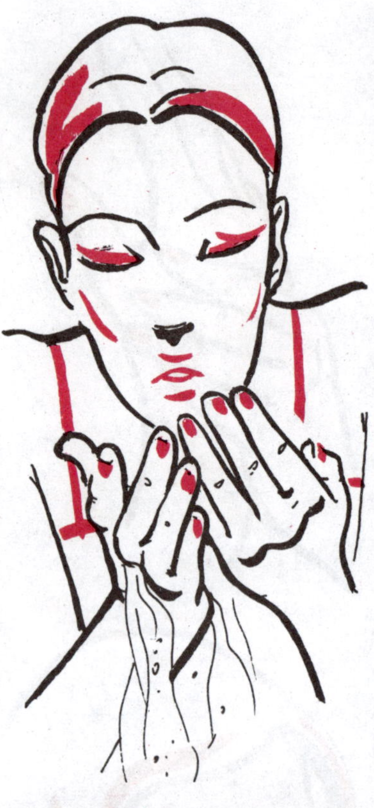

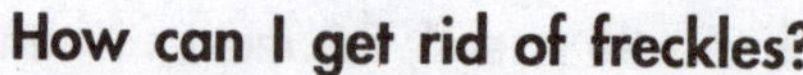

How can I get rid of freckles?

To get rid of freckles, grate a radish and extract 2-tablespoon of juice. Mix with equal quantity of buttermilk and apply on the face. Wash off with warm water, after an hour. Use it daily.

For a quick relief from freckles, grate half a white radish; mix with 2-teaspoons of lime juice and tomato juice. Apply on the face and keep it on for 20 minutes. Wash it off with lukewarm water. A regular application will ensure a freckle free face for you.

I had smallpox during my childhood. It has left scars on my face. How can I get rid of the scars?

Tender coconut water applied on the skin regularly for six months, removes smallpox scars.

Do you have any herbal solution for my pimples?

Mix an equal quantity of eau-de-cologne with boiled and cooled lemon juice. Apply the solution over pimples. They will disappear leaving your skin soft and smooth.

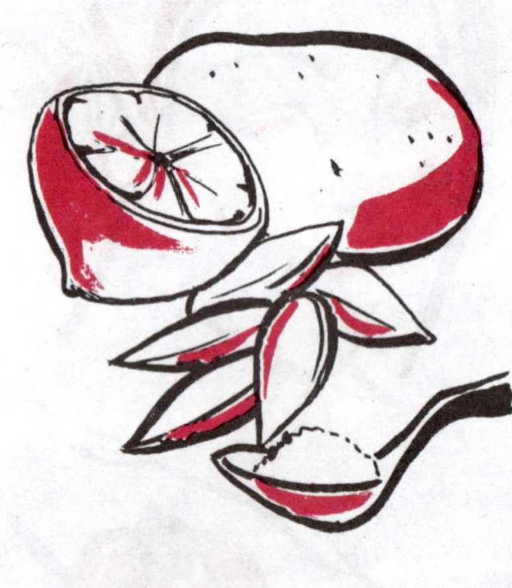

Papaya pulp when applied regularly on the face cures pimples and blackheads.

For instant cure of pimples, apply a paste of chalk and water on them. They will disappear by evening.

To reduce pimples and blackheads, rub the scrapings of bitter gourd on infected portions of the face.

A mixture of finely powdered dry tulsi leaves, 1-tablespoon of milk and almond oil helps clear pimples

Can I get rid of the dark circles under the eyes by using something from the kitchen, which is easily available?

Place pumpkin slices on your eyes and the dark circles will get erased.

For dark circles around the eyes, grind 5 almonds, 1-teaspoon fresh cream, juice of half a lemon, $^{1}/_{2}$-teaspoon Fuller's earth and $^{1}/_{2}$ grated potato, to a thick paste. Apply it around the eyes. Wipe off with cotton wool dipped in warm milk.

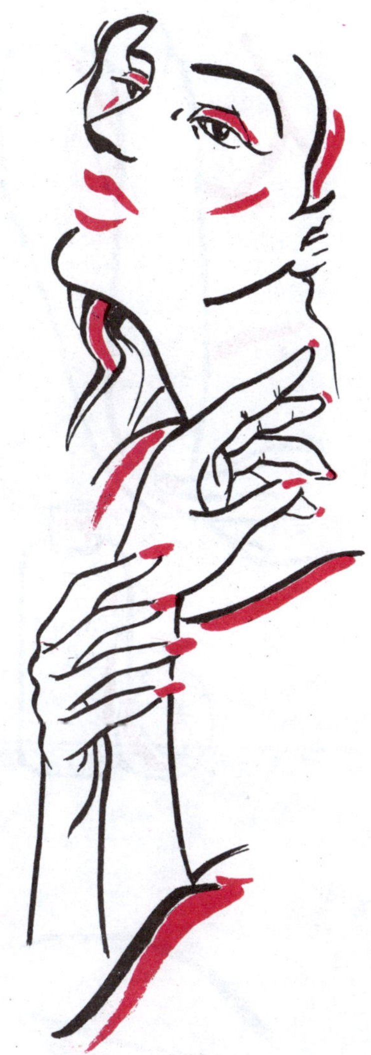

How can I get a soft and glowing complexion? Please suggest some homemade recipe for a clear complexion.
For a clear complexion, apply sour whey to your face and keep it on for at least 15 minutes. Wash off with lukewarm water. Follow this routine for 15 days.

To rejuvenate your face, put papaya pulp on it. To make your face glow, apply fresh orange juice.

Please give me a herbal recipe for making a bath scrub?
Make a bath scrub at home by mixing together 1-teaspoon each of sandalwood powder, Fuller's earth and dried orange peel powder.

A full body scrub once a week does wonders for the body. Mix 2-teaspoon flour, 1-teaspoon gramflour, a little raw milk, 1 pinch turmeric powder and 1-teaspoon honey. One can also use lemon and cream for the body.

I have very dark lips although I have never smoked. How can I lighten the colour of my lips?
To lighten the colour of dark lips, apply a mixture of honey and lime juice over the lips for a few days.

For soft lips, apply a mixture of glycerine, lime juice and rose water mixed in equal quantities.

Smear fresh cream over discoloured lips and leave it on to dry. Use regularly for at least a month to bring back a healthy colour to the lips.

For dull and dark lips, apply the juice of coriander leaves, before going to bed, for 15 days.

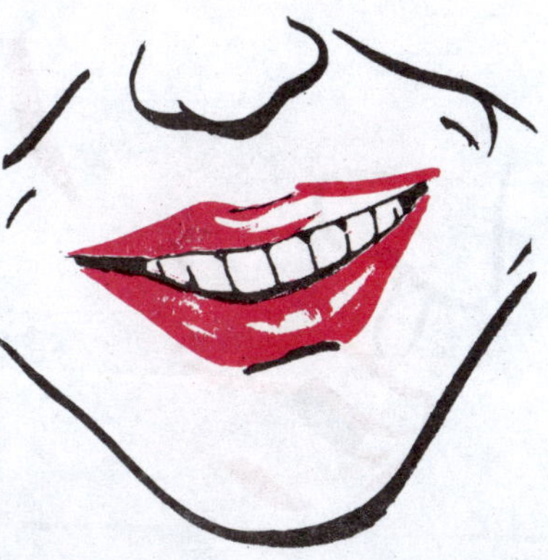

My skin becomes dry and scaly during the winter. What can I apply on my face to give me a good complexion during the winter?
For a smooth and soft complexion during winter months, apply a mixture of fresh cream and honey on your face and neck.

For dry skin, apply a mixture of glycerine, fresh cream and honey. It will keep the complexion glowing. This is a good treatment for cracked heels, too.

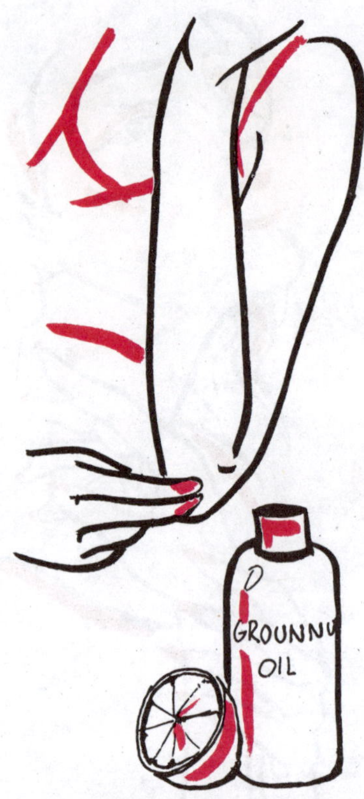

Extract some cabbage juice and mix it with a little yeast and one tablespoon of honey. Apply this mixture on the face and wash after about 20 minutes with lukewarm water. This pack helps in combating dry skin and wrinkle formation.

My elbows are dark and rough. They look quite terrible. How can I lighten the colour on my elbows?

If your elbows have become dark and rough, apply groundnut oil mixed with lemon.

I have very scanty eyelashes. How can I make them thick and dark?

To acquire seductive eyelashes, carefully apply a thin coat of pure castor oil on them, every night before retiring to bed. Castor oil is full of vitamin A, which strengthens the lashes and cools your eyes.

Can you give me a method for preparing a body lotion which can be applied before bathing?

For a smooth and shiny skin apply a mixture of 100-ml coconut oil to which 4 camphor pieces have been added. Apply it on your body before bathing.

Smear the body with equal quantities of vaseline and glycerine 10 minutes prior to bathing. This prevents the skin from drying.

Mix equal proportions of vitamin E oil, vaseline and glycerine. Cover the entire body with this paste and leave it on for an hour. Wash off with cold water for a lovely and soft skin.

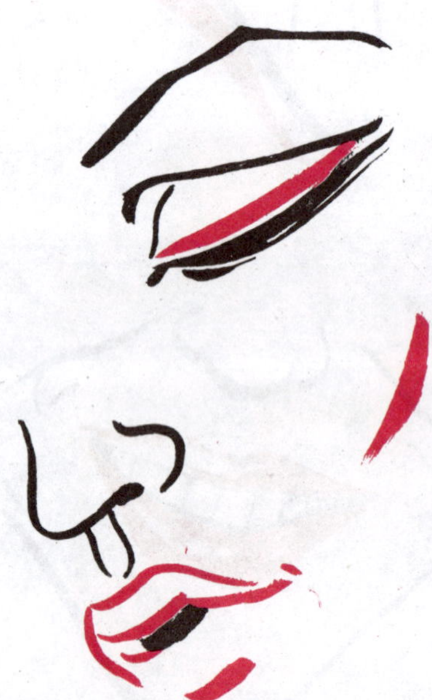

Can you suggest some good bath preparations to make the skin smooth and velvety?

If you have an itchy, dry skin, add a cup of vinegar to the bath water. This is effective. Oatmeal and bran contain oils and vegetable hormones, which soothe and soften the skin. Use one tablespoon of oatmeal in the bath.

Adding a spoonful of honey to the bath, will not only relieve tiredness but will leave the skin smooth and satiny.

A few tablespoons of laundry starch and a teaspoon of glycerine added to the bath water leaves your skin smooth, tight and soft.

How can I make a body massage oil at home?
Mix $^1/_2$ cup almond oil, $^1/_2$ cup castor oil and 1-teaspoon camphor oil. Use this to massage your body.

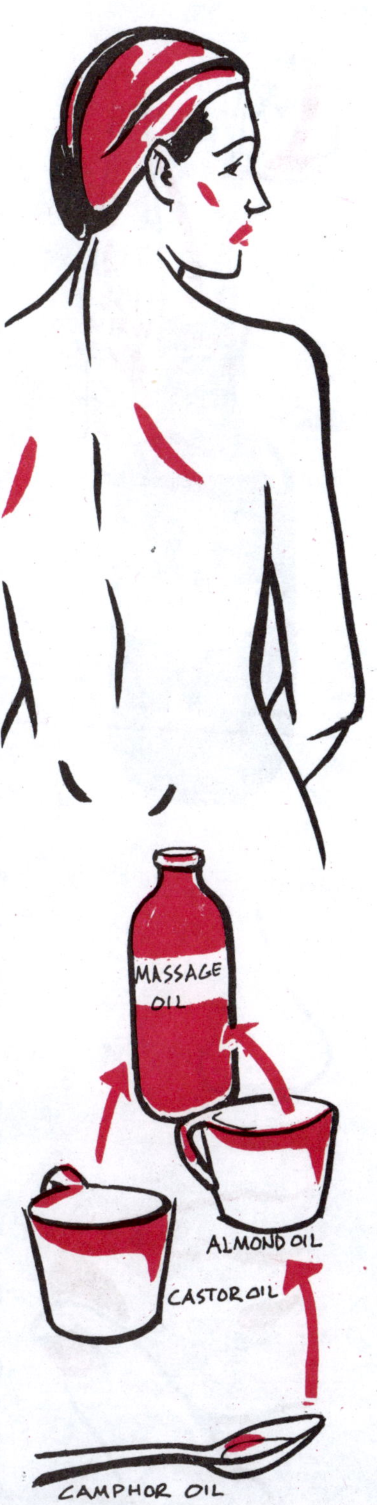

Is it possible to make a nourishing cream at home?
It is possible to make various types of nourishing creams at home. Here is a very simple method for the preparation of an oily nourishing cream, specially meant for dry skin.

Take 3-tablespoons of coconut oil, 2-tablespoons olive oil, and 1-tablespoon olive oil and $^1/_2$-teaspoon beeswax. Melt these ingredients in a double boiler.

In a separate bowl dissolve $^1/_2$-teaspoon of borax in 3-tablespoons of warm water. Slowly add the water to the oils and stir continuously until a creamy consistency is formed. Cool and bottle.

This cream is quite effective if warding off dryness of the skin.

Do you have a suggestion as to how the formation of wrinkles can be delayed?
To keep wrinkles at bay, apply a mixture of curd and gram flour to the face and leave it on for 15 minutes before washing it off.

To prevent wrinkles, mix equal proportions of cold cucumber juice with rose water and lemon juice. Cover the region around the eyes with a cotton wool soaked in this mixture.

A face mask made by blending egg white and a little lemon juice is an excellent way to prevent wrinkles. Wash off the face pack after 20 minutes with cold water.

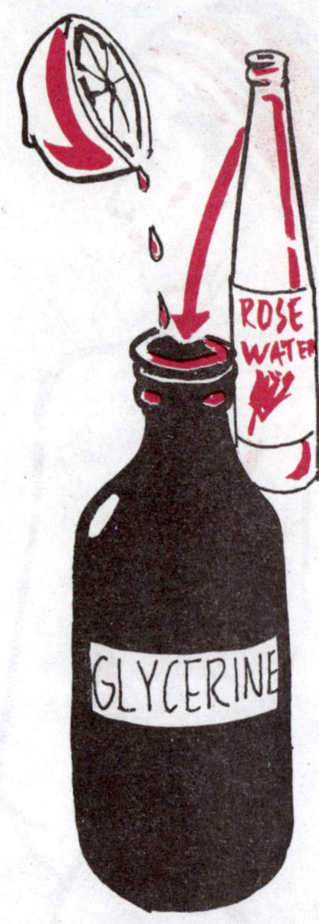

How can I achieve a nice and healthy skin and glowing complexion?

Glycerine mixed with rose water and lemon juice is the best remedy for dry skin. Glycerine retains moisture and the lemon juice cleanses the skin. For a soft and rosy complexion, grind a few fresh or dry rose petals with a dash of milk or fresh cream. Add a teaspoon of gram flour and a few drops of rose water to it. Apply the mixture liberally all over the face and neck. It will help you in reviving a tired and dull skin.

For a glowing skin, mash a banana in a teaspoon of milk and apply the paste on the face.

I am troubled by my blackheads. Is there any method by which I can get rid of them?

Getting rid of blackheads is quite easy if you try this remedy. Apply a paste of gram flour and curd on the affected area. When the mixture hardens and dries up, gently scrape off with your fingertips and wash the face.

Please give me a recipe for a home-made face scrub.

You can make a great scrub at home by grinding equal quantities of chana, moong and masoor dals and mix with milk or curd or honey.

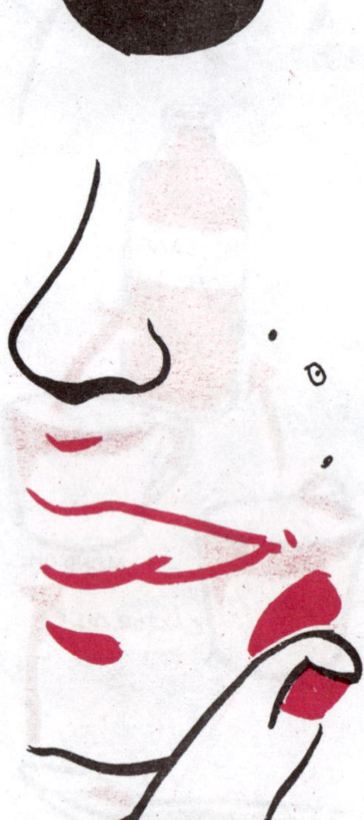

How can I make face packs at home? Please give me the recipe for making some packs?

For an excellent face pack, use grated potatoes and honey.

A pack made by mixing a tablespoon each of coarsely ground 'moong dal' powder, orange rind and milk prevents the skin from drying in winter.

Boil carrot and turnip and blend it to make a paste. Apply this for 10-15 minutes and rinse off with milk. This is an excellent face mask, which leaves the skin feeling fresh, and clean.

Can a toner be made at home?

You can make your own skin toner by making mixture of 2-tablespoon each cucumber and carrot juice. This is an excellent toner for the skin, especially during winters.

Vodka makes a good pore-tightening astringent cum toner for oily skins.

To tighten skin pores, cover the body with a mixture of 2″ piece cucumber, 2-tablespoon mint, $^1/_2$-teaspoon lemon juice and 2-3 drops of vinegar.

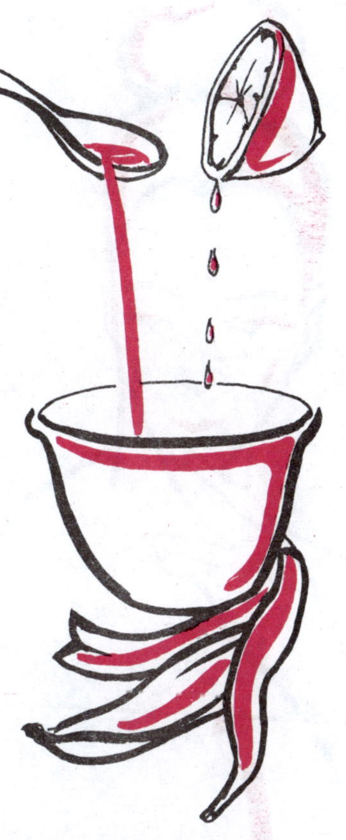

How can I get rid of the blemishes on my skin?

For removing blemishes, apply the juice of grated cucumber, potato or watermelon to the face. To remove blackheads, chop a tomato and apply on the affected area regularly.

My facial skin looks tired and dull. How can I revive it give it a fresh look?

Mash a ripe banana and mix it with 1-teaspoon honey and a few drops of lemon. This makes an excellent face pack for tired skin.

Can you suggest a method for making a hand and foot lotion, at home?

For a hand and foot lotion, mix together $^1/_2$ cup rose water, $^3/_4$ cup glycerine, $^3/_4$ cup aftershave lotion, $^3/_4$-tablespoon white vinegar.

Rubbing lime juice and sugar between the palms till the sugar dissolves will keep the palms smooth.

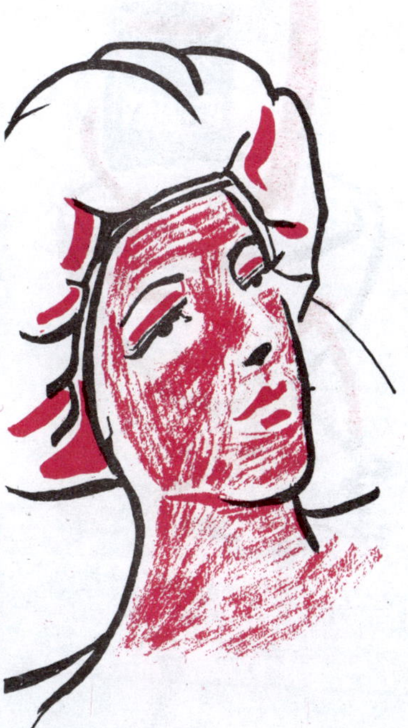

How can I get rid of stretch marks on my stomach?

To remove stretch marks acquired during pregnancy, use $^1/_2$-teaspoon of aloe, $^1/_2$-teaspoon papaya pulp, 1-teaspoon rose water, 1-teaspoon sandalwood paste, 10 drops of almond oil and 2 drops of lavender oil. Add 2-teaspoon milk cream to this and make a paste. Apply over the affected skin and massage gently before a bath. Doing this twice a week will take care of the marks.

Please suggest some home products for a facial?

For a home facial, smear fresh, unboiled cold milk on the face for five minutes. Then cover the face with chilled rose water mixed with milk cream. Wash with warm water. Finally

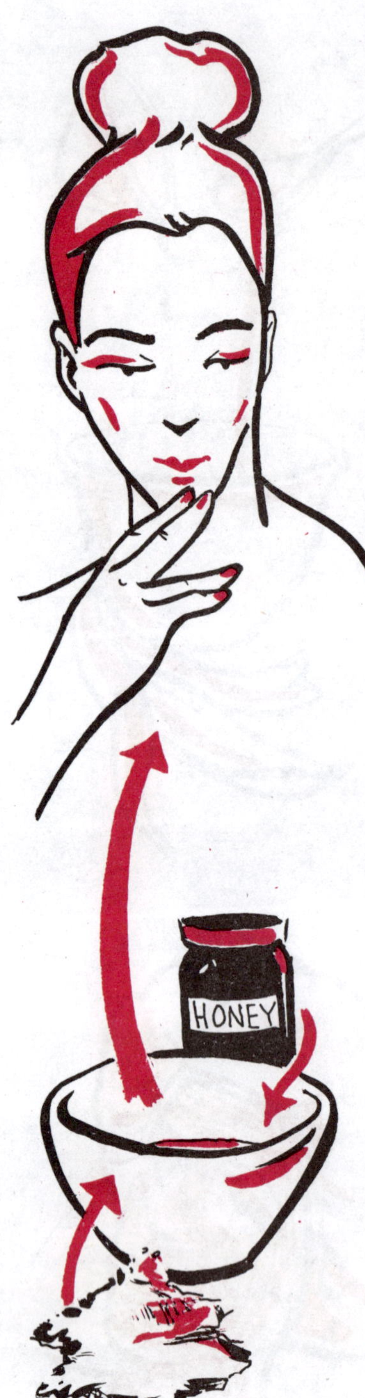

cover the face with a pack made of sandalwood and rose water and place slices of cucumber on the eyes. Wash off after 15 minutes.

Could I make an effective face mask at home?

Mix together 1 cup each of green gram flour and rice flour, $^1/_2$ cup wheat flour, $^3/_4$ cup milk powder, 3-teaspoon turmeric, 4-teaspoon semolina, 2-teaspoon granulated sugar, 4-5-teaspoon red sandalwood powder and 1-teaspoon henna. Mix lemon juice to this mixture and use as a face mask for normal skin.

How can I treat the black as well as the whiteheads on my face?

Mix 1-teaspoon honey with $^1/_2$-teaspoon rice powder and rub all over the face, especially on the chin and nose. This removes the black as well as the white heads.

To get rid of blackheads, cover the area with a mixture of green gramflour, curd and turmeric powder. Leave it for 10 minutes. Scrub off, using cold water.

In a thick-bottomed pan, heat a mixture of egg white and lemon juice till thick. Cool, smear this mixture over the face to get rid of blackheads permanently.

Can you give me a common treatment for removing skin blemishes?

Mash a few mint leaves, neem leaves and a banana. Apply the paste all over the face and neck, avoiding the eyes. Wash off when dry. This face pack removes scars, freckles and minor skin blemishes.

How can I make an exfoliant at home?

Alpha hydroxy acid (AHA) which is found in citrus fruits, sugarcane and milk that has gone sour, is extremely effective as a natural exfoliant. It can be used to remove dead cells.

While washing the face, add a little powdered sugar to the soap lather. It will help in exfoliating the dead cells from your face.

I am besieged with the problem of acne. Is there any herbal recipe for getting rid of acne?

Take 1-teaspoon neem powder and mix it with 1-teaspoon Fuller's earth and 1-teaspoon curd. Apply this mixture twice or thrice a week. Leave it on the face for half an hour and then scrub your face with cold water.

Mix 1-teaspoon wheat flour in a little water and apply on the face. Scrub with moist fingertips lightly after it is dry.

Take the white of an egg. Mix it with 1-teaspoon of rava. Apply this mixture on the face. After it is dry, dip your fingertips in milk and scrub the face with light upward movements. Wash off. Doing this twice a week should take care of the acne problem.

How can I get a beautiful and clear complexion?

Mashed peaches applied on the face brighten and deep cleanse a sallow and dull complexion.

Applying a paste of sandalwood and rose petals on the face, everyday, will make the skin soft and glowing. Wash off after 10 minutes.

I have bags under my eyes and this makes them look puffy. How could I get rid of the problem?

Wrap ice cubes in a thin cloth and rub lightly all over the face and the neck. This helps in reducing the puffiness around the eyes and the face.

I have become dark due to constant exposure to the sun. How can I lighten my complexion?

Grate and squeeze out the juice from a tender cucumber. To this add an equal quantity of milk and use over darkened patches of skin. This serves as an excellent whitening tonic.

To get rid of unwanted tan, mix together equal quantities of olive oil and vinegar. Apply on the effected area, 15 minutes before the bath.

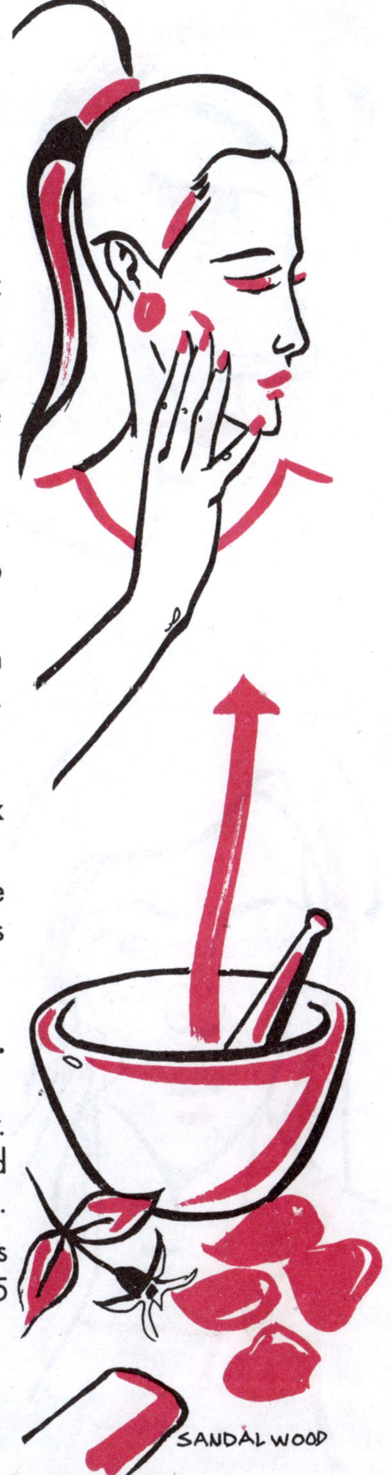

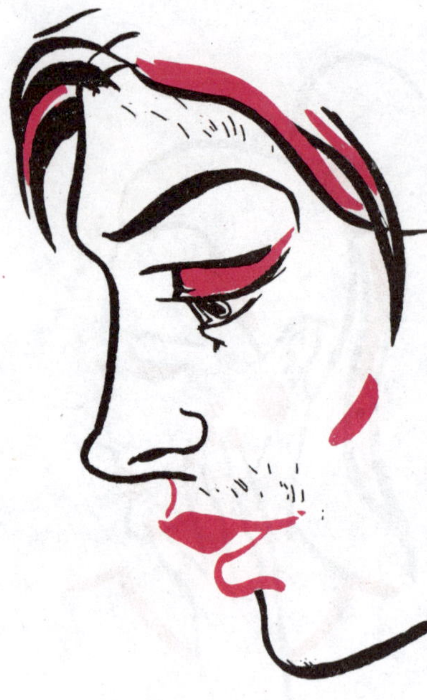

Is there any method by which I can get rid of the superfluous hair on my chin?

To get rid of facial hair, apply a mixture of fenugreek powder and green gram powder on the unwanted facial hair. Let it dry before scrubbing off.

Please give an idea about making cleansing milk at home.

You can make an effective cleanser at home by mixing a tablespoon of rice flour with 2-tablespoons of curd. This is an effective cleansing milk, which removes stale make up and opens up the pores.

I want a few home-made recipes for winter care of the skin. Could you please help?

To prevent a dry skin during the winters, moisturise it with a mixture of 1″ piece of mashed banana, $^1/_2$ a teaspoon milk cream, 5 drops glycerine and 2 drops of vitamin E oil.

To stop the skin from dehydrating during the winter, minimise the use of soap. Instead, use a mixture of 1-tablespoon each of gram flour and beaten curd, $^3/_4$-teaspoon of orange peel powder and 1-teaspoon olive oil.

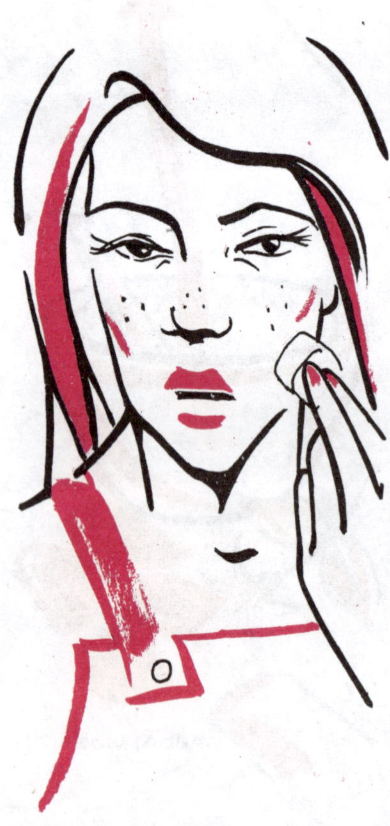

Are there any methods by which the pores of the facial skin can be tightened? How can the skin be prevented from sagging?

Beat a raw egg and apply it on the face and neck. Relax for 20 minutes and rinse it off with warm water. Eggs help tighten the skin pores and nourish the skin.

A pack made from 3-teaspoon each of cucumber juice, coconut water, lemon juice and sandalwood powder, prevents skin from sagging.

Can I have a recipe for making a moisturiser at home? Please advise how pimple marks can be removed?

Use the residue of spoilt milk as a moisturiser for dry skin.

To remove marks left by pimples, mix radish juice with equal quantity of buttermilk, apply on face. Wash off after an hour.

I have been plagued by pigmented skin for quite some time now. How can I get rid of the problem?
To get rid of pigmented skin, mix 1-teaspoon each of lemon juice and honey to papaya pulp. Rub this granular paste on the face and wash off after it dries.

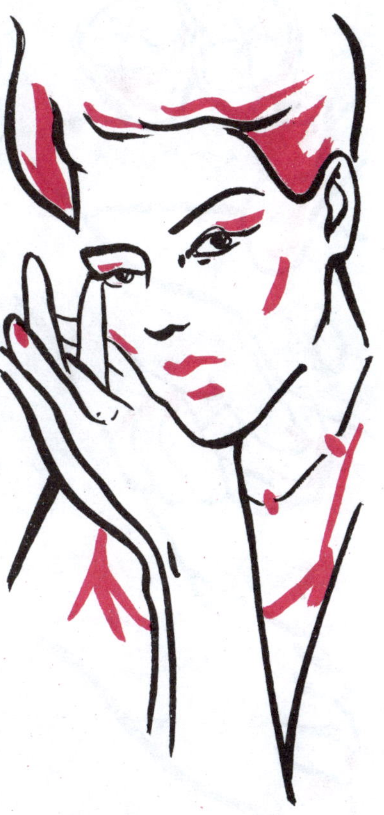

Please give me a method for making an astringent at home. I also want to know how I can make a cleanser for my face?
Mix equal parts of fresh tomato juice and cucumber juice, add a dash of rose water and refrigerate. It makes an excellent astringent for all types of skin.

Make a cleanser with 2 cups dried, powdered green peas, 1-cup gram flour, 1 cup dried orange powder and 1 cup of powdered almonds.

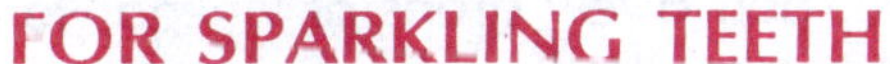

FOR SPARKLING TEETH

How can I make my teeth sparkle?
Sprinkle a little salt on the toothpaste while brushing the teeth to make them sparkle.

For sparkling teeth, rub them with bay leaf once or twice a week.

For shining white teeth, take dry lemon peel and powder it. Add a little bit of salt and 2-3 drops of mustard oil. Mix well and use this to clean your teeth. It keeps the bad breath away, too.

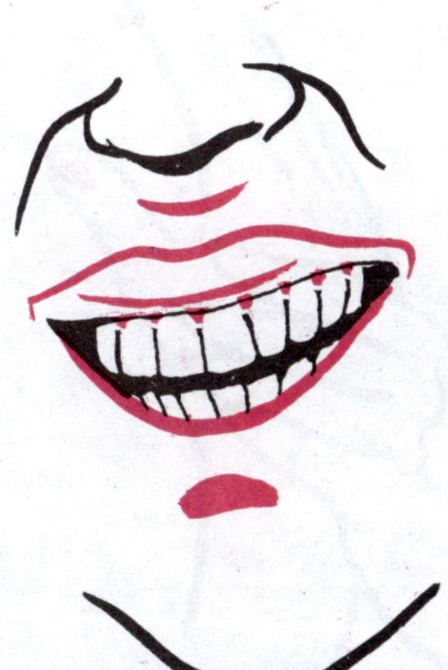

How can I remove yellow stains on my teeth?
Add a drop of clove oil to the toothpaste before brushing your teeth to remove stains on them.

Please give me a method for making mouthwash at home.
For a home made mouthwash, boil guava leaves in water for ten minutes. Cool, strain and use as mouthwash.

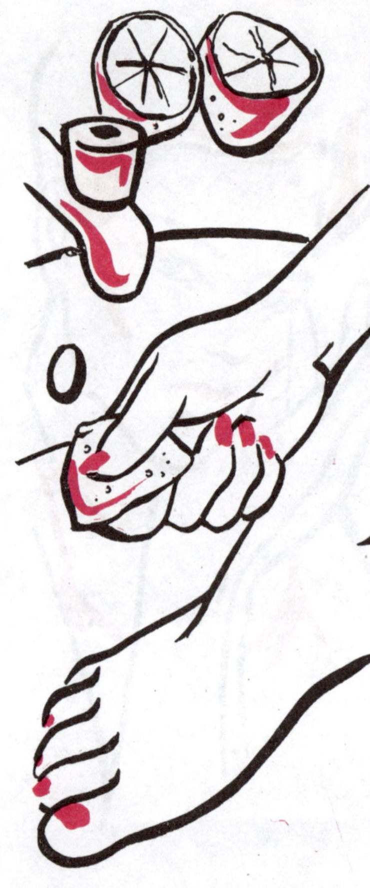

FOR PEDICURE AND MANICURE

Can you suggest some simple ingredients that can be used for a pedicure at home? Also give me a method by which I can get rid of the cracks on my heels.

To soften tough calluses on soles of feet, coat with a mixture of 6 crushed aspirin tablets and half cup each of water and lemon juice. Wrap feet with a warm towel and scrub the calluses with a pumice stone after ten minutes. Within a few days the calluses will soften and can be easily removed.

Roast an onion and make a paste. Use this on the cracks on your feet. The cracks will disappear within a month's time.

After a bath, massage the feet with a few drops of mustard oil for 5 minutes. Pour 2 mugs of water over them. A daily treatment will make your feet soft.

For a quick pedicure, add a few drops of vinegar to $^3/_4$ cup curd and rub this mixture well on the feet, ankles, and heels and between the toes. After 10 minutes, wash off with warm water. This removes dead tissues and the skin becomes softer, too.

Apply a paste made of 2-tablespoon of heated mustard oil and 15 gms wax, leave overnight on cracked heels. The cracks will vanish.

I have very rough hands. How can I make them soft?

Soak rough and scaly hands in a bowl of warm water to which 1-teaspoon of cornstarch has been added. This regular 5-minute treatment will soften the hands.

Apply some petroleum jelly on your nails if you are about to do a messy job. It will prevent the dirt from getting lodged.

Another good method of improving circulation while exfoliating the hands is to rub them with sugar and lime juice. The sugar granules will exfoliate while the lime juice will lighten the skin and soften it, too.

POPULAR SCIENCE

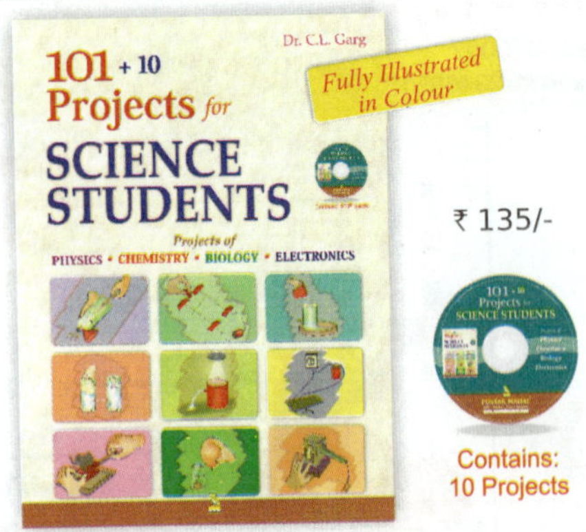

₹ 135/-

Contains: 10 Projects

2215 S

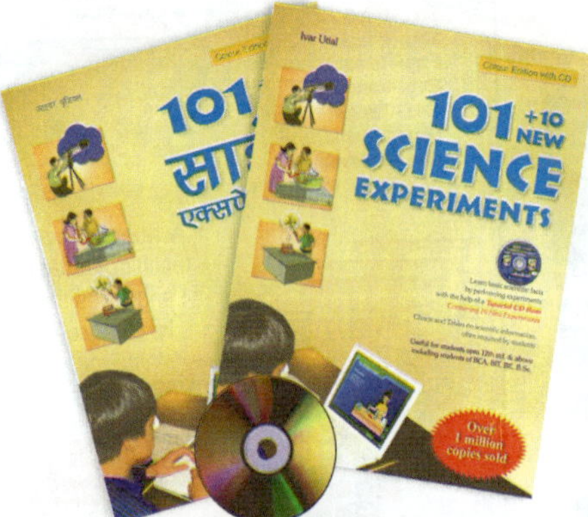

2213 S
Rs. 135/- (Colour)

2214 S
Rs. 135/- (Colour)

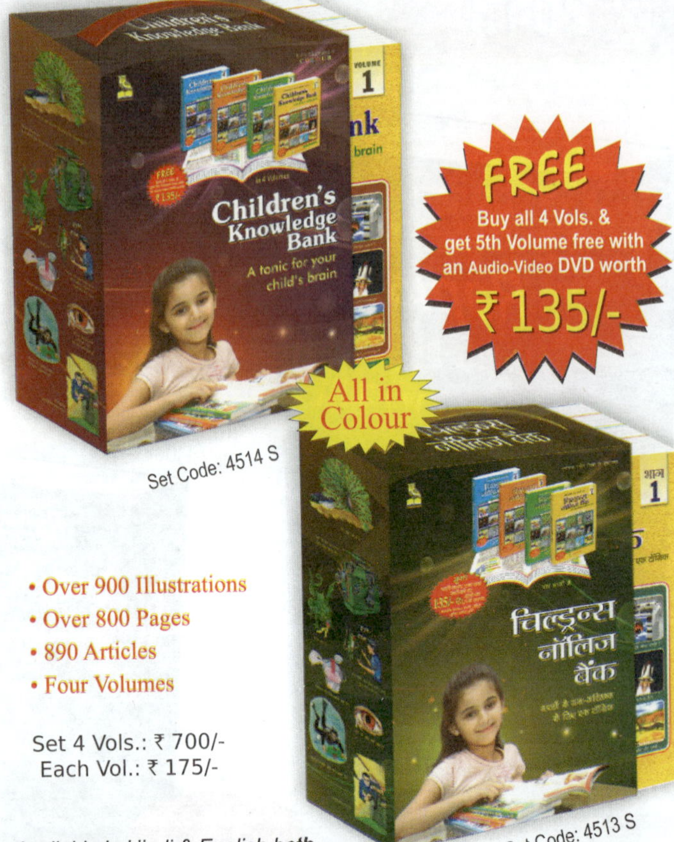

FREE Buy all 4 Vols. & get 5th Volume free with an Audio-Video DVD worth ₹ 135/-

Set Code: 4514 S

- Over 900 Illustrations
- Over 800 Pages
- 890 Articles
- Four Volumes

Set 4 Vols.: ₹ 700/-
Each Vol.: ₹ 175/-

Available in Hindi & English both

Set Code: 4513 S

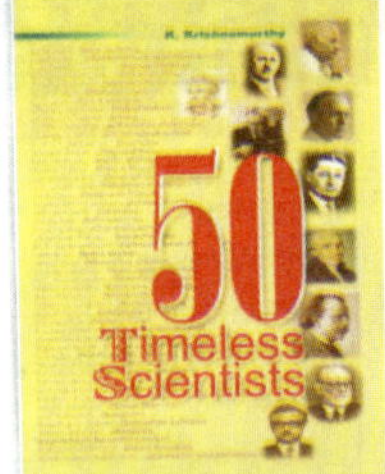

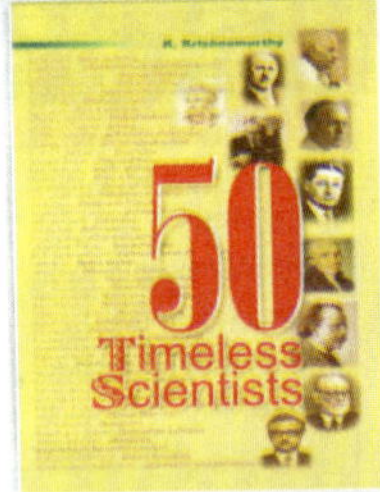

9412 C • Rs. 120/-

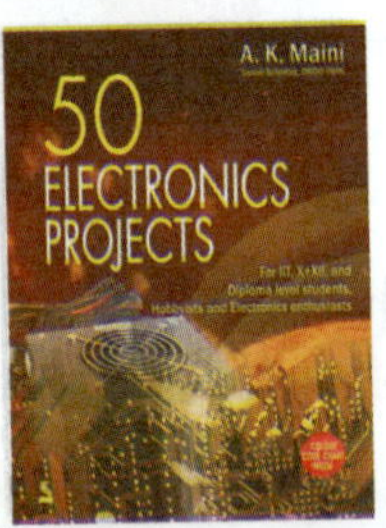

6678 D • Rs. 150/-

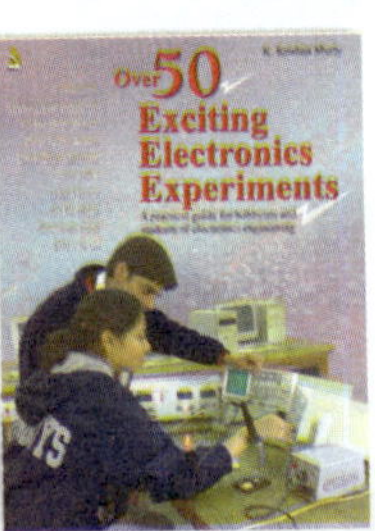

6679 A • Rs. 150/-

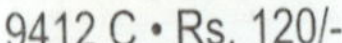

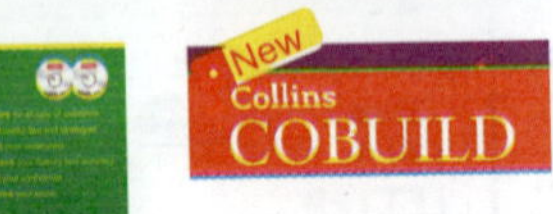

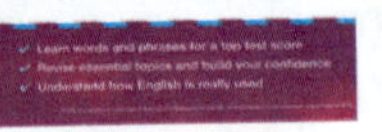

HC009 • Rs. 620/-

HC008 • Rs. 399/-

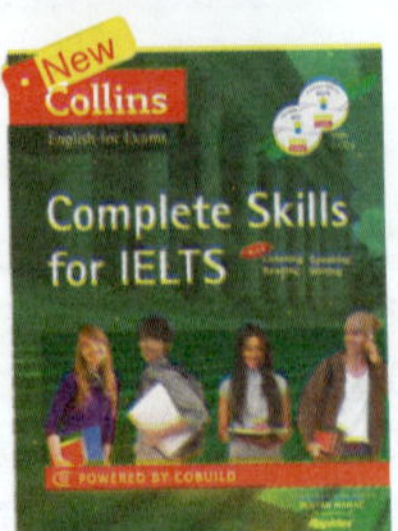

HC005 • Rs. 540/-

This Library is must for every student of a **School** or a **College**

Also equally useful for everyone else

Price: ₹ 600/-
Contains 4 books of ₹ 150/- each

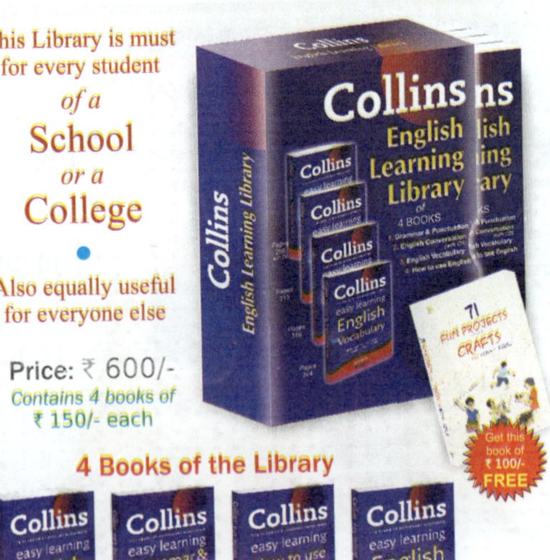

4 Books of the Library

- ₹ 150/- Page 256 (with CD) English Conversation
- ₹ 150/- Page 310 Grammar & Punctuation
- ₹ 150/- Page 316 How to use English
- ₹ 150/- Page 344 English Vocabulary

Sherlock Holmes

30 Stories in 5 Books

Price
₹ 495/-
(₹ 99/- each)

Pages each vol.
220 - 232

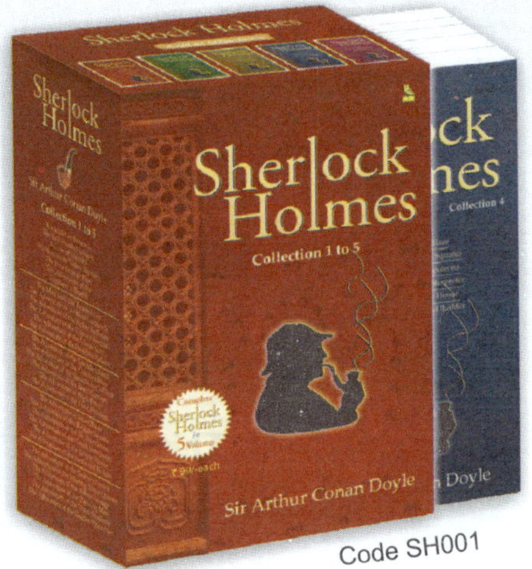

Code SH001

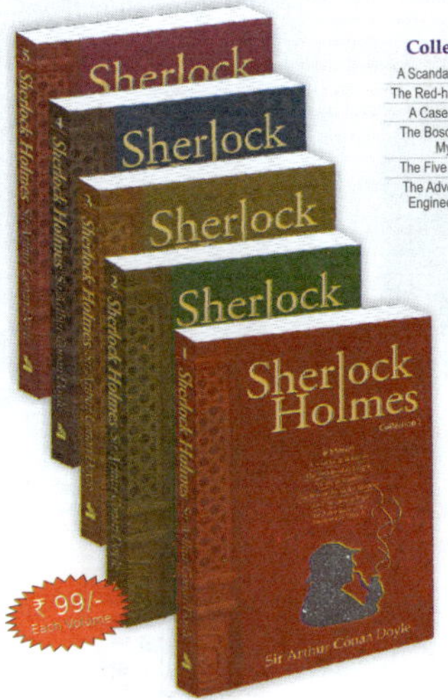

Collection 1
- A Scandal in Bohemia
- The Red-headed League
- A Case of Identity
- The Boscombe Valley Mystery
- The Five Orange Pips
- The Adventure of the Engineer's Thumb

Collection 2
- The Man with the Twisted Lip
- The Adventure of the Blue Carbuncle
- The Adventure of the Noble Bachelor
- The Adventure of the Copper Beeches
- The Adventure of the Gloria Scott
- The Adventure of the Resident Patient

Collection 3
- The Adventure of the Speckled Band
- The Adventure of the Crooked Man
- The Adventure of the Stockbroker's Clerk
- The Adventure of the Beryl Coronet
- The Adventure of Black Peter
- The Adventure of the Final Problem

Collection 4
- The Adventure of Silver Blaze
- The Adventure of the Reigate Squares
- The Adventure of the Six Napoleons
- The Adventure of the Greek Interpreter
- The Adventure of the Empty House
- The Adventure of the Norwood Builder

Collection 5
- The Adventure of the Solitary Cyclist
- The Adventure of the Missing Three-Quarter
- The Adventure of the Abbey Grange
- The Adventure of the Dancing Men
- The Adventure of the Three Students
- The Adventure of the Golden Pince-Nez

William Shakespeare

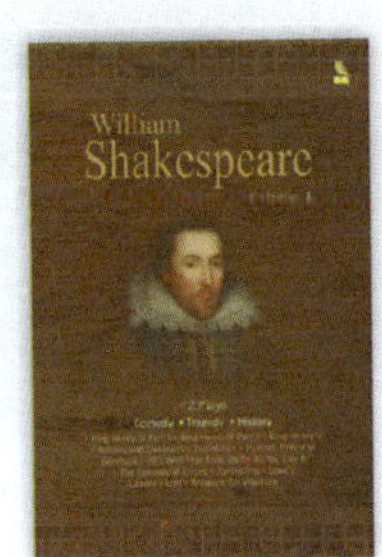

9791 C • ₹ 99/-

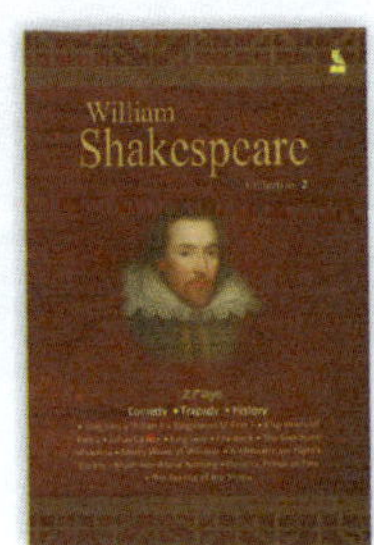

9792 D • ₹ 99/-

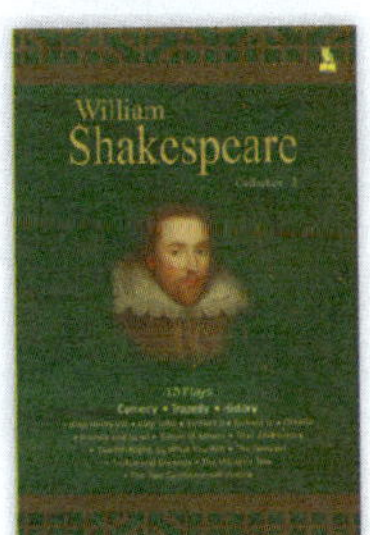

9793 E • ₹ 99/-

37 Plays in 3 Books

Price
₹ 297/-
(₹ 99/- each)

Pages each vol.
190 - 210

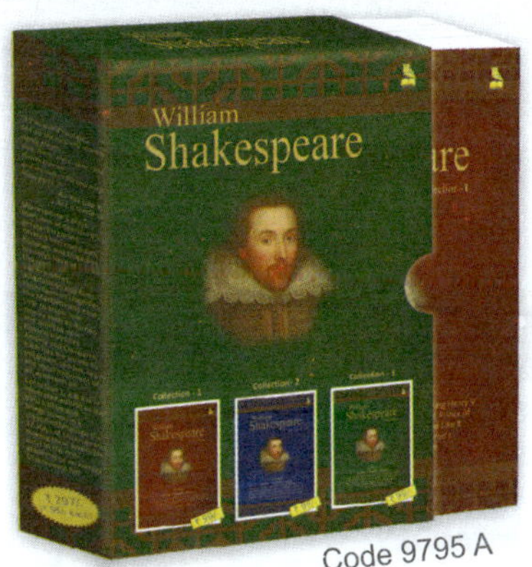

Code 9795 A

Munshi Premchand

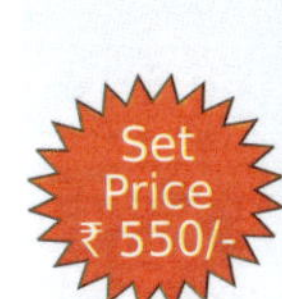

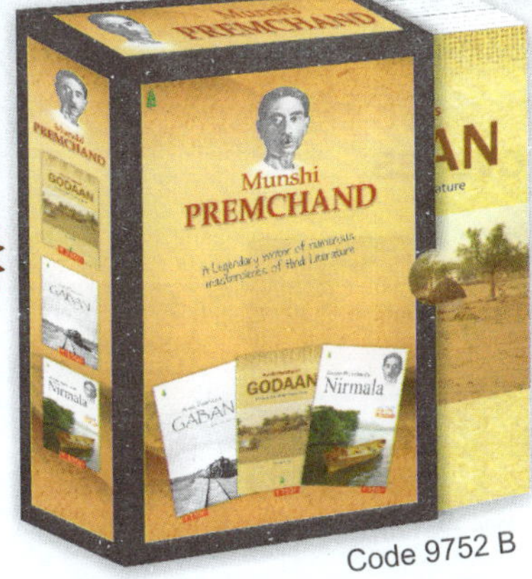

Code 9752 B

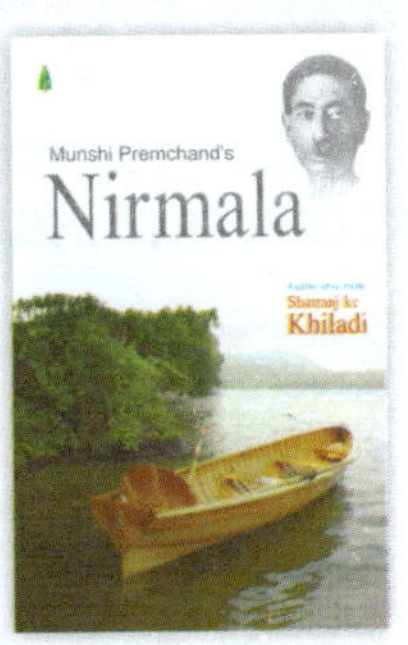

9820 H • ₹ 150/-
Pages 208

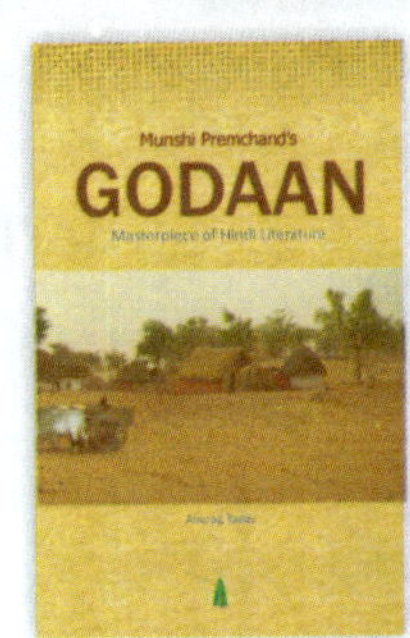

9512 D • ₹ 250/-
Pages 352

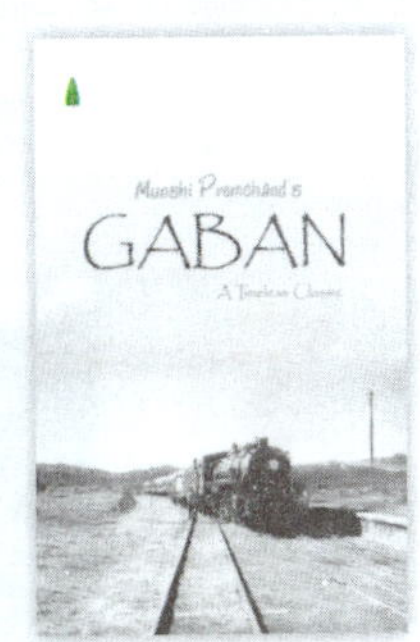

9592 H • ₹ 150/-
Pages 272

PERSONALITY DEVELOPMENT

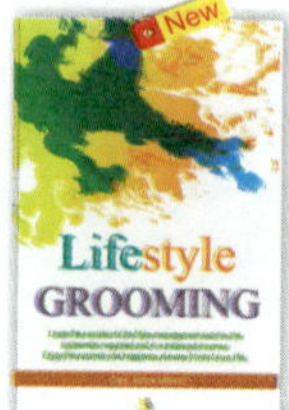

9450 B • Rs. 195/-

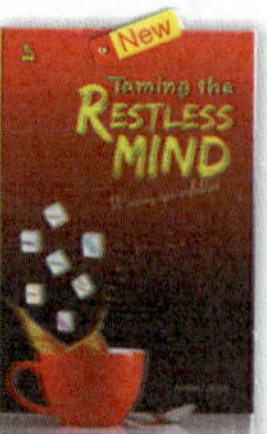

9487 E • Rs. 150/-

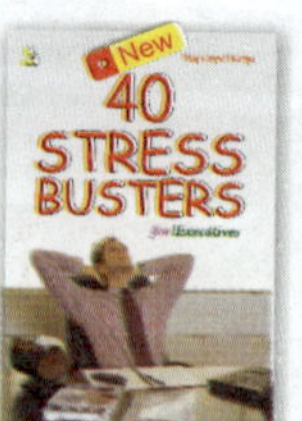

9466 T • Rs. 96/-

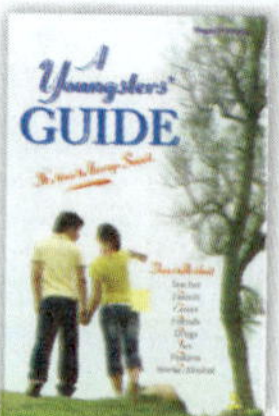

5639 B • Rs. 80/-

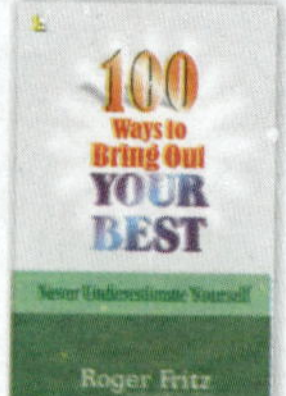

5641 A • Rs. 150/-

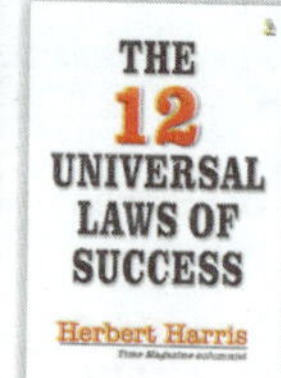

9088 C • Rs. 195/-

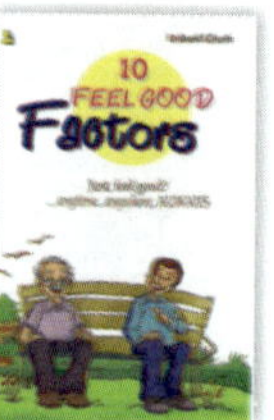

9973 B • Rs. 110/-

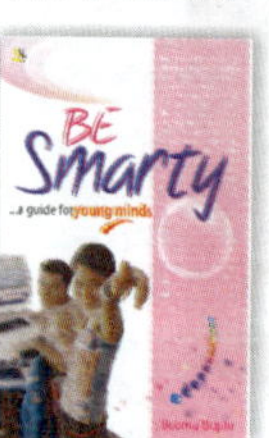

9981 B • Rs. 96/-

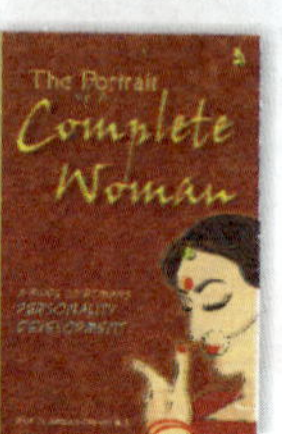

8868 D • Rs. 120/-

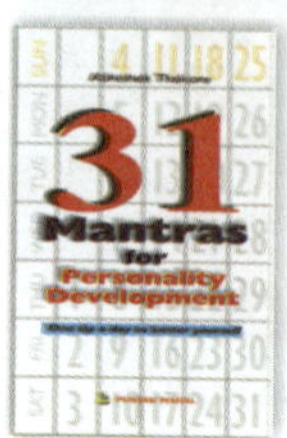

8966 E • Rs. 100/- T

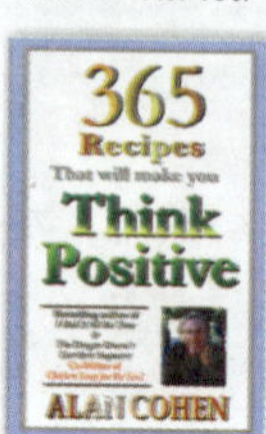

9070 B • Rs. 175/-

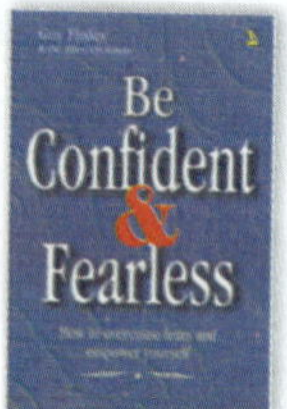

9028 D • Rs. 120/-

STUDENT DEVELOPMENT

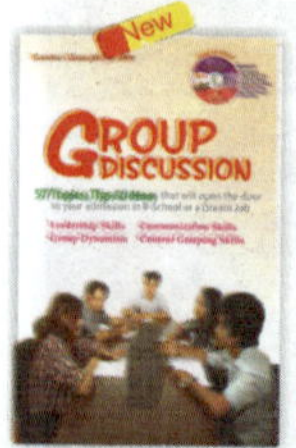

97540 D • Rs. 175/-

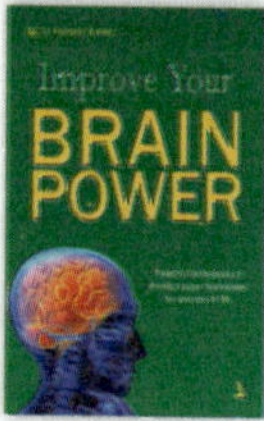

9071 D • Rs. 120/-

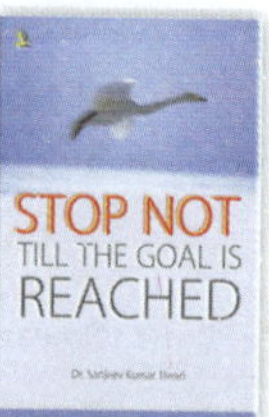

9455 C • Rs. 150/-

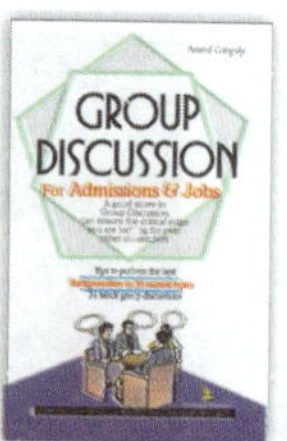

5622 A • Rs. 108/-

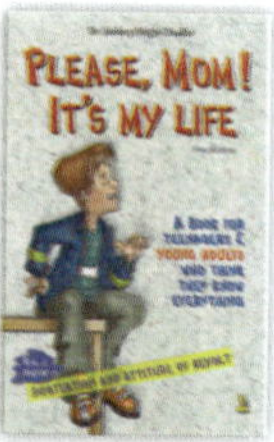

9967 C • Rs. 120/-

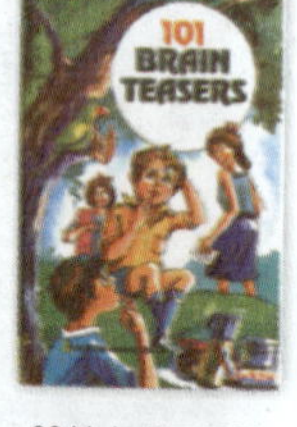

2241 J • Rs. 100/-

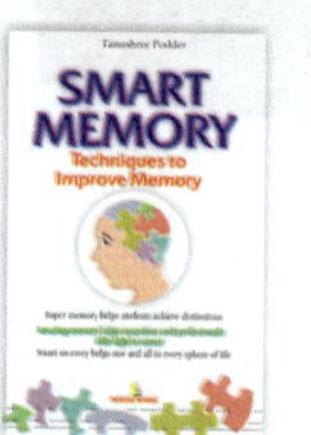

8962 A • Rs. 96/-

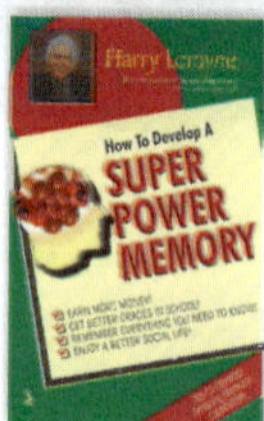

9089 D • Rs. 135/-

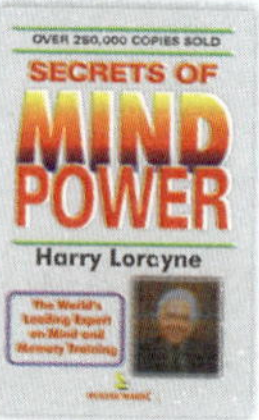

4016 D • Rs. 120/-

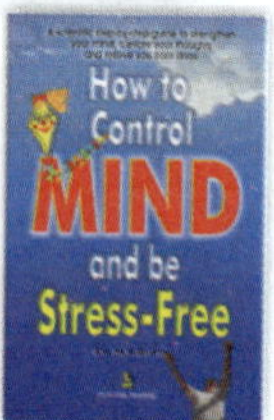

4009 K • Rs. 96/-

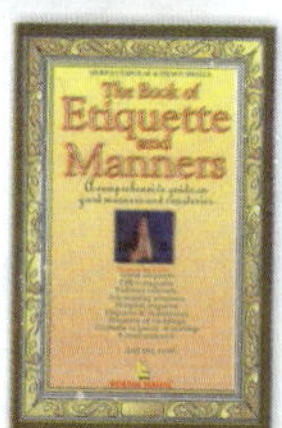

8997 B • Rs. 120/-

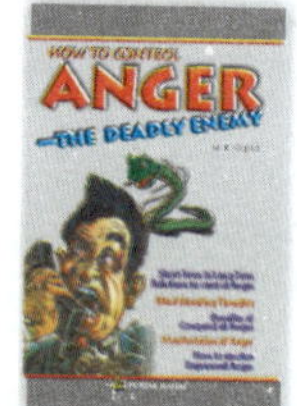

4010 L • Rs. 100/-

SAYING/QUOTATIONS/PROVERBS

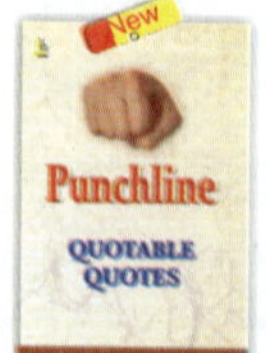

9474 F • Rs. 150/-

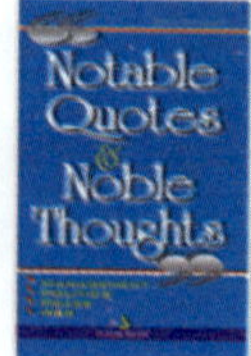

9953 A • Rs. 100/-

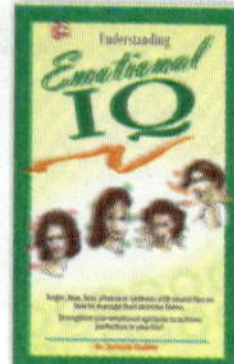

8947 E • Rs. 100/-

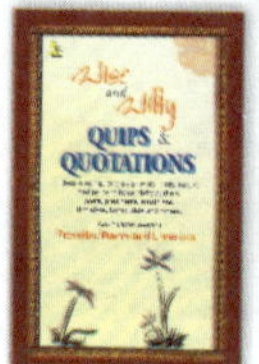

8999 D • Rs. 80/-

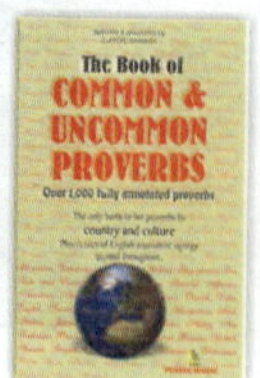

5512 A • Rs. 120/-

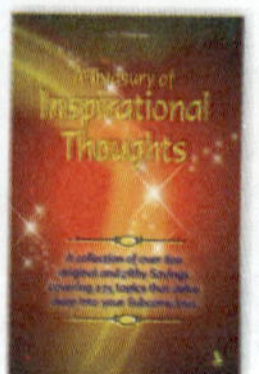

8963 B • Rs. 80/-

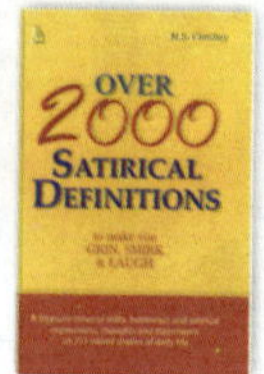

8890 D • Rs. 150/-

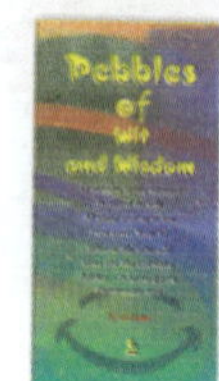

9925 A • Rs. 60/-

Rapidex Picture & Children's Dictionary

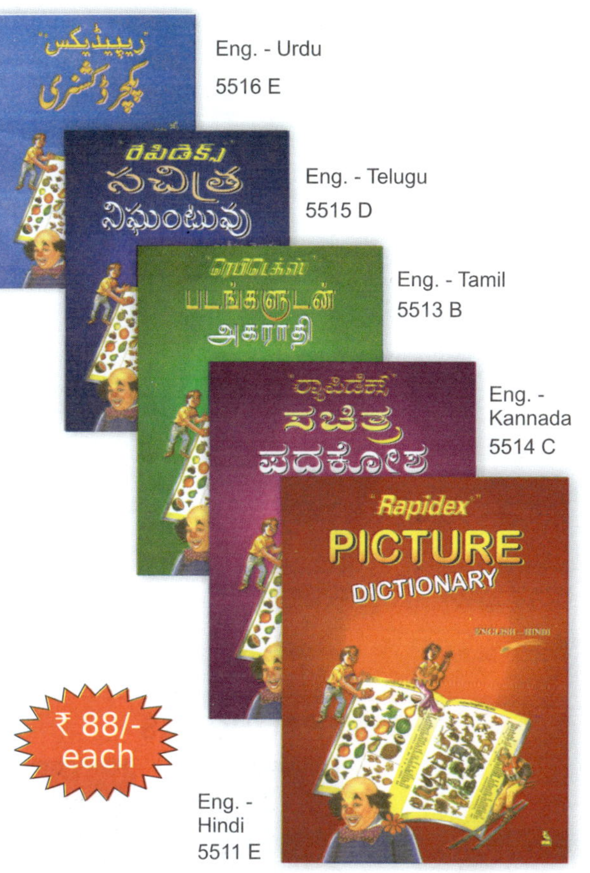

Eng. - Urdu
5516 E

Eng. - Telugu
5515 D

Eng. - Tamil
5513 B

Eng. - Kannada
5514 C

Eng. - Hindi
5511 E

₹ 88/- each

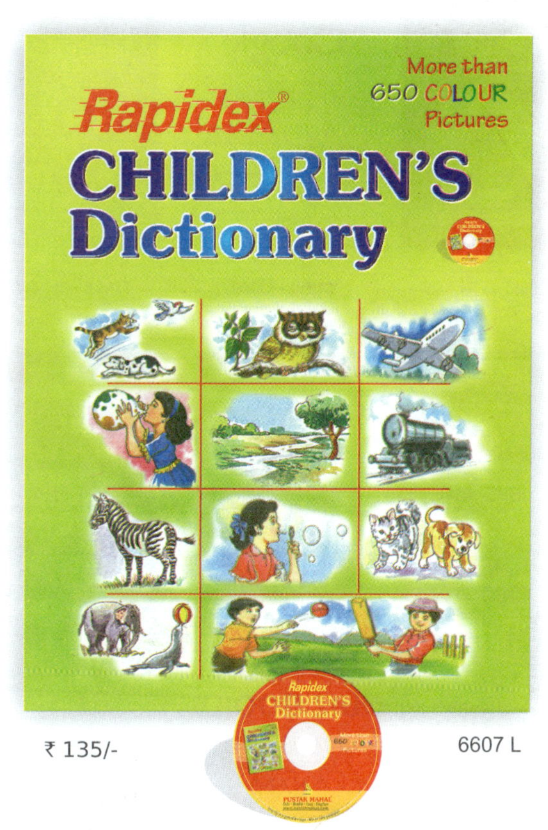

₹ 135/-

6607 L

New Releases

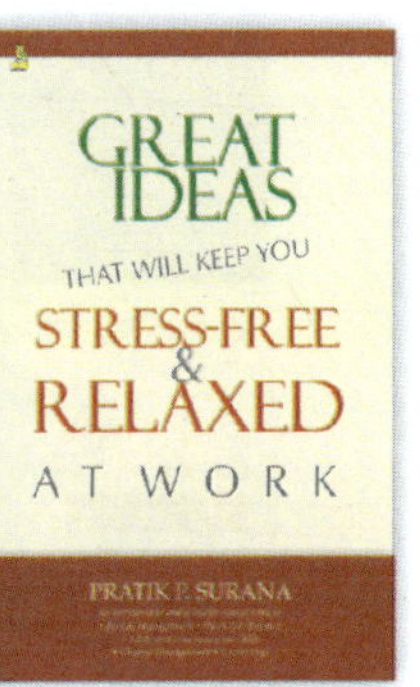

9786 M ₹ 195/-

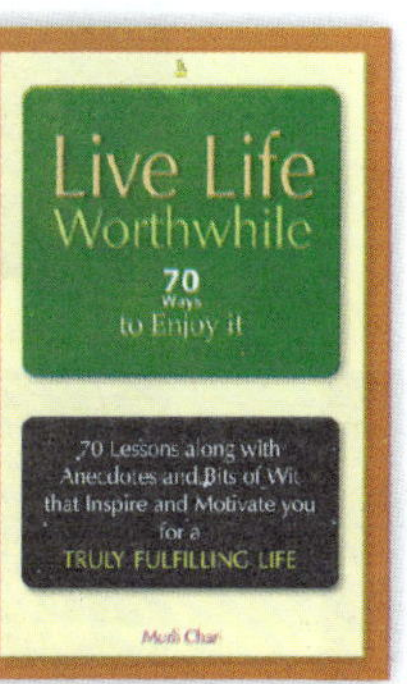

9788 R ₹ 195/-

BACK TO SCHOOL @30

9783 H ₹ 150/-

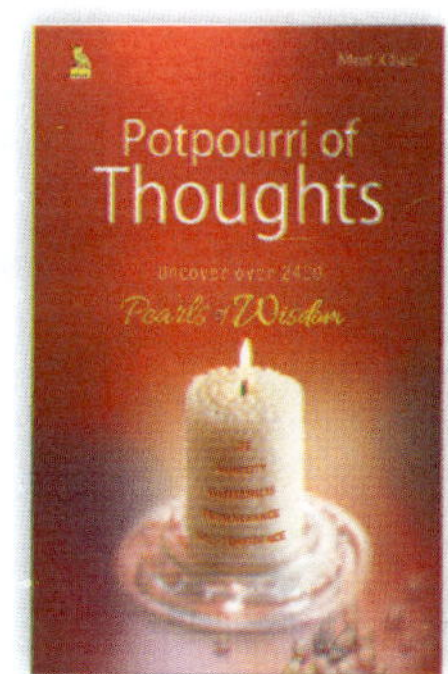

9789 A ₹ 150/-

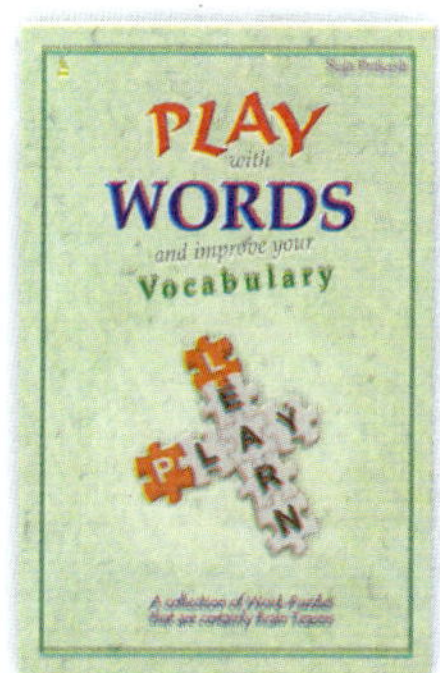

9787 P ₹ 100/-

COMPUTERS

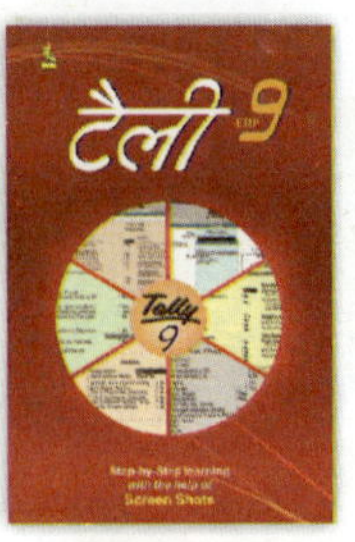

9651 A • Rs. 140/-

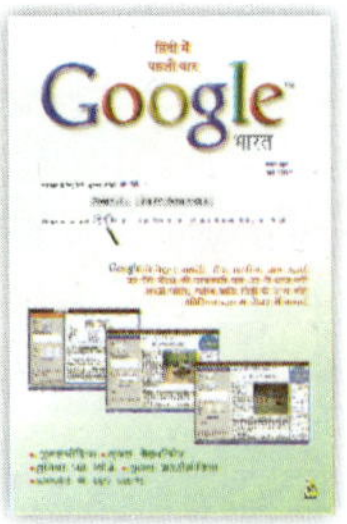

9460 J • Rs. 96/-

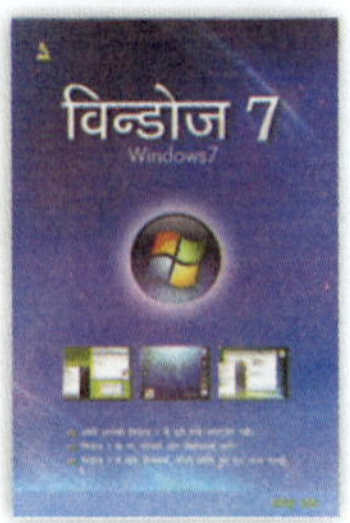

7765 B • Rs. 96/-

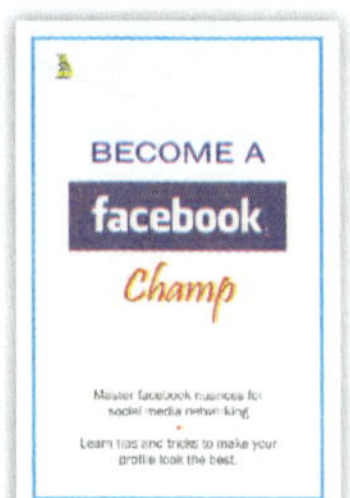

7764 A • Rs. 120/-

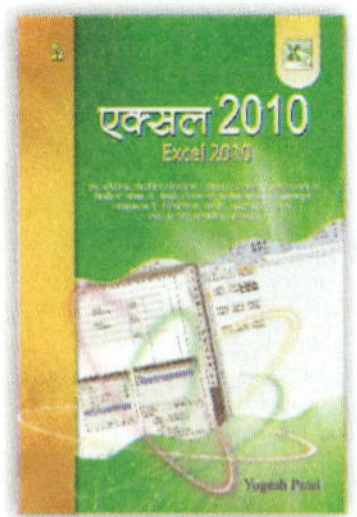

9478 K • Rs. 140/-

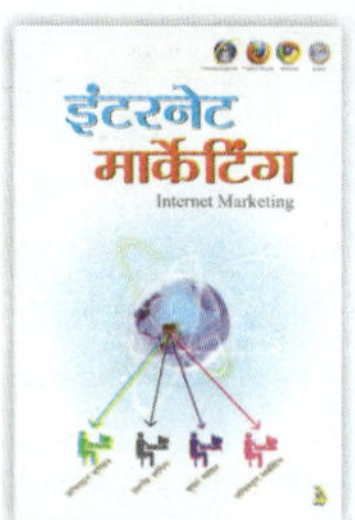

9823 B • Rs. 96/-

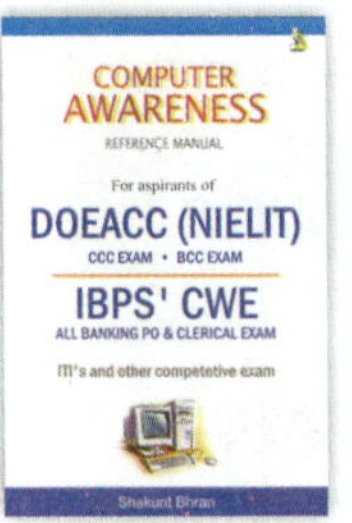

9768 C • Rs. 175/-

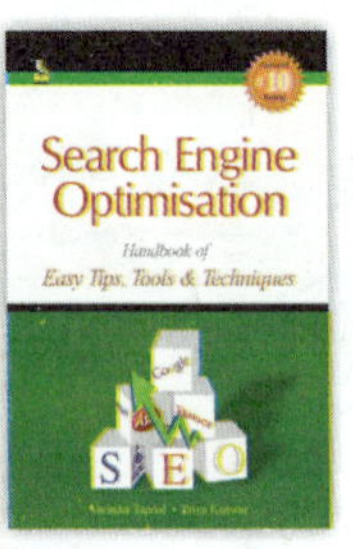

7766 A • Rs. 120/-

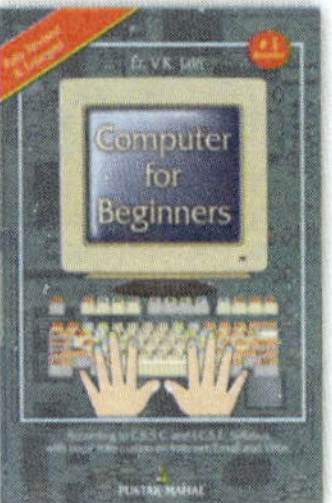

7711 J • Rs. 120/-

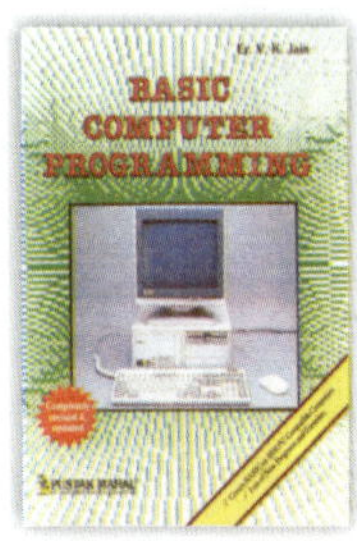

7712 K • Rs. 80/-

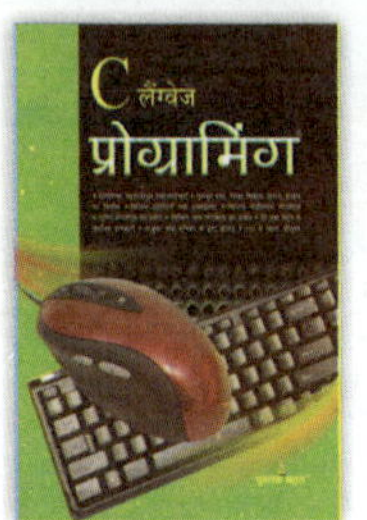

7797 C • Rs. 250/-

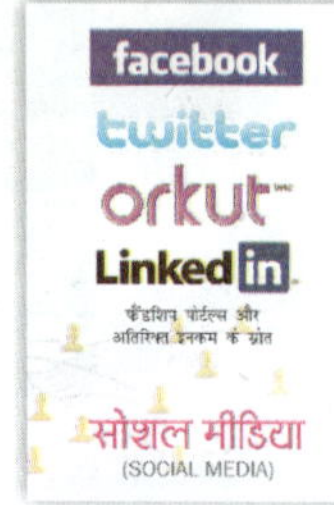

9460 J • Rs. 120/-

QUIZ BOOKS

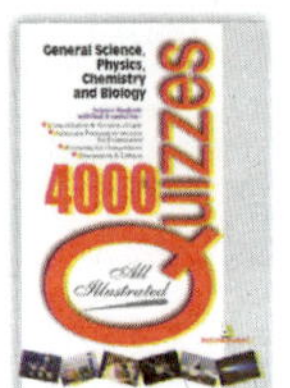

8965 D • Rs. 120/-

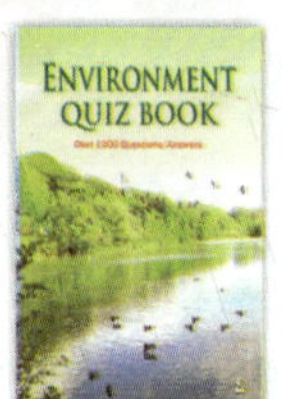

7726 K • Rs. 100/-

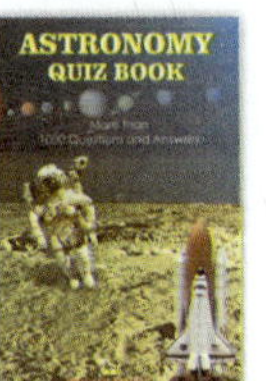

7727 L • Rs. 80/-

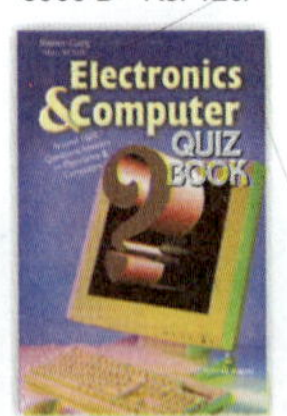

7723 F • Rs. 100/-

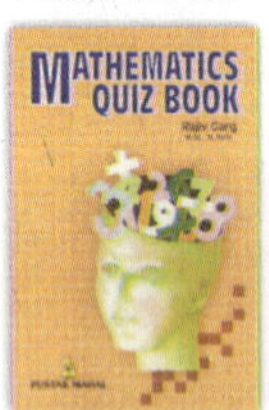

7722 E • Rs. 100/-

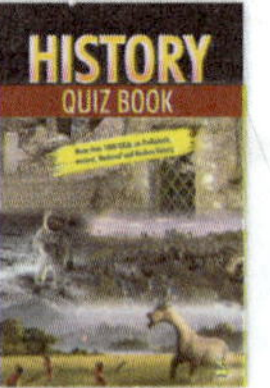

7753 G • Rs. 100/-

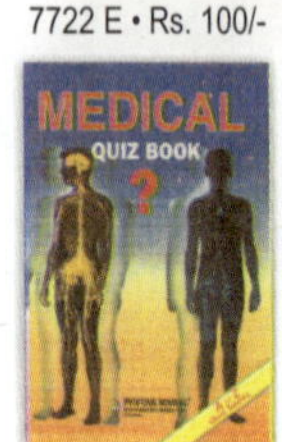

7725 B • Rs. 100/-

GENERAL BOOKS

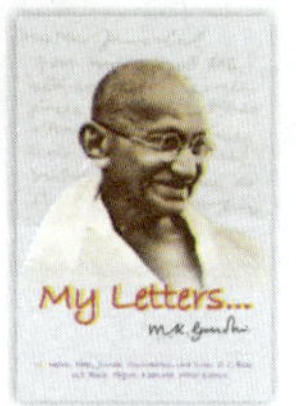

9532 D • ₹ 250/- HB

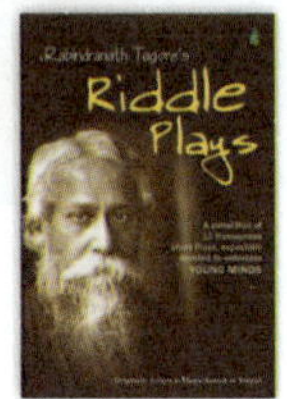

8526 B • ₹ 125/-

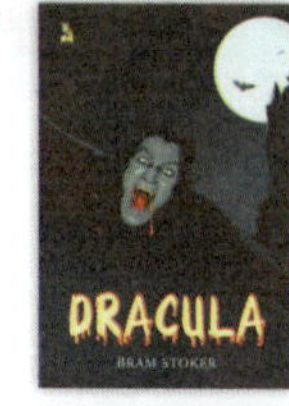

9767 B • ₹ 150/-

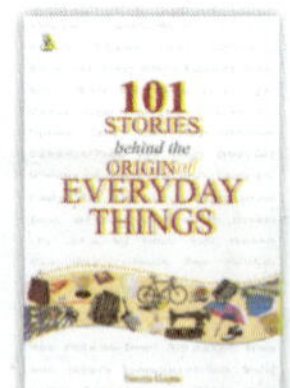

5114 B • Rs. 68/-

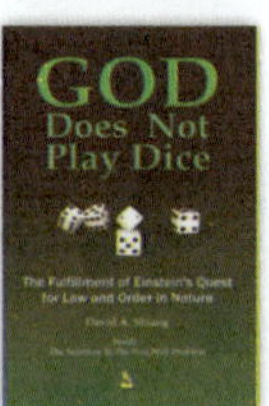

4175 A • Rs. 195/-

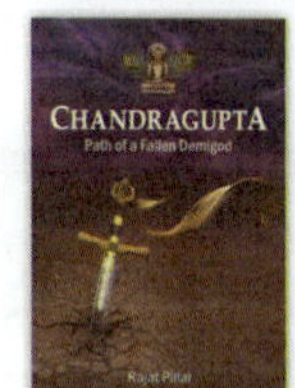

9821 K • Rs. 175/-

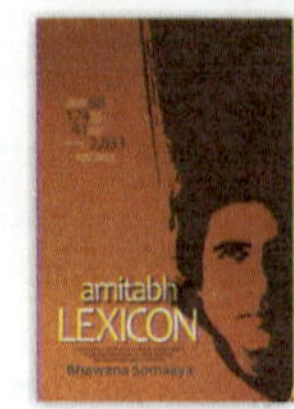

9459 H • Rs. 1000/- (HB)

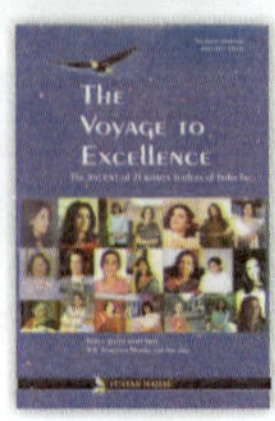

9041 A • Rs. 195/-

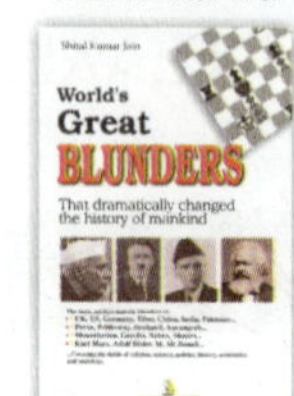

4022 D • Rs. 80/-

SELF-IMPROVEMENT

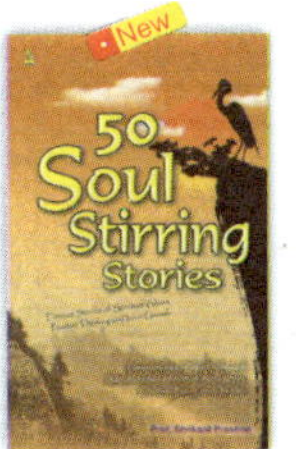

9491 J • Rs. 100/-

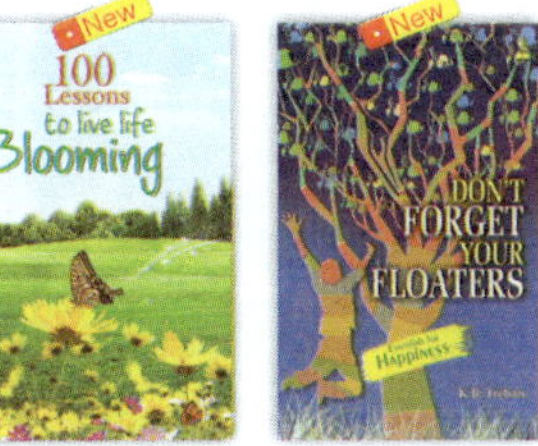

9498 C • Rs. 180/-

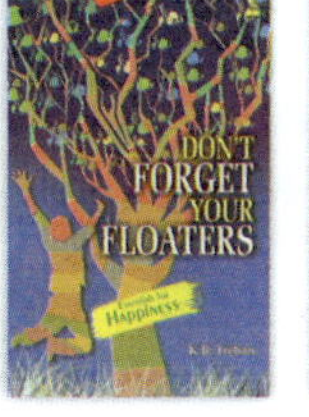

9490 H • Rs. 175/-

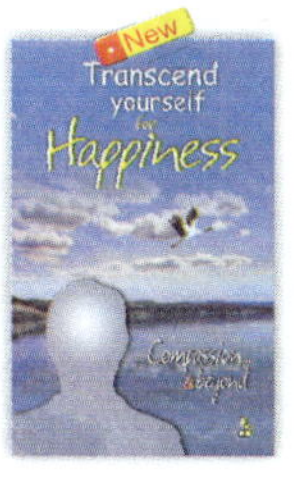

9464 R • Rs. 80/-

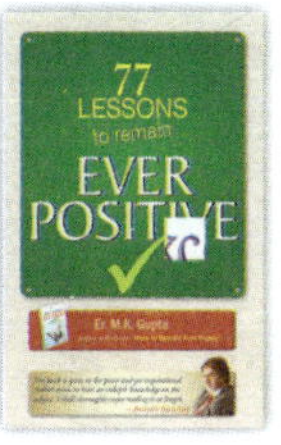

9096 B • Rs. 120/-

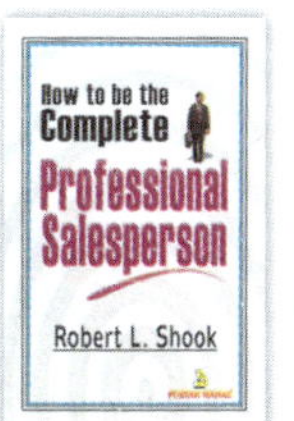

5614 E • Rs. 150/-

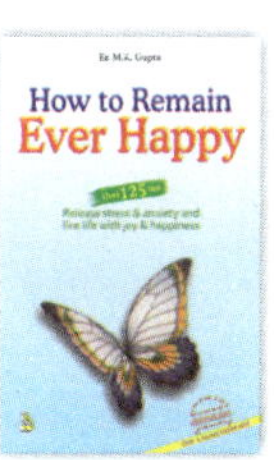

4008 J • Rs. 120/-

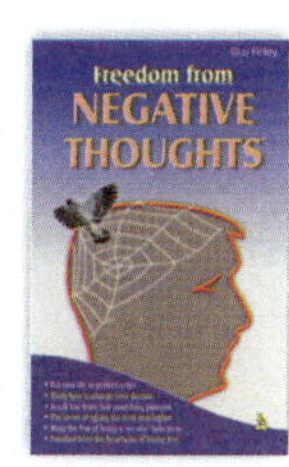

9026 D • Rs. 120/-

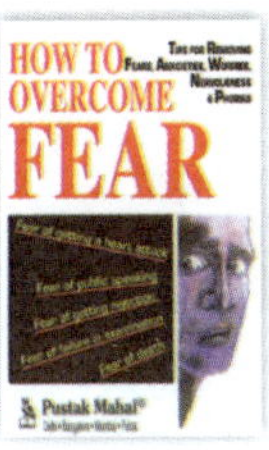

8885 D • Rs. 80/-

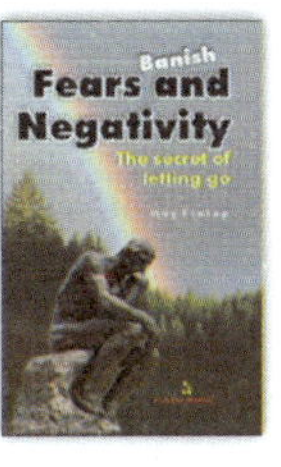

9027 D • Rs. 120/-

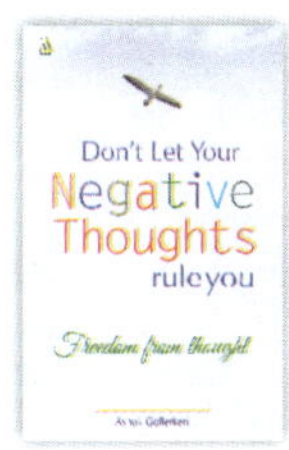

9081 D • Rs. 150/-

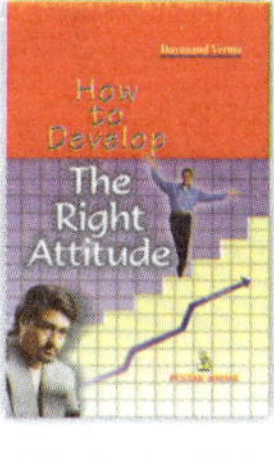

9091 B • Rs. 120/-

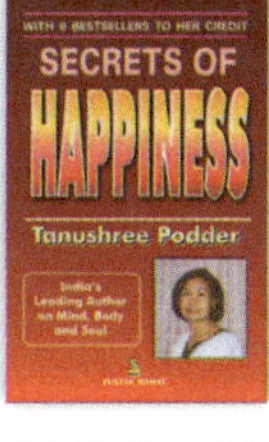

9060 B • Rs. 120/-

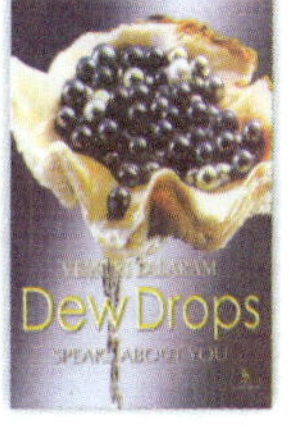

9969 A • Rs. 96/-

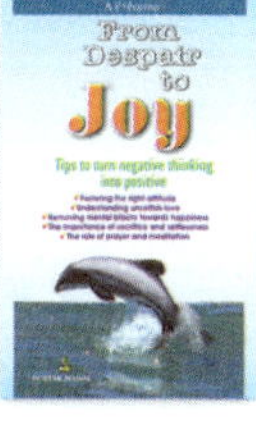

8928 D • Rs. 80/-

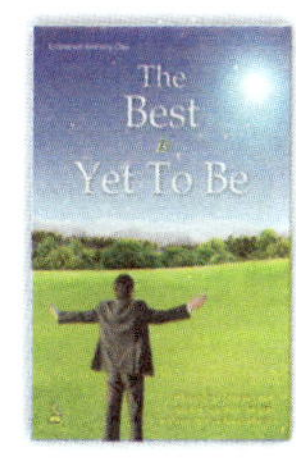

9449 A • Rs. 195/-

MANAGEMENT/JOB/CARRIER/BUSINESS & PROFESSION

All Time Bestsellers

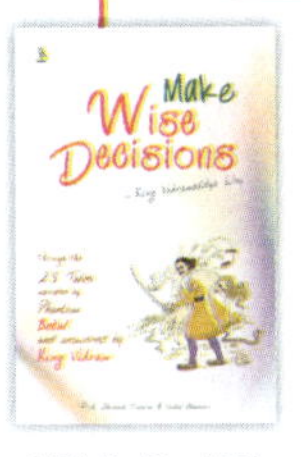

9461 K • Rs. 135/-

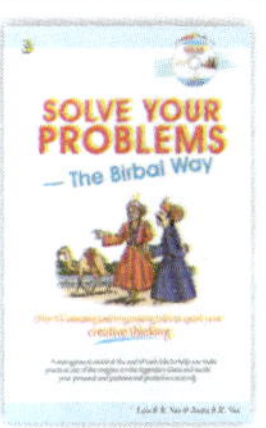

5338 A • Rs. 135/- with CD

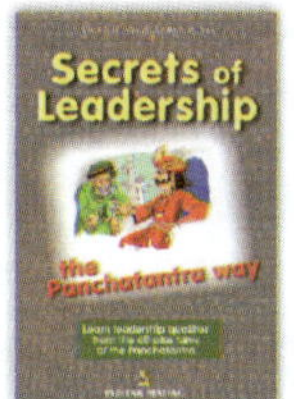

8979 A • Rs. 96/-

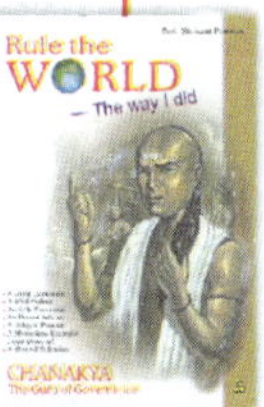

9406 B • Rs. 150/-

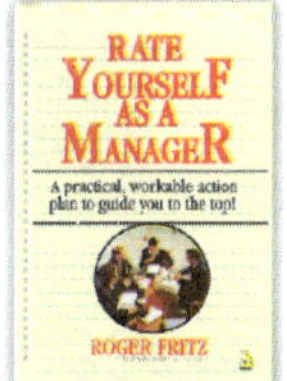

5441 D • Rs. 195/-

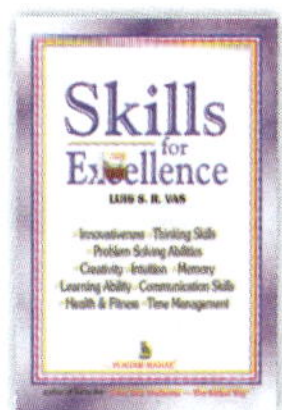

8883 D • Rs. 120/-

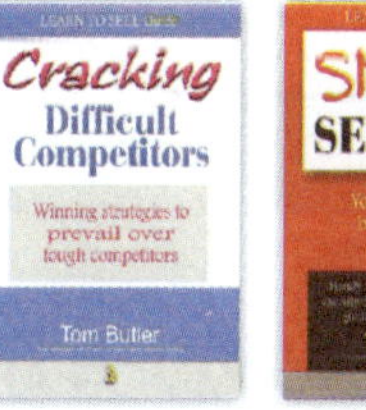

9402 B • Rs. 195/-

3403 C • Rs. 195/-

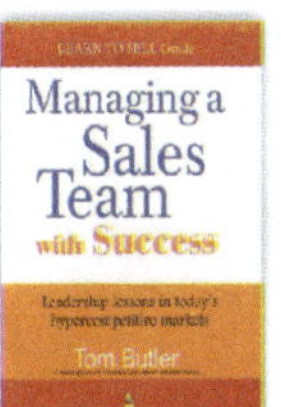

9404 D • Rs. 195/-

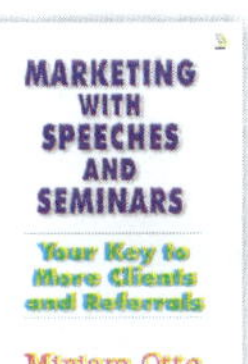

9313 D • Rs. 150/-

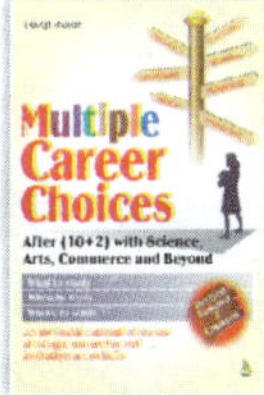

5623 B • Rs. 195/-

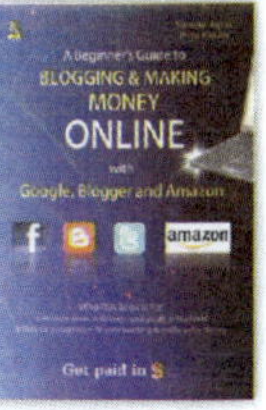

9439 L • Rs. 150/-

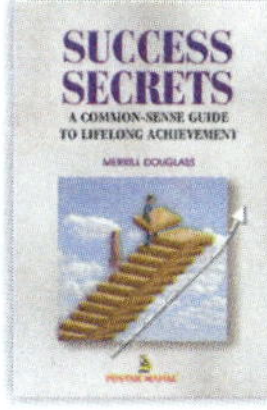

4017 D • Rs. 120/-

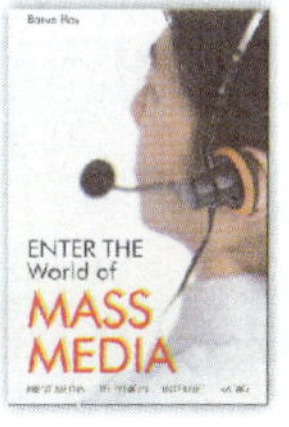

9431 C • Rs. 175/-

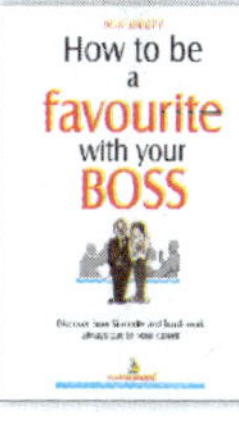

4004 D • Rs. 88/-

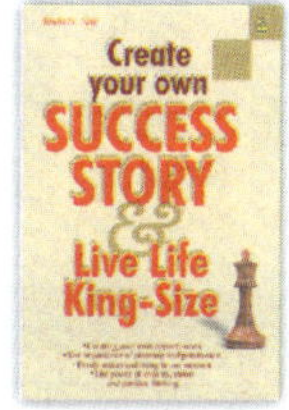

8990 C • Rs. 96/-

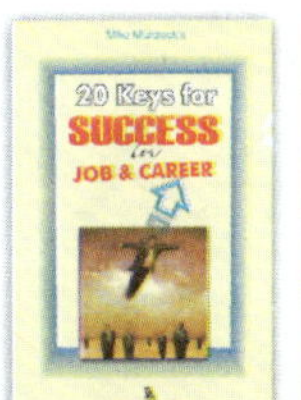

4018 D • Rs. 80/-

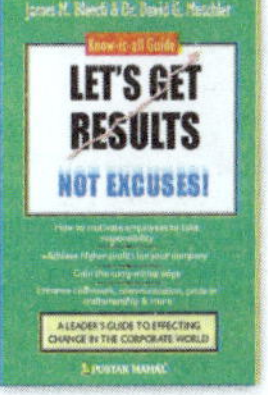

9079 B • Rs. 195/-

5618 D • Rs. 120/-

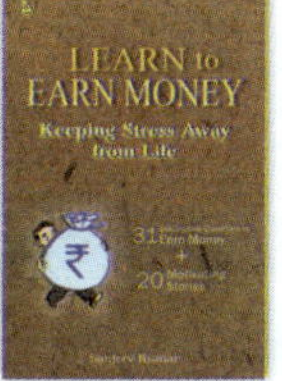

5640 C • Rs. 120/-

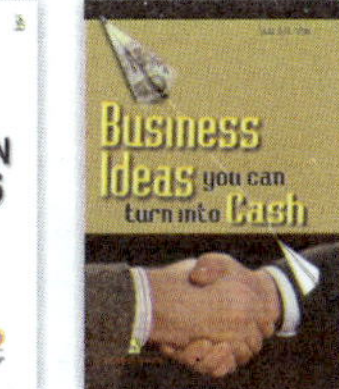

5615 D • Rs. 150/-

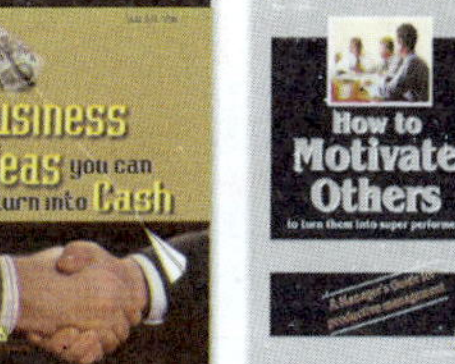

8972 C • Rs. 80/-

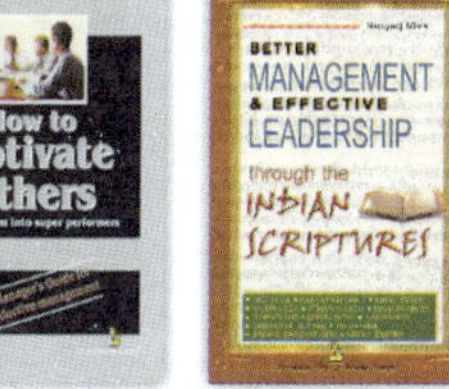

4001 A • Rs. 150/-

5646 A • Rs. 225/-

ALTERNATIVE THERAPIES

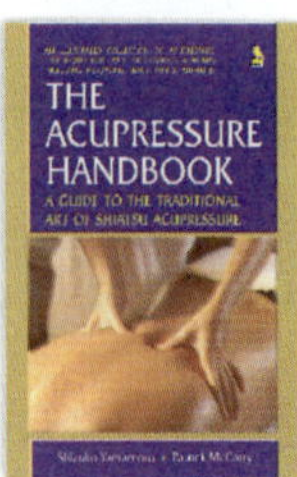

8882 F • Rs. 180/-

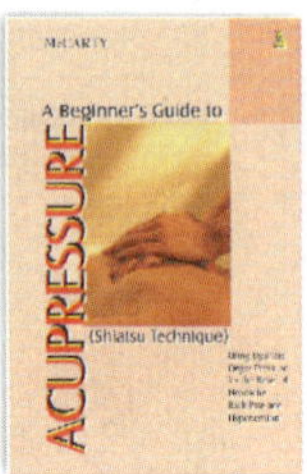

8879 C • Rs. 60/-

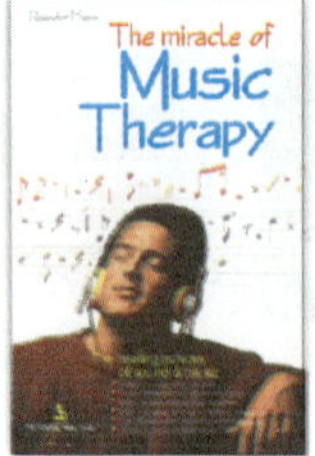

8983 E • Rs. 100/-

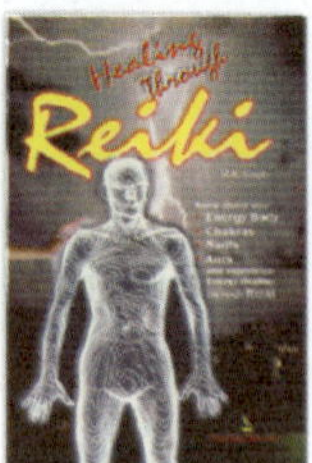

8842 D • Rs. 100/-

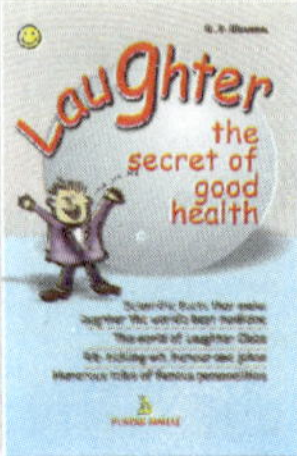

2317 E • Rs. 60/-

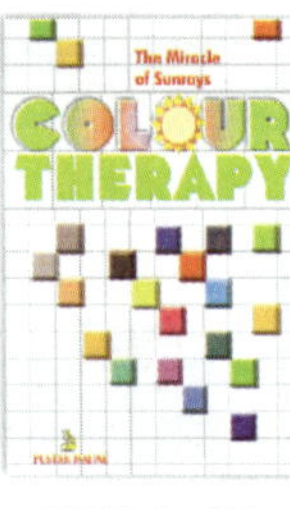

8889 D • Rs. 80/-

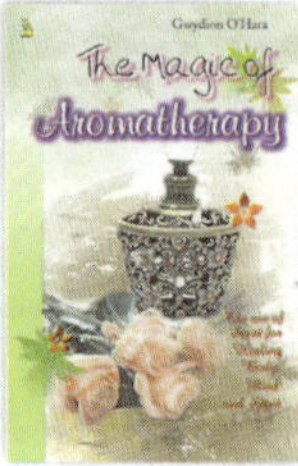

8836 D • Rs. 135/-

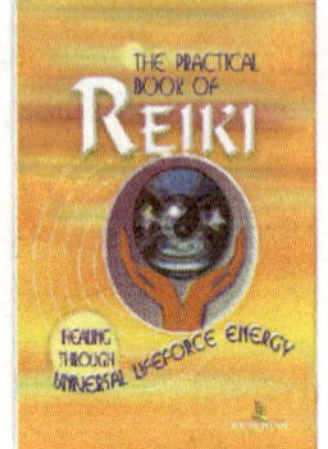

9935 F • Rs. 120/-

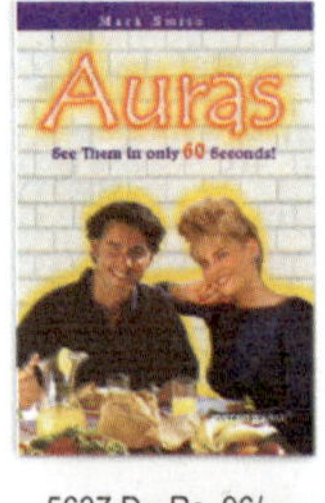

5637 D • Rs. 96/-

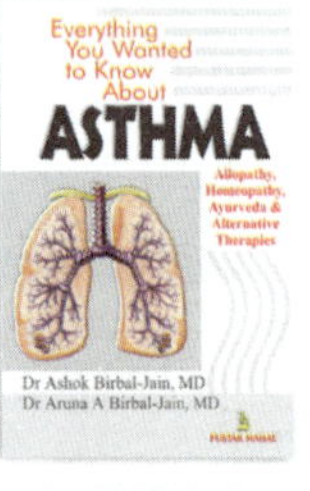

8281 A • Rs. 80/-

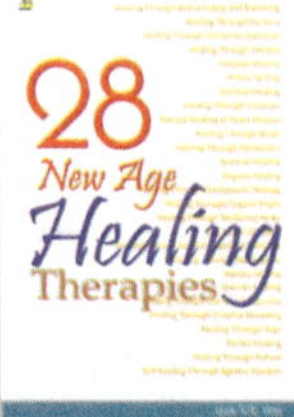

9950 B • Rs. 120/-

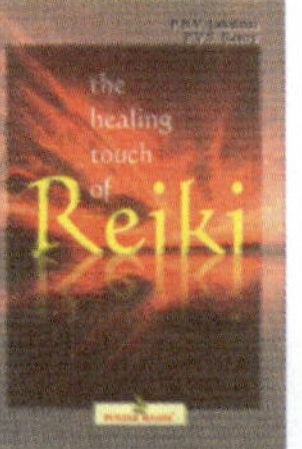

8941 A • Rs. 80/-

GENERAL HEALTH

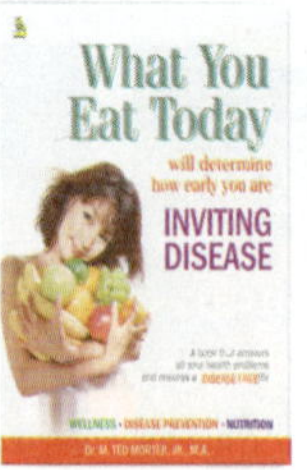

9075 C • Rs. 225/-

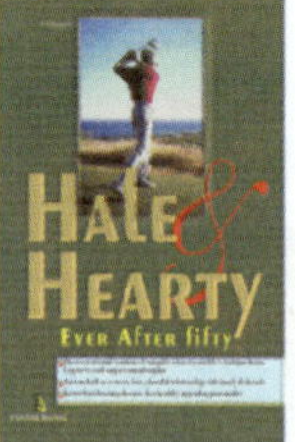

8939 D • Rs. 88/-

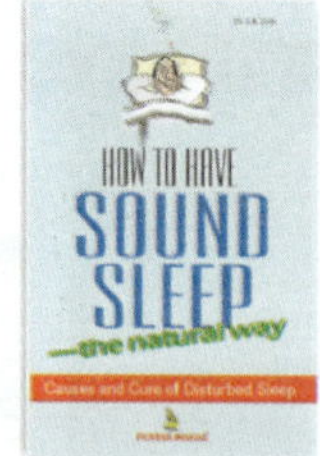

9039 D • Rs. 68/-

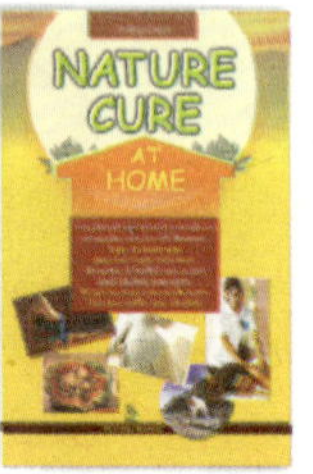

8859 G • Rs. 80/-

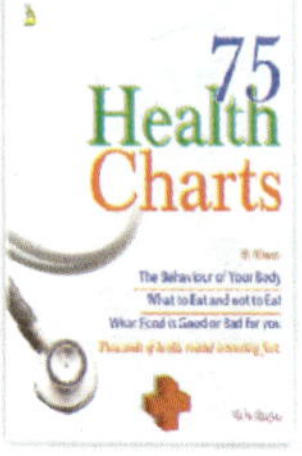

8877 A • Rs. 120/-

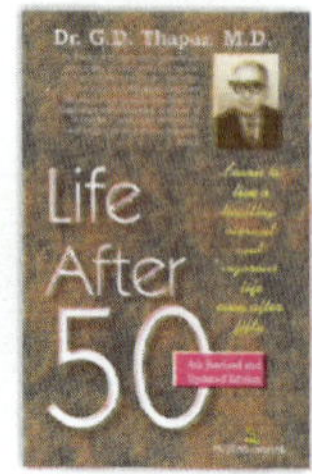

9940 D • Rs. 150/-

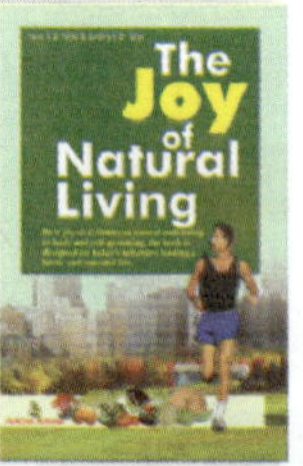

8948 A • Rs. 96/-

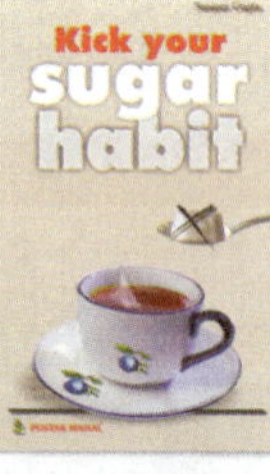

9038 A • Rs. 68/-

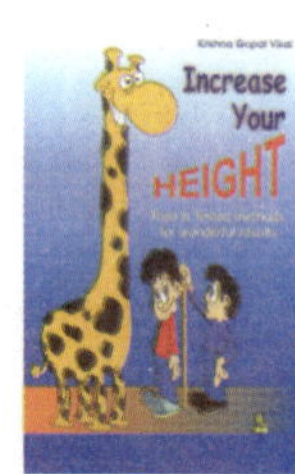

8847 M • Rs. 100/-

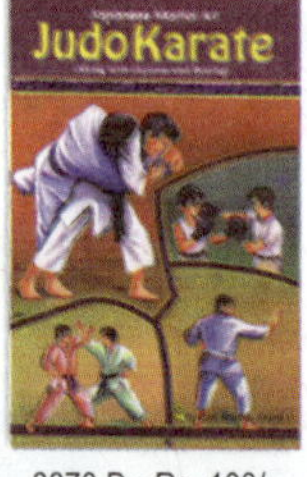

8870 D • Rs. 100/-

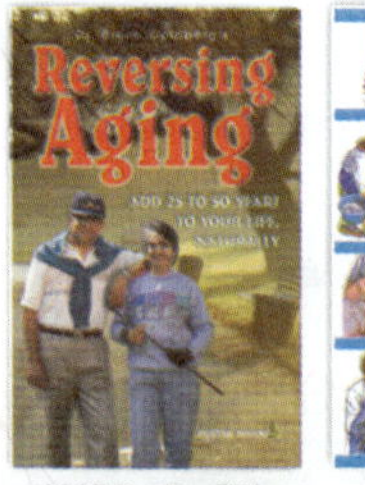

9025 D • Rs. 80/-

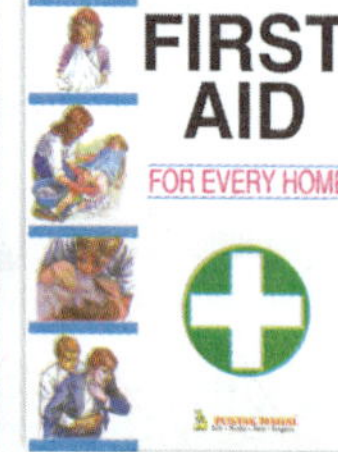

9902 F • Rs. 120/-

COMMON AILMENTS & DISEASES

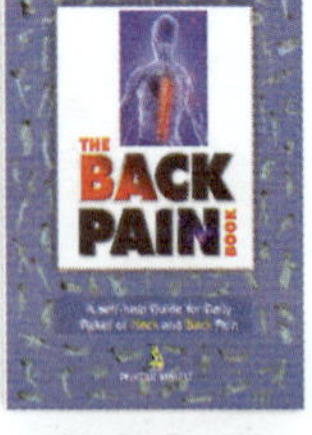

8891 D • Rs. 120/-

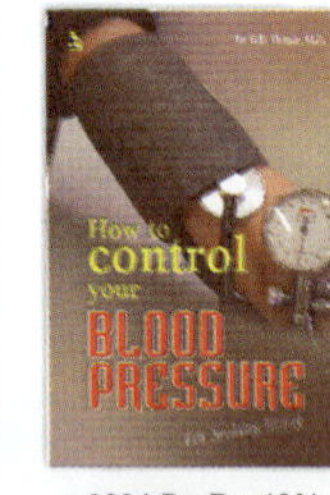

8094 D • Rs. 120/-

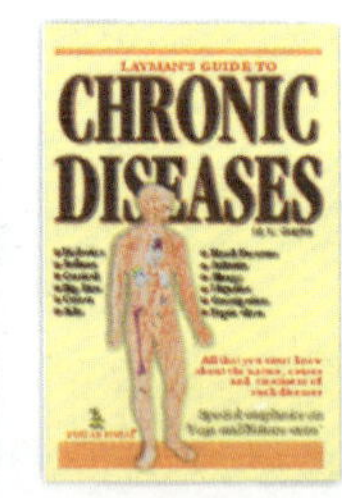

8848 D • Rs. 96/-

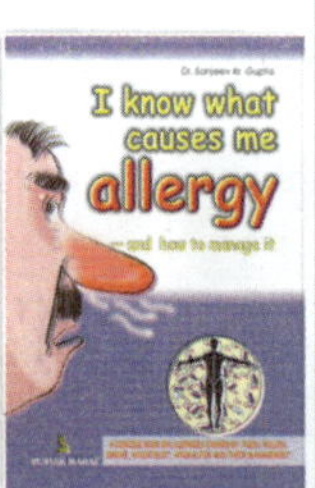

8915 D • Rs. 40/-

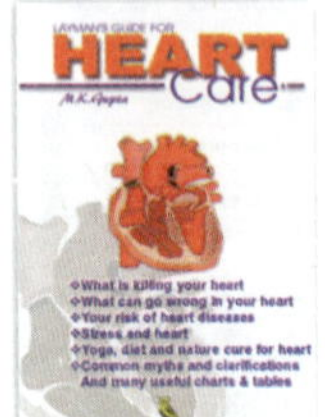

8888 D • Rs. 96/-

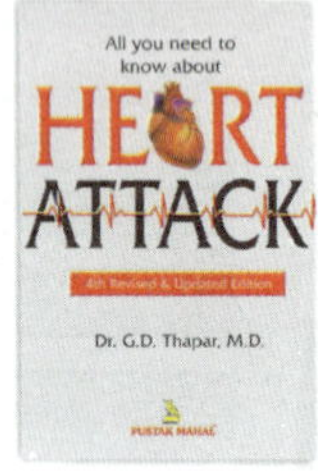

8908 D • Rs. 120/-

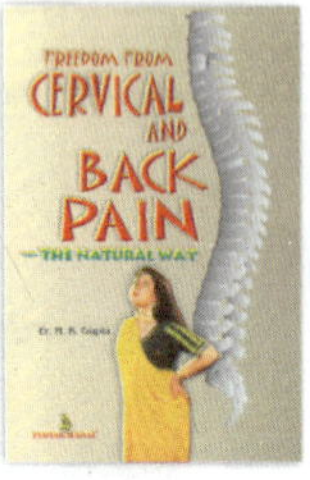

8878 B • Rs. 80/-

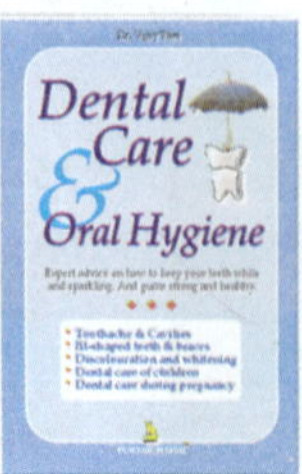

8964 C • Rs. 96/-

SLIMMING & FITNESS

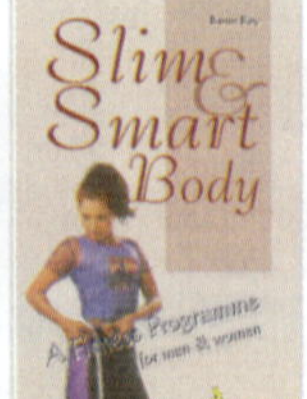

8277 B • Rs. 120/-

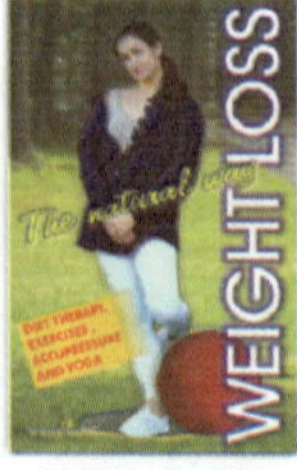

8875 K • Rs. 120/-

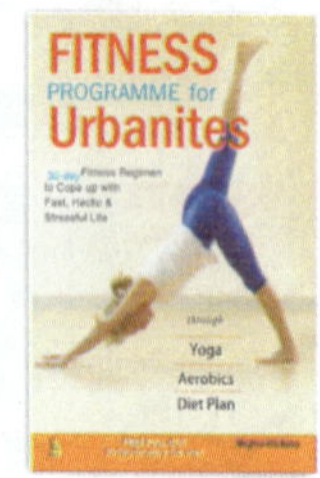

9445 A • Rs. 150/-

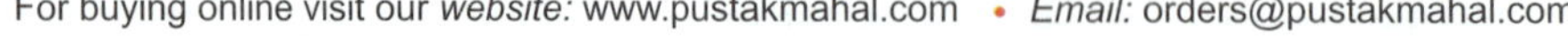

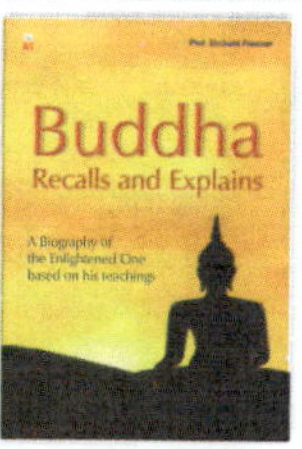

9770 E • Rs. 150/-

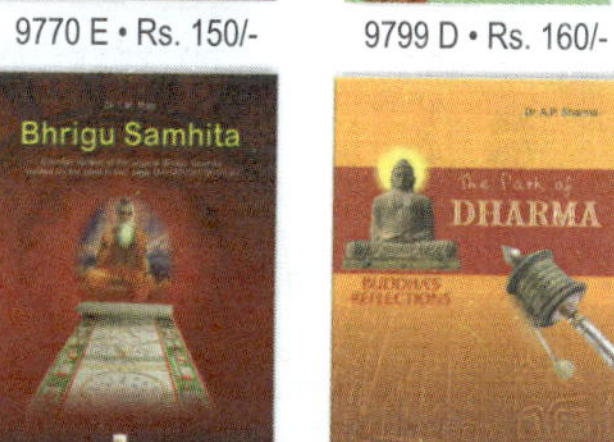

9799 D • Rs. 160/-

9453 A • Rs. 195/-

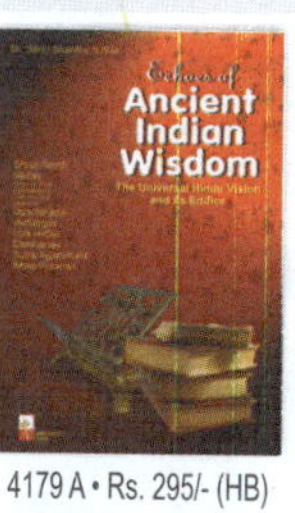

4179 A • Rs. 295/- (HB)

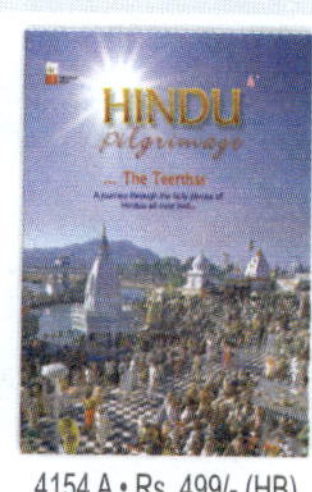

4154 A • Rs. 499/- (HB)

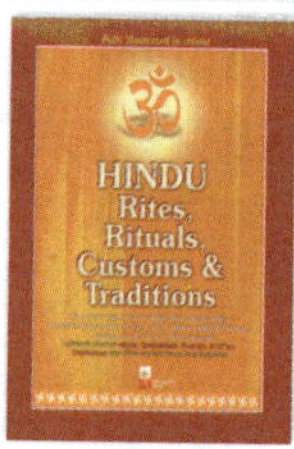

4128 D • Rs. 250/- (HB)

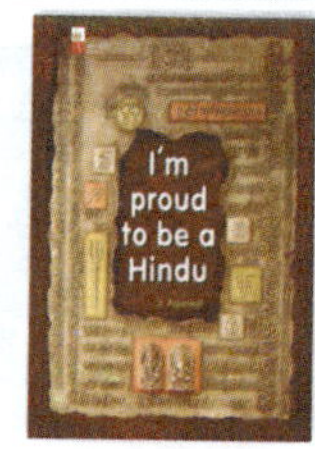

4181 C • Rs. 195/-

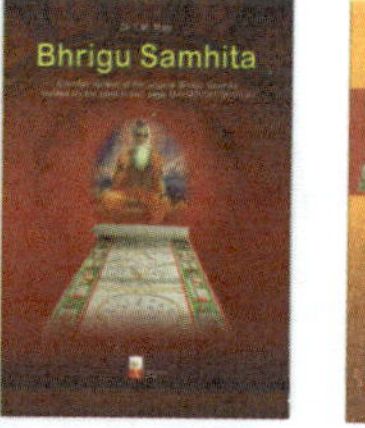

4177 B • Rs. 195/-

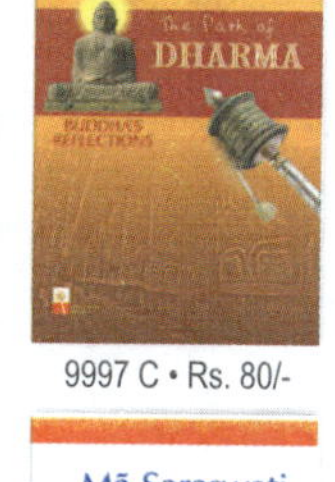

9997 C • Rs. 80/-

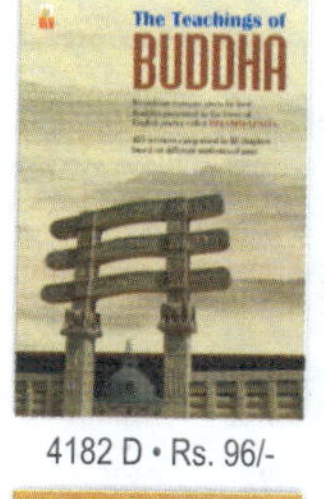
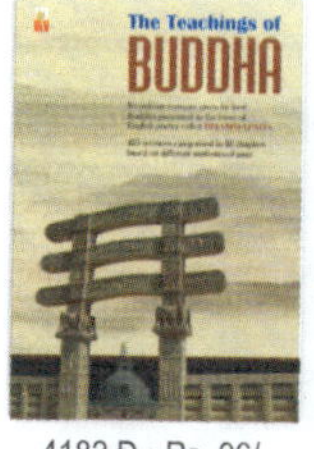

4182 D • Rs. 96/-

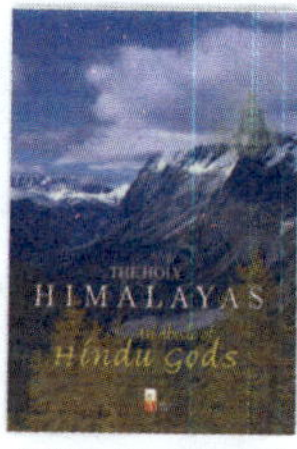

9984 E • Rs. 399/- (HB)

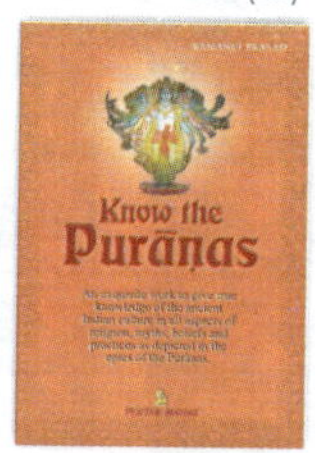

4130 B • Rs. 120/-

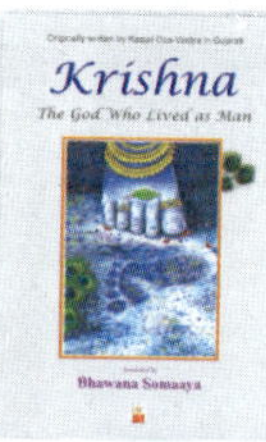

4183 A • Rs. 350/- (HB)

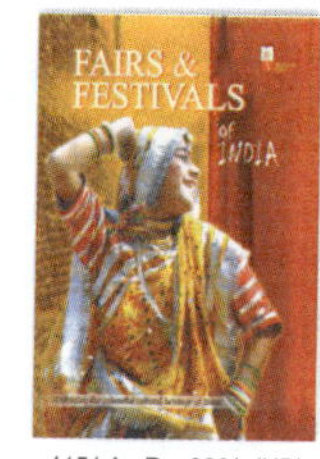

4151 A • Rs. 399/- (HB)

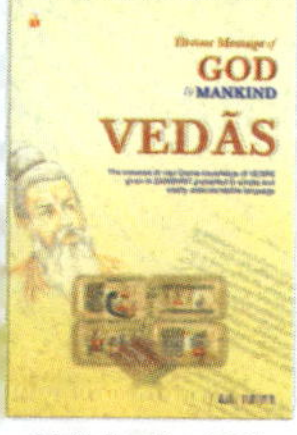

9811 P • Rs. 120/-

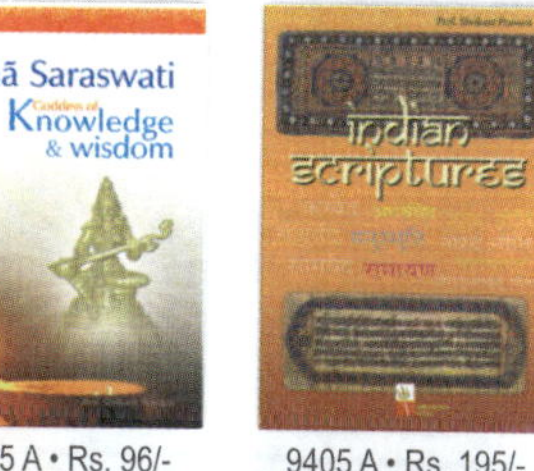

9585 A • Rs. 96/-

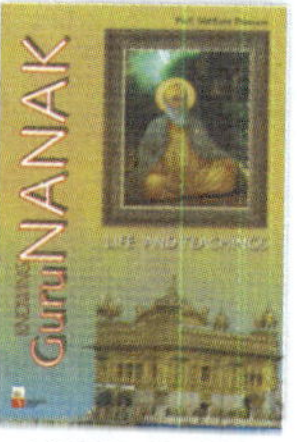

9405 A • Rs. 195/-

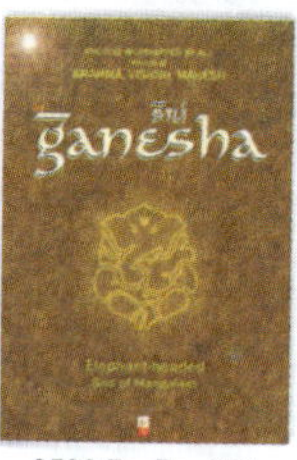

9989 D • Rs. 96/-

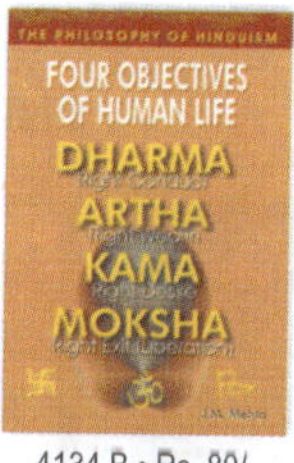

9508 D • Rs. 95/-

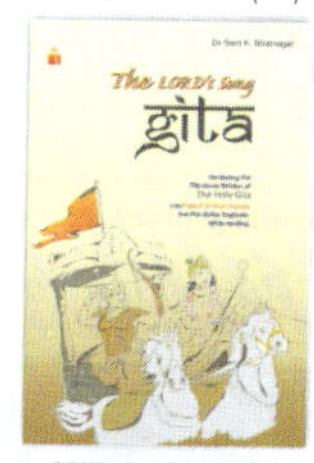

4134 B • Rs. 80/-

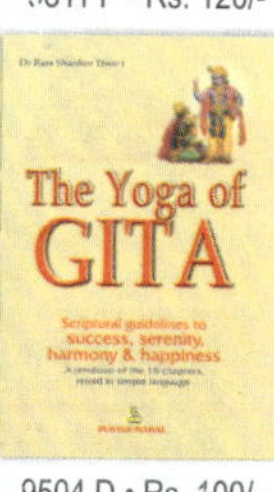

4188 A • Rs. 160/-

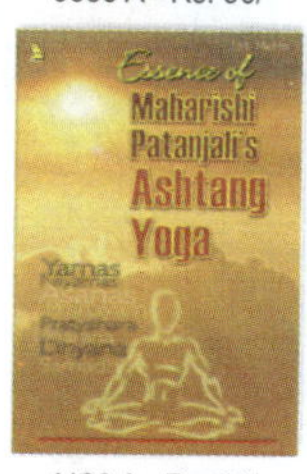

9504 D • Rs. 100/-

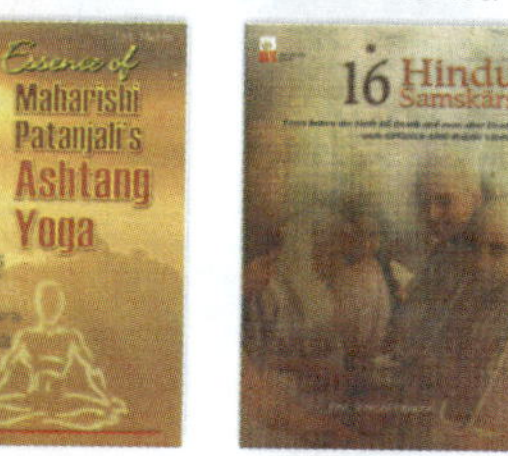

4133 A • Rs. 60/-

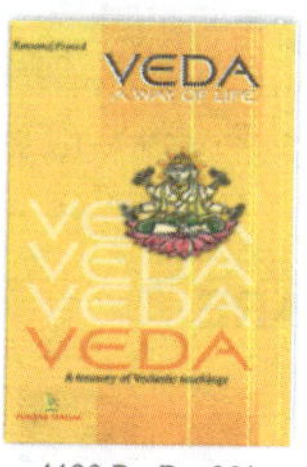

9513 A • Rs. 195/-

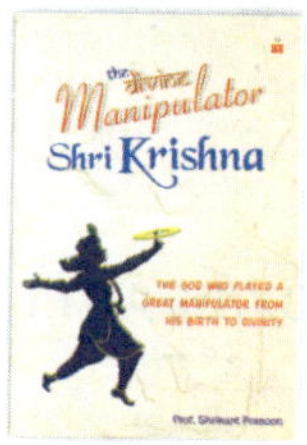

4126 B • Rs. 96/-

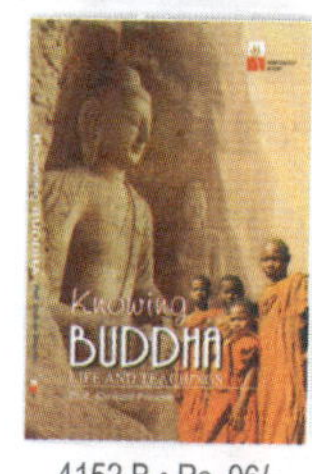

9812 R • Rs. 120/-

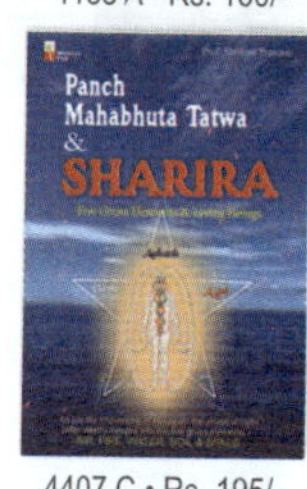

4152 B • Rs. 96/-

4407 C • Rs. 195/-

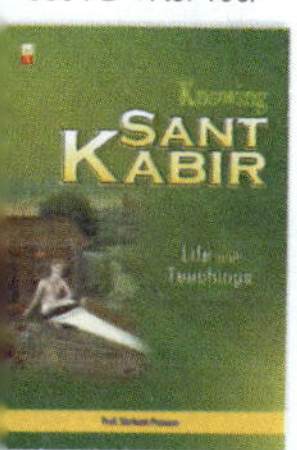

9504 D • Rs. 100/-

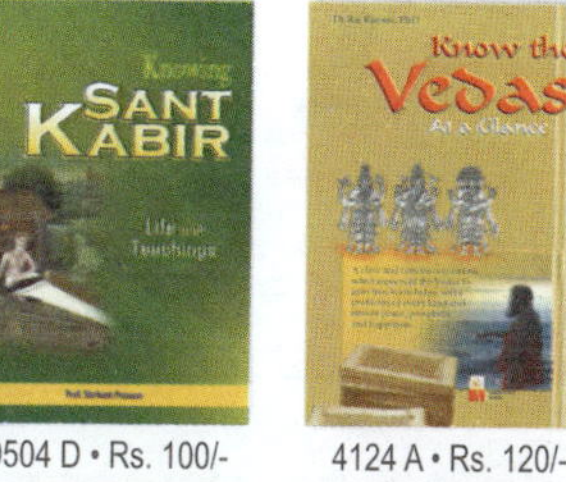

4124 A • Rs. 120/-

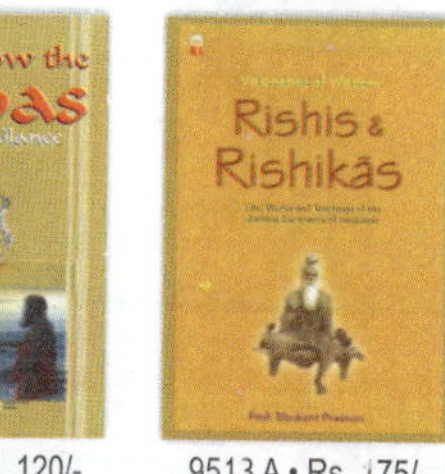

9513 A • Rs. 175/-

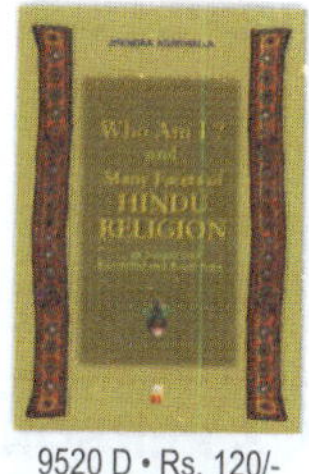

9520 D • Rs. 120/-

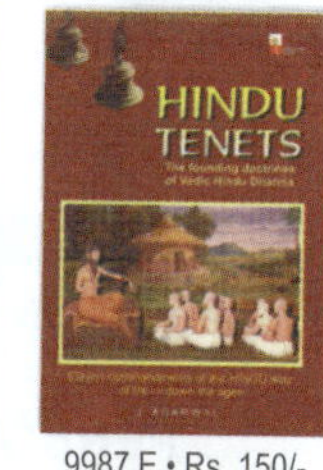

9987 E • Rs. 150/-

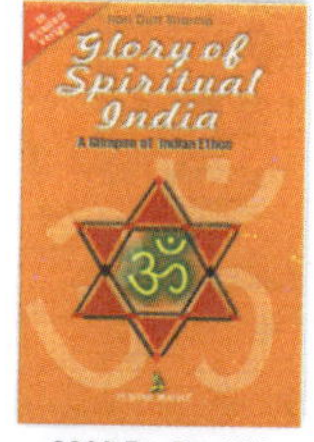

8898 D • Rs. 80/-

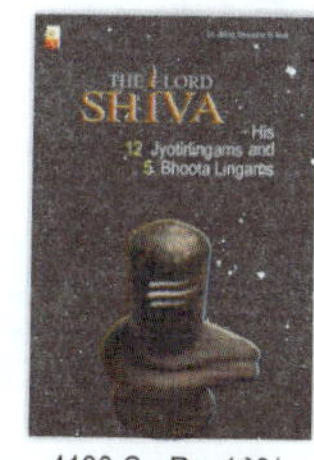

4190 C • Rs. 160/-

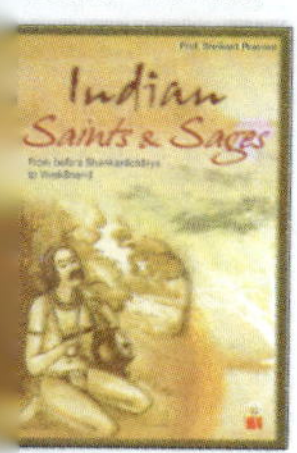

9509 A • Rs. 150/-

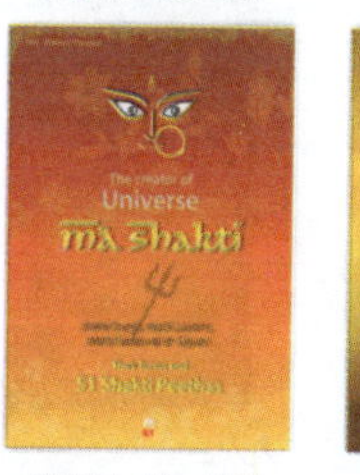

9525 A • Rs. 150/-

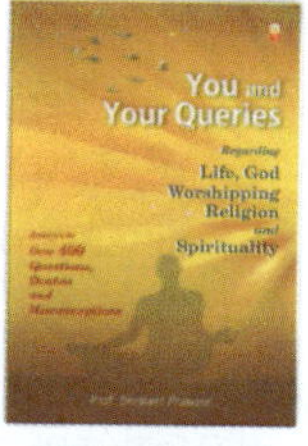

9540 D • Rs. 150/-

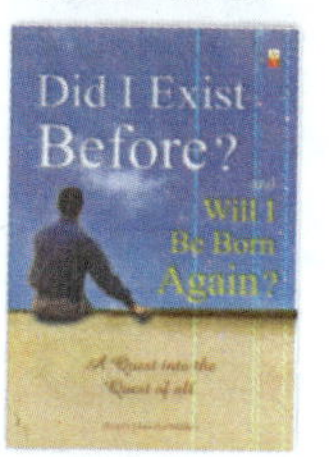

9542 B • Rs. 150/-

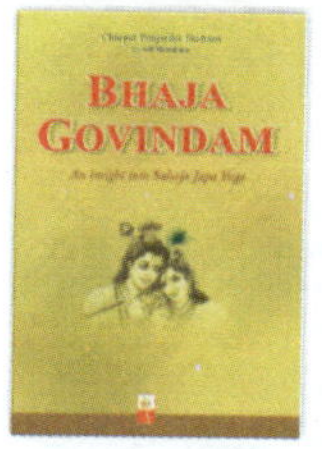

9514 B • Rs. 60/-

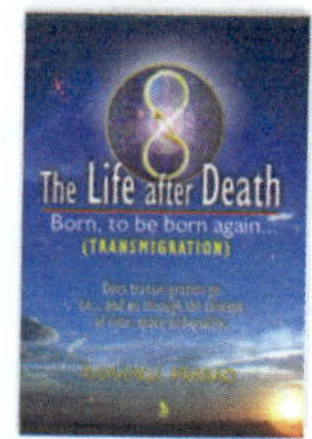

4132 D • Rs. 100/-

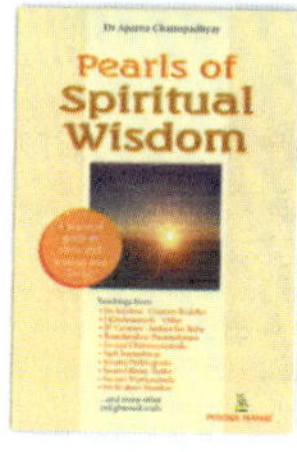

9069 A • Rs. 80/-

ASTROLOGY/VASTU/HYPNOTISM/PAMISTRY

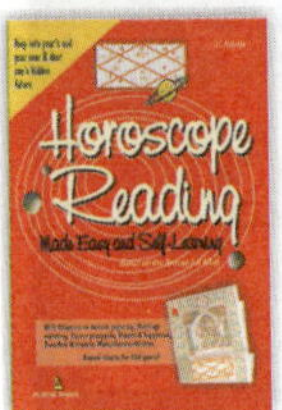
2127 D • Rs. 150/-

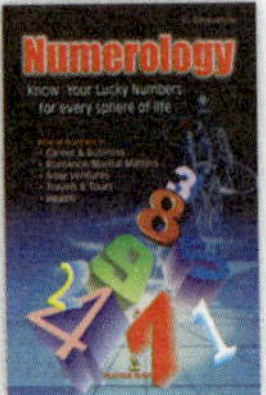
2109 F • Rs. 100/-

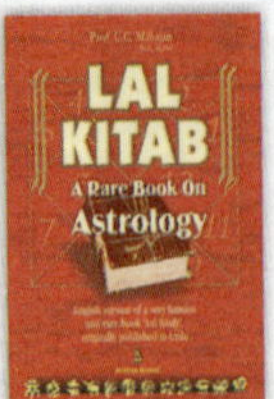
9086 A • Rs. 295/- HB

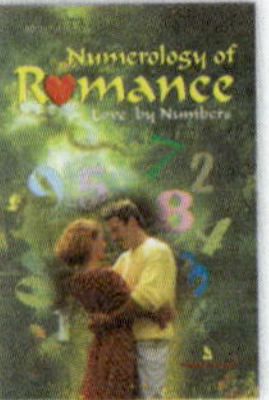
2125 D • Rs. 80/-

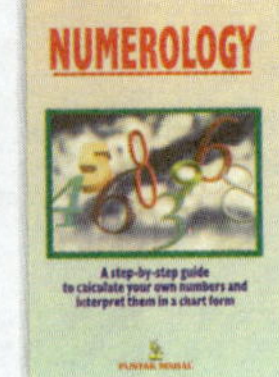
2109 F • Rs. 120/-

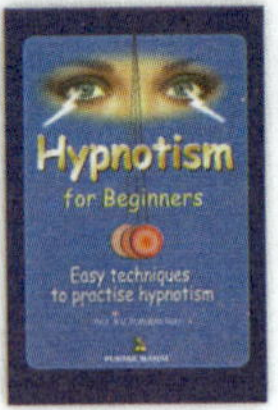
2112 D • Rs. 120/-

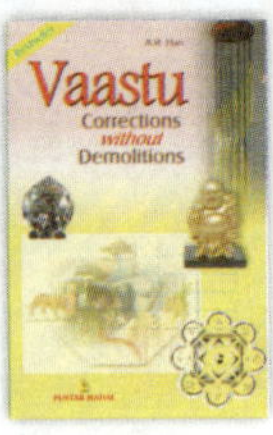
3110 B • Rs. 100/-

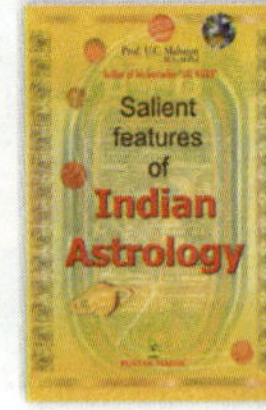
2133 B • Rs. 96/-

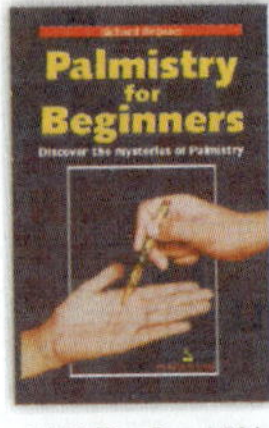
2116 D • Rs. 150/-

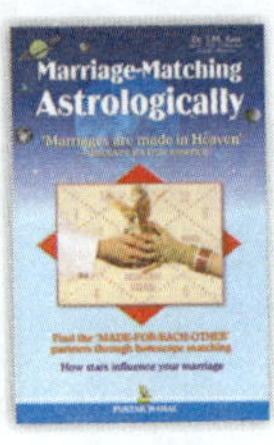
8259 D • Rs. 88/-

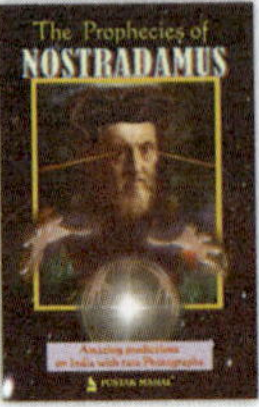
2108 E • Rs. 80/-

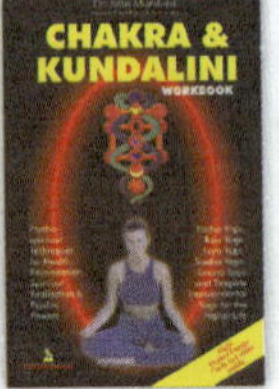
8899 D • Rs. 110/-

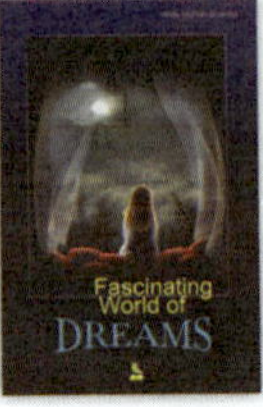
8925 D • Rs. 96/-

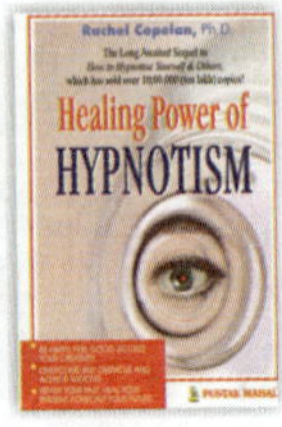
2132 A • Rs. 150/-

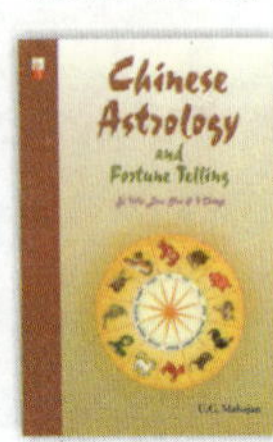
9432 D • Rs. 150/-

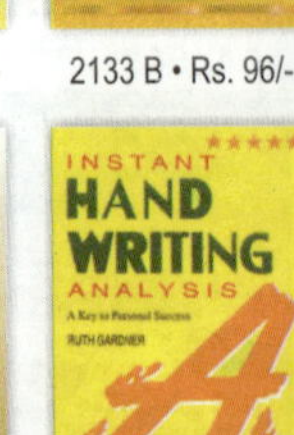
2120 D • Rs. 96/-

ENGLISH IMPROVEMENT

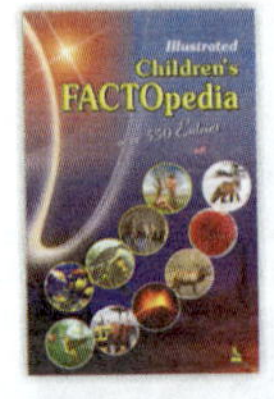
9496 A • Rs. 120/-

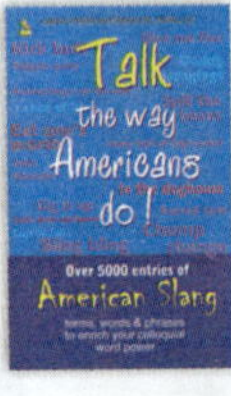
5541 C • Rs. 196/-

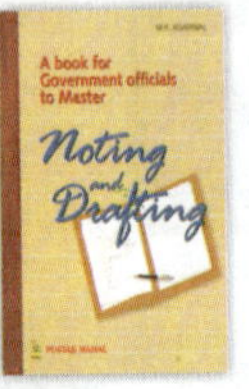
6651 E • Rs. 175/-

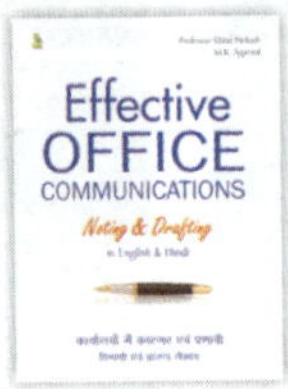
9448 D • Rs. 175/-

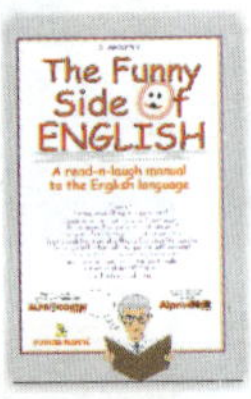
9056 A • Rs. 96/-

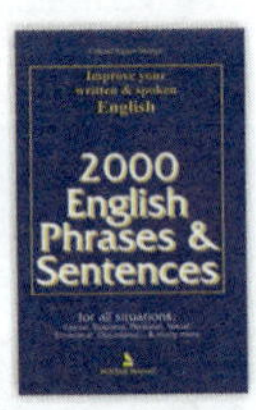
5538 D • Rs. 80/-

PARENTING

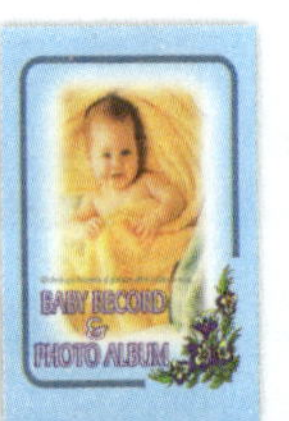
9906 J • Rs. 175/- (HB)

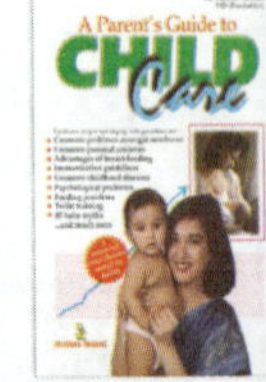
8261 D • Rs. 180/

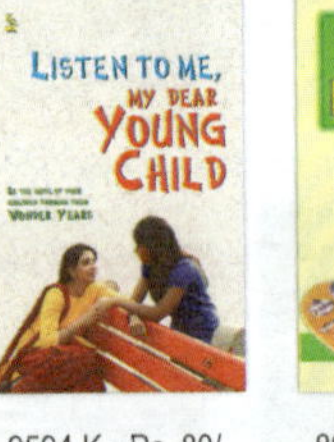
9594 K • Rs. 80/-

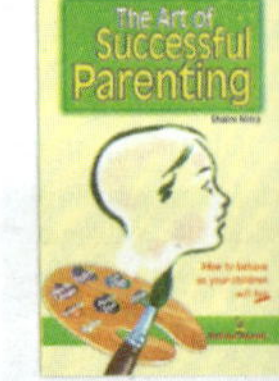
8917 D • Rs. 96/-

BODY/BEAUTY CARE

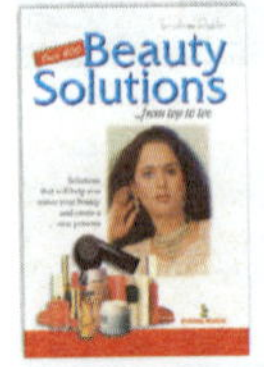
8093 D • Rs. 150/-

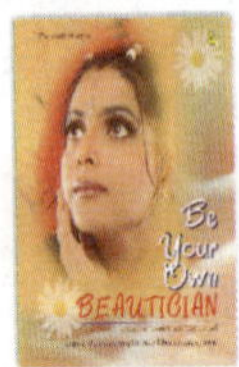
9986 B • Rs. 150/-

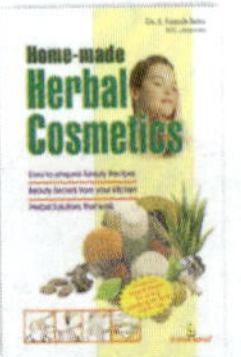
8971 B • Rs. 120/-

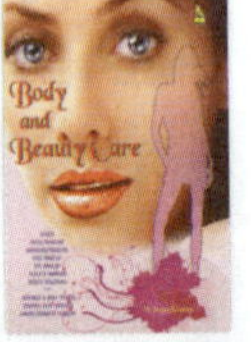
9922 F • Rs. 120/-

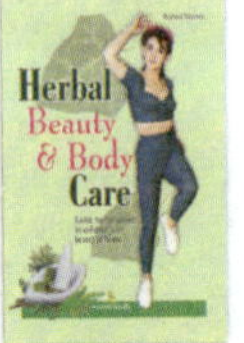
8865 F • Rs. 120/-

PERSON & PERSONALITIES

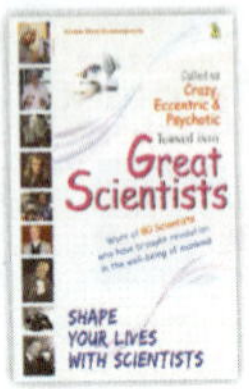
9825 E • Rs. 150/-

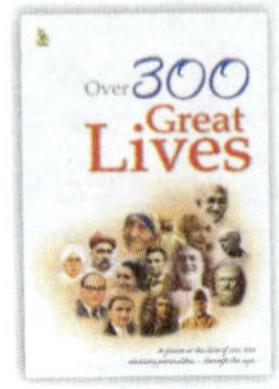
2113 D • Rs. 175/-

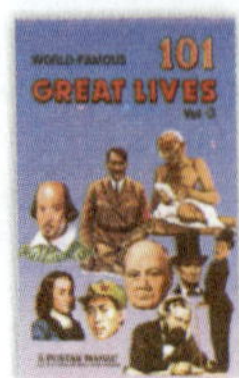
51102 L • Rs. 100/-

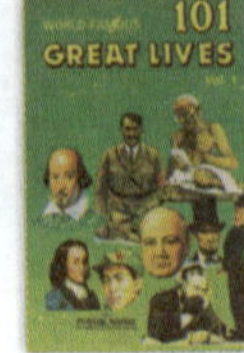
5122 L • Rs. 100/-

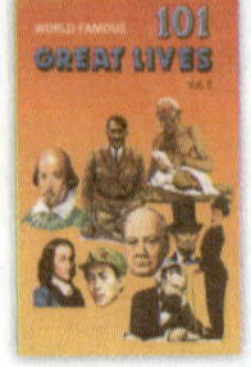
5178 E • Rs. 100/-

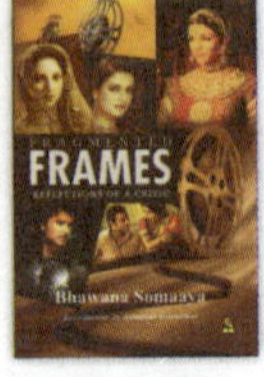
4170 B • Rs. 395/- (HB)

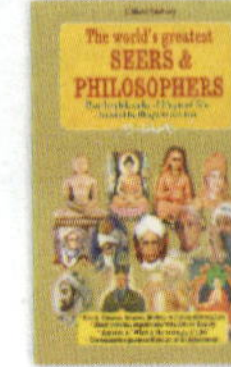
8991 D • Rs. 12(

FUN, FACTS, MAGIC & MYSTERIES

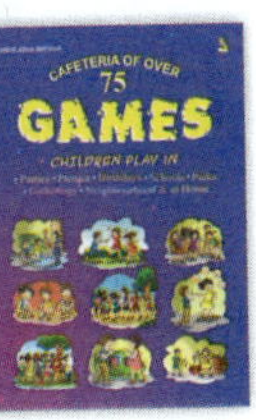

9484 B • Rs. 150/-

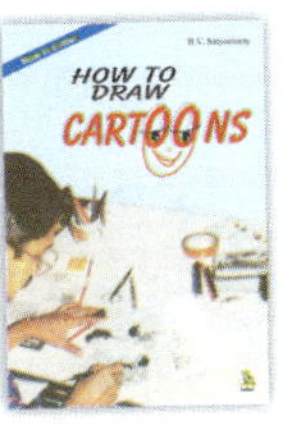

2275 D • Rs. 120/-

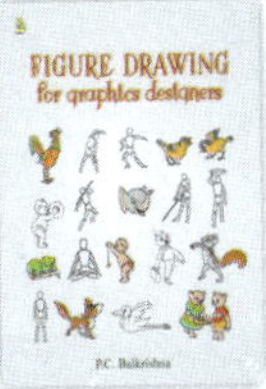

9479 M • Rs. 120/-

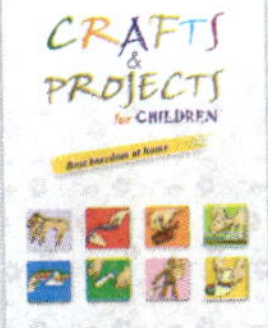

9470 B • Rs. 100/-

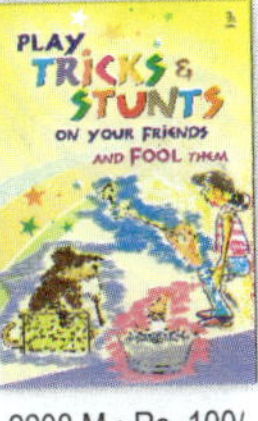

2208 M • Rs. 100/-

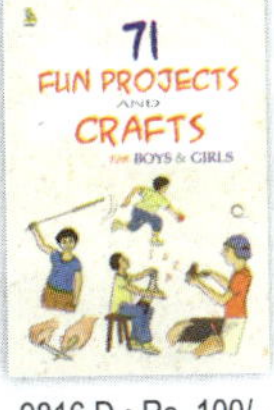

9816 D • Rs. 100/-

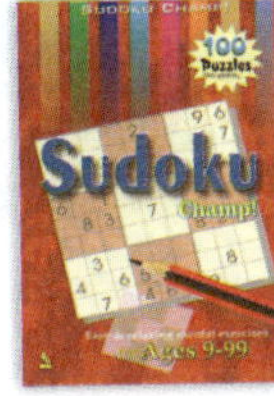

2328 G • Rs. 50/-

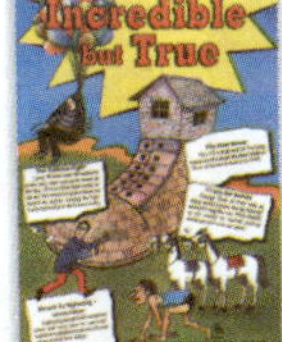

2247 F • Rs. 60/-

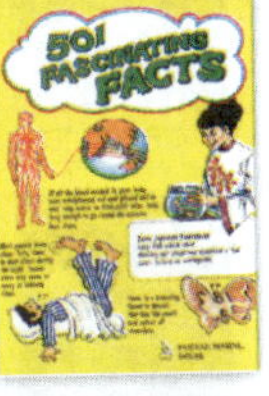

2211 F • Rs. 80/-

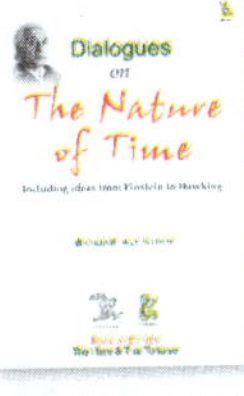

9467 E • Rs. 150/-

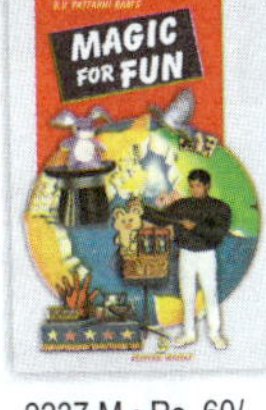

2237 M • Rs. 60/-

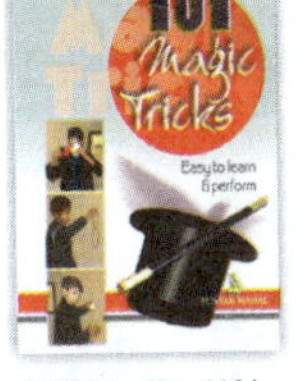

2250 A • Rs. 110/-

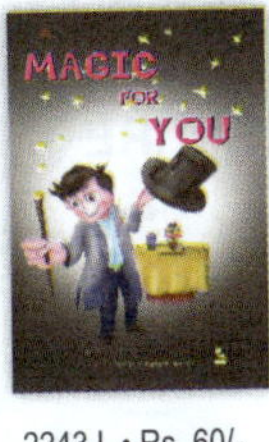

2243 L • Rs. 60/-

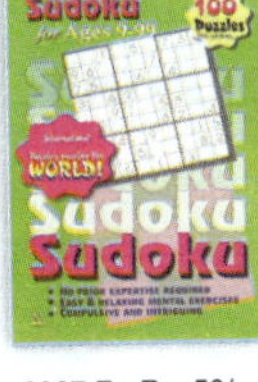

2327 F • Rs. 50/-

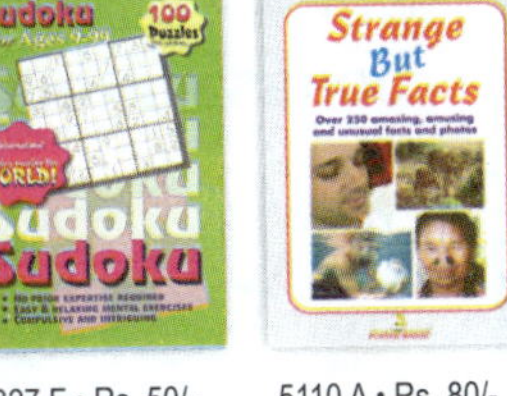

5110 A • Rs. 80/-

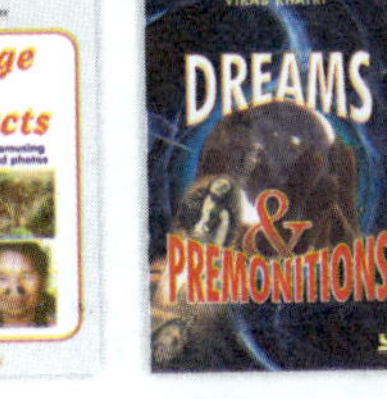

2335 A • Rs. 80/-

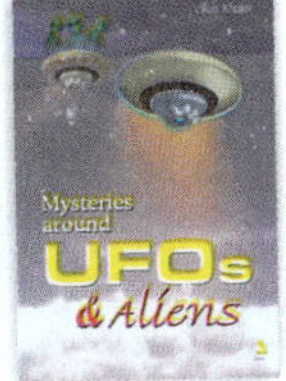

2337 C • Rs. 96/-

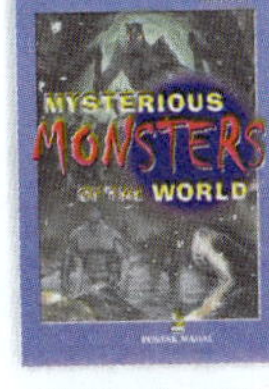

9977 B • Rs. 100/-

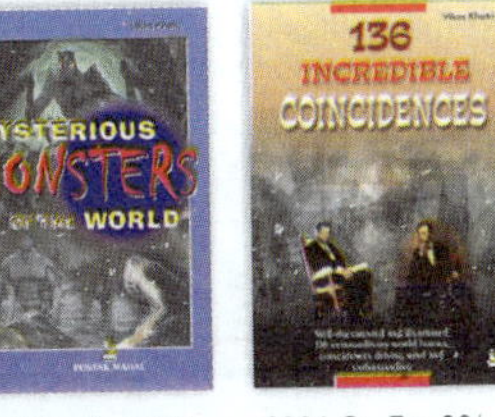

2331 C • Rs. 80/-

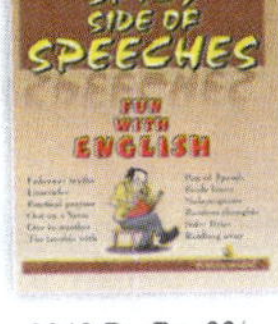

9040 D • Rs. 60/-

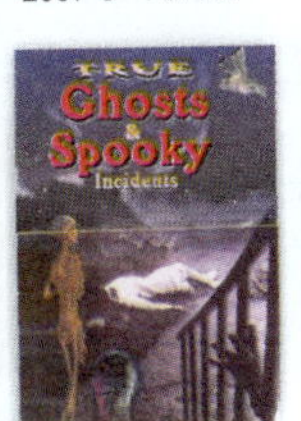

2336 B • Rs. 100/-

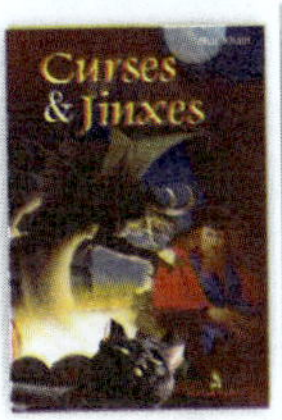

9985 A • Rs. 80/-

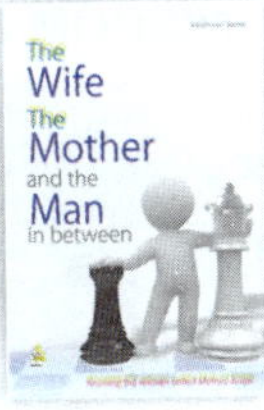

9458 G • Rs. 80/-

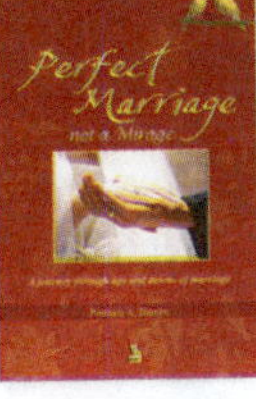

9438 B • Rs. 150/-

COOKERY BOOKS

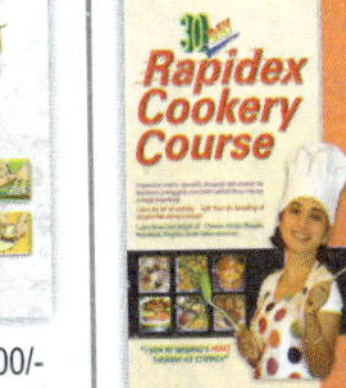

1237 B • Rs. 695/-
Fully Coloured (HB)

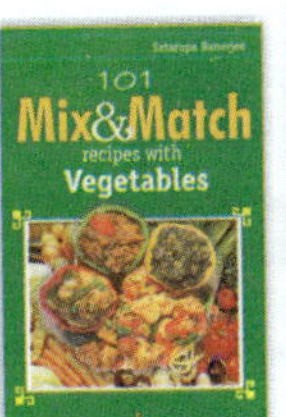

9942 D • Rs. 80/-

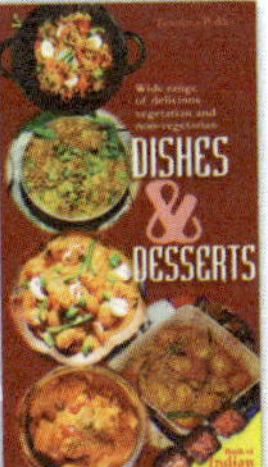

9936 D • Rs. 120/-

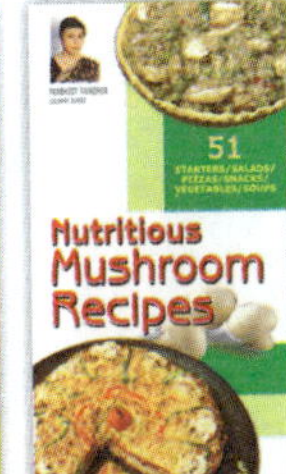

9962 C • Rs. 125/-

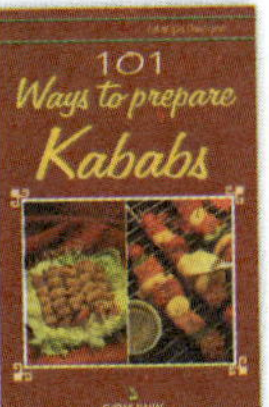

9948 D • Rs. 80/-

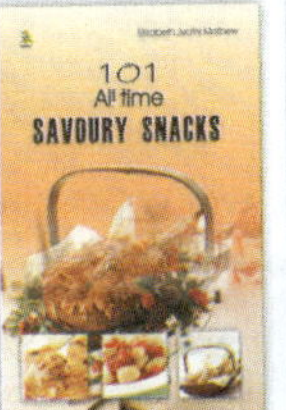

9943 D • Rs. 80/-

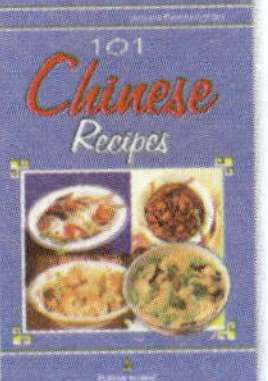

9944 D • Rs. 80/-

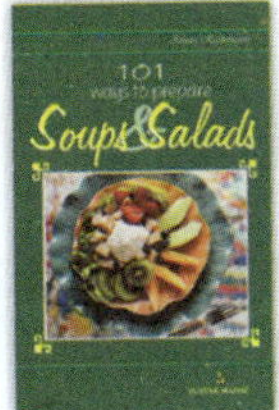

9938 D • Rs. 100/-

HOME MAKING / GRILL & RAILINGS

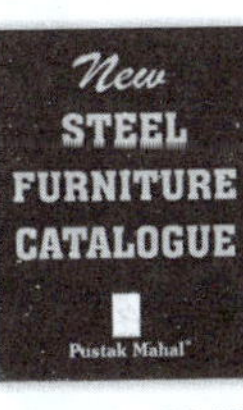

3102 K • Rs. 195/- (HB)

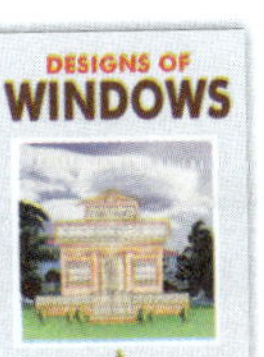

3106 E • Rs. 88/-

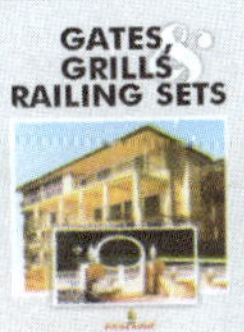

3104 M • Rs. 60/-

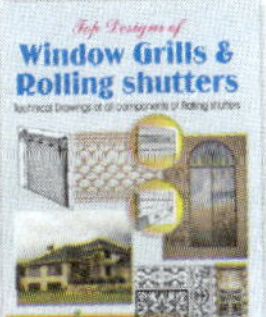

3103 L • Rs. 72/-

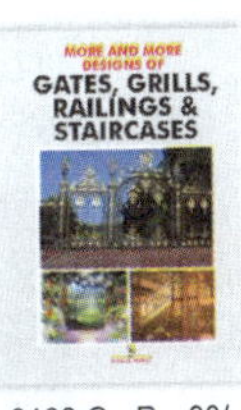

3108 G • Rs. 90/-

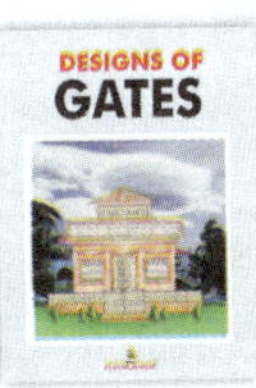

3105 D • Rs. 88/-

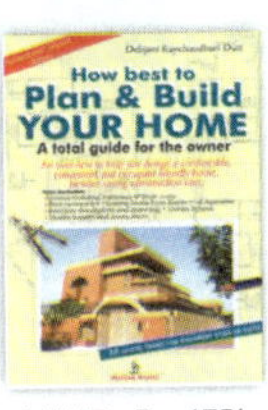

3111 E • Rs. 175/-

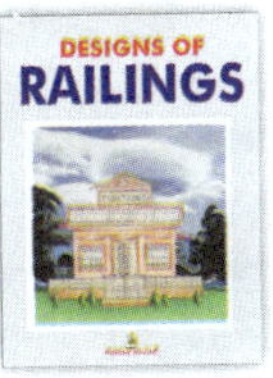

3107 F • Rs. 88/-

RELATIONSHIP

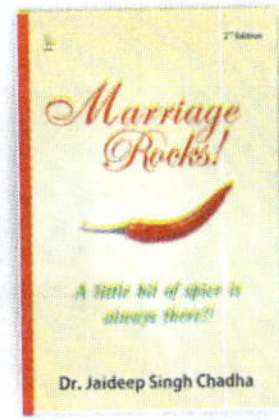

9994 E • Rs. 120/-

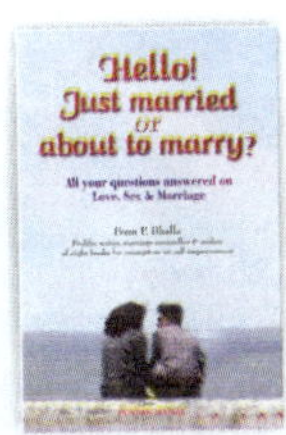

9065 A • Rs. 80/-

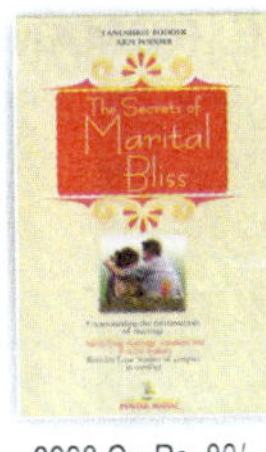

8998 C • Rs. 80/-

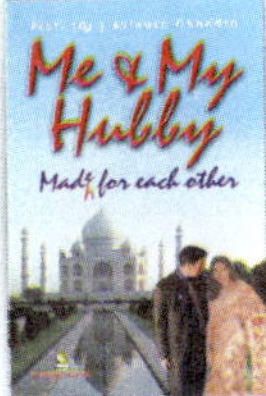

9031 D • Rs. 96/-

YOGA & MEDITATION

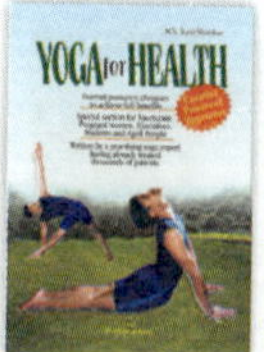
8269 A • Rs. 195/-

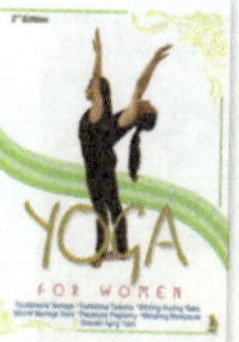
9998 D • Rs. 120/-

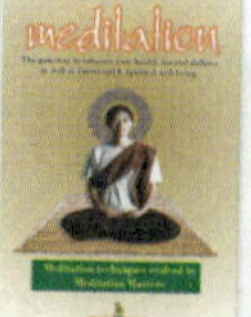
8939 D • Rs. 96/-

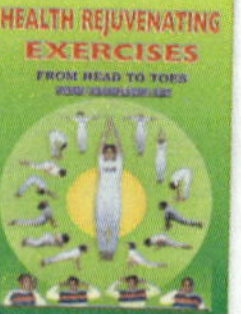
9080 C • Rs. 24/-

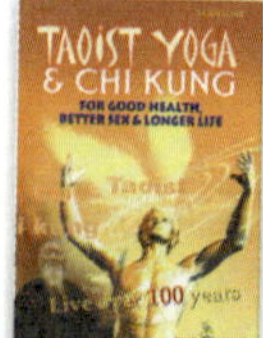
8867 D • Rs. 120/-

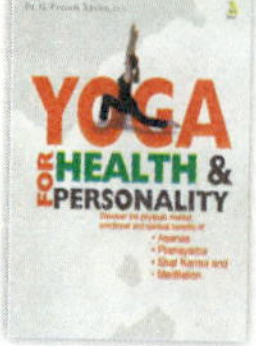
9958 S • Rs. 160/-

9087 B • Rs. 120/-

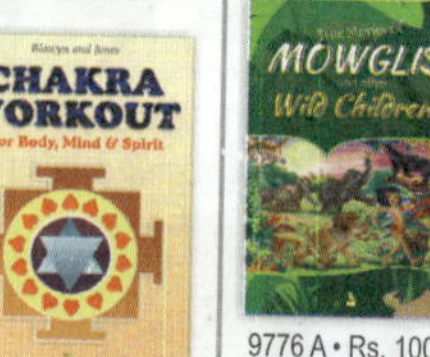
2118 F • Rs. 120/-

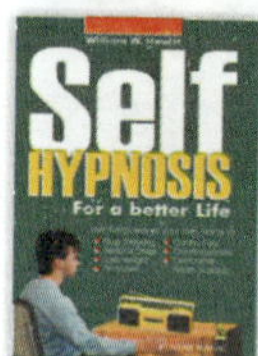
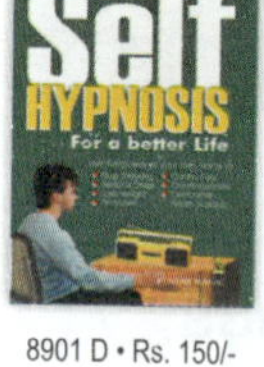
8901 D • Rs. 150/-

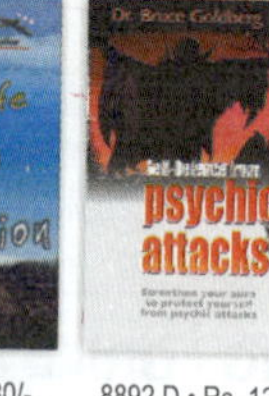
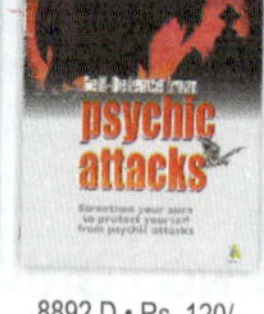
8099 D • Rs. 80/-

8892 D • Rs. 120/-

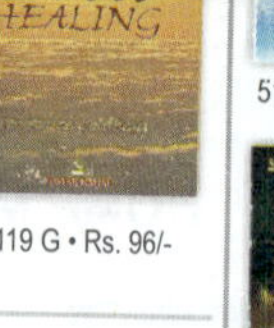
2119 G • Rs. 96/-

HOMEOPATHY, AYURDEDA

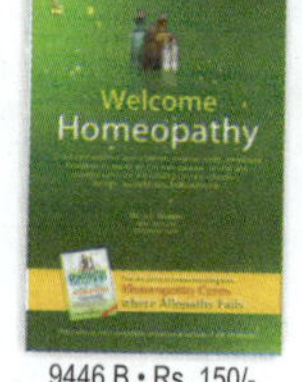
9446 B • Rs. 150/-

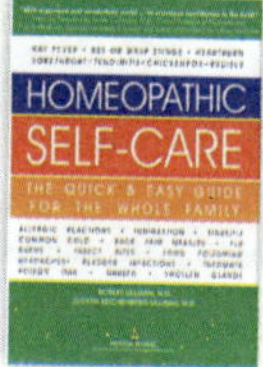
8887 D • Rs. 175/-

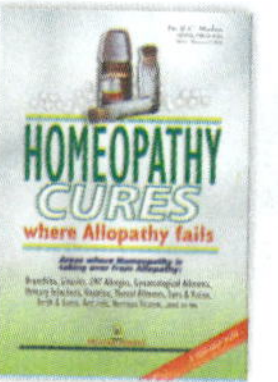
8270 B • Rs. 165/-

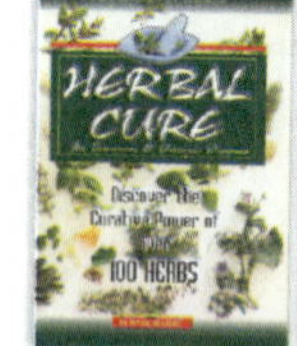
8010 D • Rs. 96/-

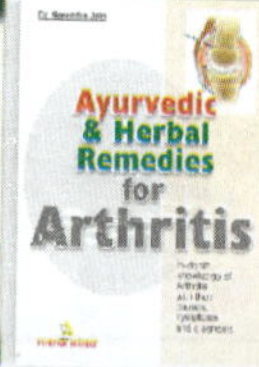
9094 E • Rs. 96/-

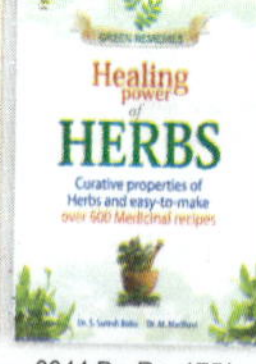
8944 D • Rs. 175/-

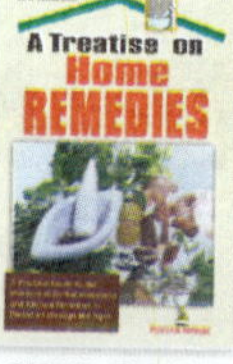
8923 D • Rs. 150/-

LOVE, ROMANCE & SEX

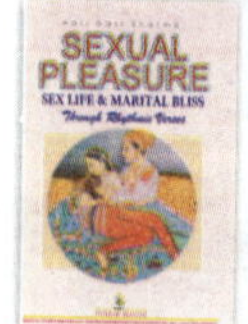
8260 D • Rs. 96/-

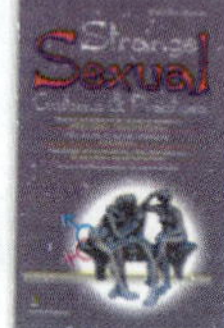
8266 D • Rs. 80/-

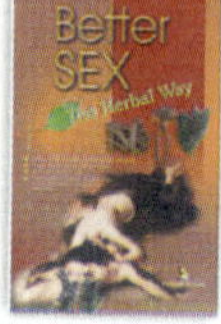
8278 C • Rs. 100/-

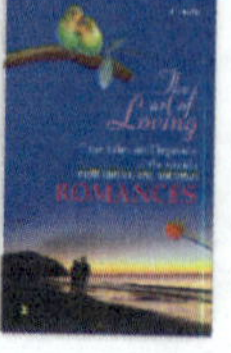
8916 D • Rs. 120/-

WORLD FAMOUS SERIES

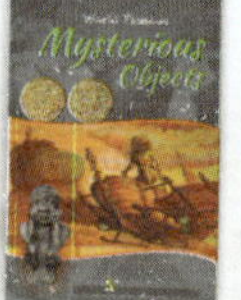
9775 M • Rs. 100/-

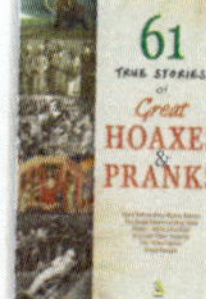
9766 A • Rs. 100/-

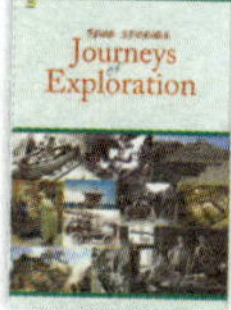
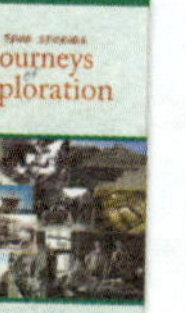
9765 S • Rs. 100/-

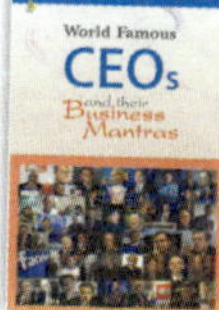
9761 M • Rs. 100/-

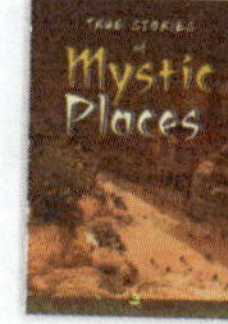
9769 D • Rs. 100/-

9776 A • Rs. 100/-

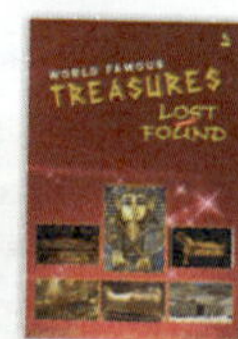
9492 K • Rs. 100/-

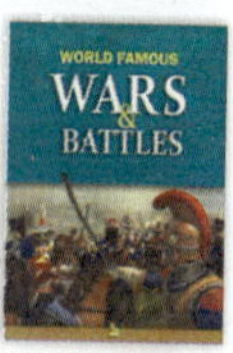
9755 E • Rs. 100/-

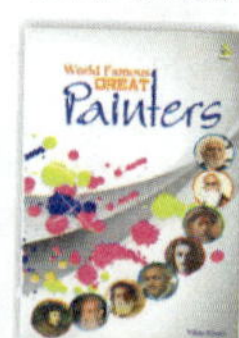
9483 A • Rs. 100/-

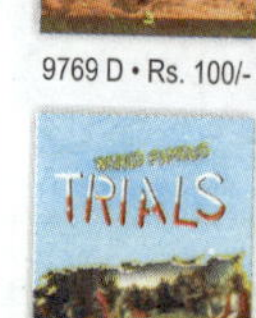
9489 G • Rs. 100/-

5121 K • Rs. 100/-

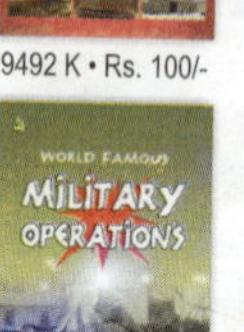
5175 K • Rs. 100/-

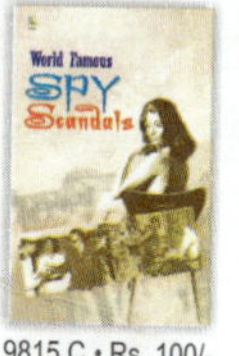
9815 C • Rs. 100/-

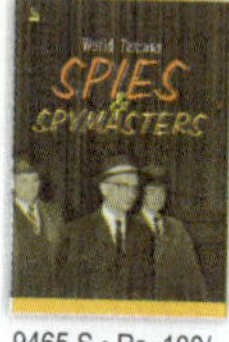
9465 S • Rs. 100/-

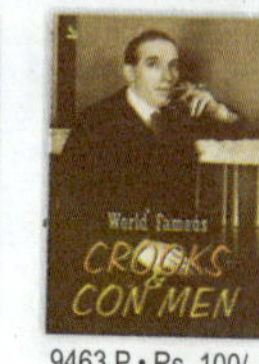
9463 P • Rs. 100/-

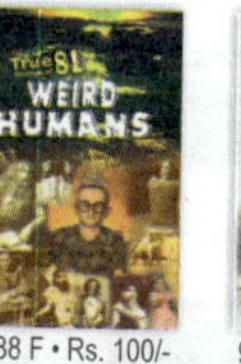
9488 F • Rs. 100/-

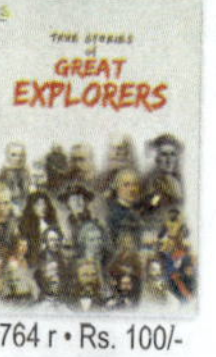
9764 r • Rs. 100/-

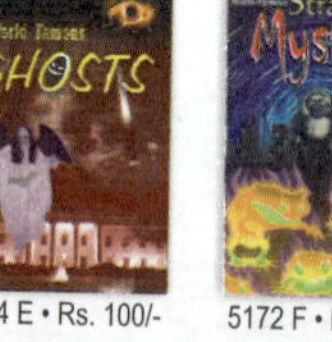
5164 E • Rs. 100/-

5172 F • Rs. 100/-

51107 • Rs. 100/-

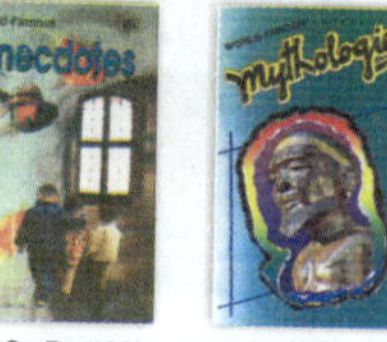
5151 G • Rs. 100/-

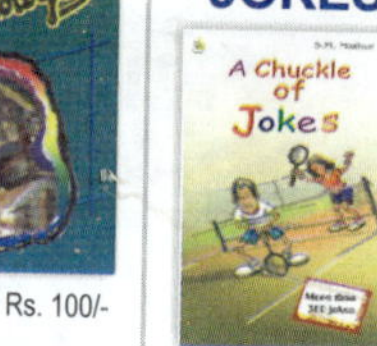
5156 D • Rs. 100/-

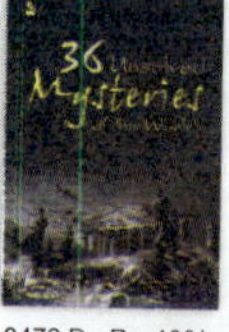
9472 D • Rs. 100/-

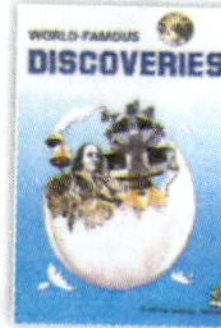
5116 D • Rs. 100/-

JOKES HUMOUR & SATIRE

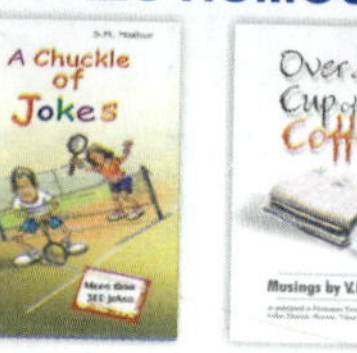
2341 B • Rs. 60/-

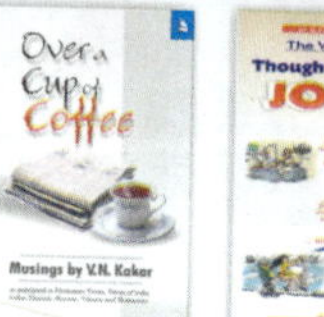
2326 E • Rs. 120/-

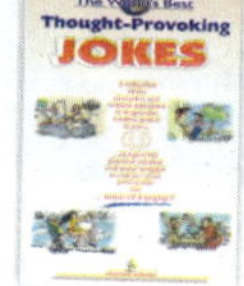
2318 A • Rs. 96/-

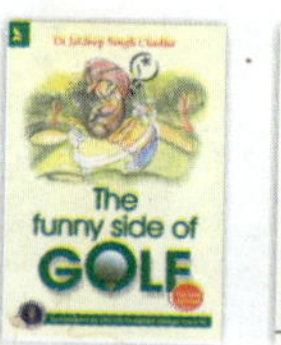
2338 D • Rs. 120/-

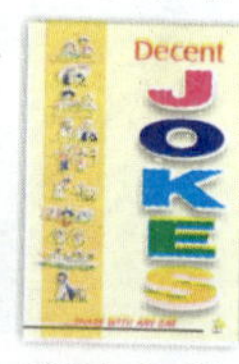
2330 B • Rs. 80/-

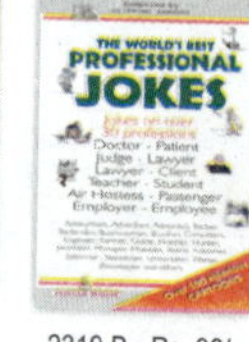
2319 B • Rs. 96/-

MORAL, WISDOM & FAIRY TALES

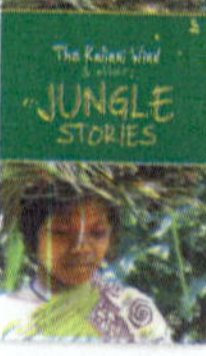
9486 D • Rs. 250/-

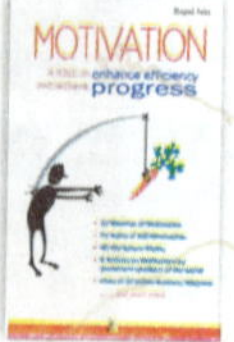
9763 P • Rs. 150/-

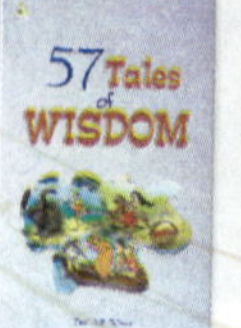
8967 F • Rs. 80/-

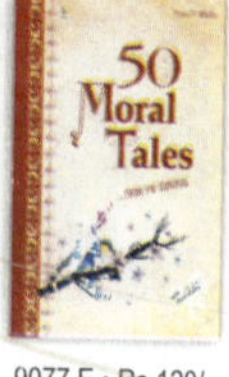
9077 E • Rs.120/-

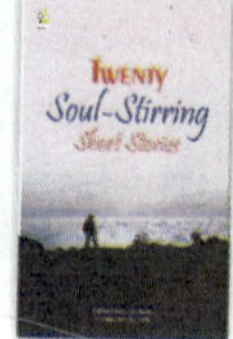
9563 N • Rs. 125/-